PRINCIPLES OF PSYCHOPHARMACOLOGY FOR MENTAL HEALTH PROFESSIONALS

PRINCIPLES OF PSYCHOPHARMACOLOGY FOR MENTAL HEALTH PROFESSIONALS

Jeffrey E. Kelsey, MD PhD
Georgia Institute of Mood and Anxiety Disorders

D. Jeffrey Newport, MD
Charles B. Nemeroff, MD PhD
Department of Psychiatry and Behavioral Science
Emory University School of Medicine

A JOHN WILEY & SONS, INC., PUBLICATION

Published by John Wiley & Sons, Inc., Hoboken, New Jersey
Published simultaneously in Canada

For general information on our other products and services or for technical support, please contact our Customer Care Department within the United States at 877-762-2974, outside the United States at 317-572-3993 or fax 317-572-4002.

Wiley also publishes its books in a variety of electronic formats. Some content that appears in print may not be available in electronic formats. For more information about Wiley products, visit our web site at www.wiley.com.

Library of Congress Cataloging-in-Publication Data:

Principles of psychopharmacology for mental health professionals / Jeffrey E. Kelsey.
p. cm.
Includes index.
ISBN-13: 978-0-471-25401-0 (paper)
ISBN-10: 0-471-25401-0 (cloth)

Printed in the United States of America

10 9 8 7 6 5 4 3 2 1

To my wife Marlene, my children Stephen, Lauren, and Alexander, my parents, and especially to my patients who have taught me the art of medicine.

—Jeffrey K

To my wife, Deborah, the most courageous woman I have ever known.

—Jeffrey N

To my patients, students, colleagues, and friends for their support and understanding and for all they have taught me and most of all to my family, Gayle, the most loving and understanding wife anyone could hope for, and our children, Michael, Mandy, Ross, and Gigi, and finally to my sister who has been there for me the longest of all.

—Charles

CONTENTS

PREFACE

Why buy a book about psychopharmacology if you don't prescribe medications? Ask yourself, how many of your clients tell you about the medications they are taking or wonder if they should be taking, for whatever disorder they are receiving treatment for from you. Or, do they tell you that they appreciate having more time with you than they get with the person who prescribes their medications so they can ask their questions in a less hurried environment? This is the feedback from many mental health professionals, psychologists, social workers, therapists, and nurses, that we have received.

Our purpose with this book is to provide a background into the what, why, how, and when questions of psychotropic medications. Recognizing that this conversation cannot exist in a vacuum, we also review diagnostic issues, treatment goals, and ways to integrate psychotherapy with pharmacotherapy and then intersperse this information with clinical examples. It is this combination, the "bio" with the "psychosocial" that optimizes care for so many of the people we treat.

We hope that you enjoy this book, but more importantly, we hope that should we meet, you will tell us that this book improved the outcome and quality of life for those that you work with in treatment.

JEFFREY E. KELSEY, M.D., Ph.D.
D. JEFFREY NEWPORT, M.D., M.S., M.Div
CHARLES B. NEMEROFF, M.D., Ph.D.

FACULTY DISCLOSURE

Jeffrey E. Kelsey, M.D., Ph.D.

Research Support

- Abbott Laboratories
- Bristol-Meyers Squibb
- Cyberonics
- Eli Lilly
- Forest Pharmaceuticals, Inc.
- GlaxoSmithKline
- Merck
- Mitsubishi
- Organon
- Pfizer
- Wyeth

Speakers Bureau

- Bristol-Meyers Squibb
- Eli Lilly
- Forest Pharmaceuticals, Inc.
- GlaxoSmithKline
- Pfizer
- Shire
- Wyeth

Consultant

- Bristol-Meyers Squibb
- Eli Lilly
- Wyeth

D. Jeffrey Newport, M.D., M.S., M.Div.

Grants/Research

- Eli Lilly
- GlaxoSmithKline
- Janssen Pharmaceutica
- NARSAD
- NIMH
- Wyeth

Speakers Bureau
- Eli Lilly
- GlaxoSmithKline
- Pfizer

Charles B. Nemeroff, M.D., Ph.D.

Grants/Research
- Abbott Laboratories
- AFSP
- AstraZeneca
- Bristol Meyers Squibb
- Forest Laboratories
- GlaxoSmithKline
- Janssen Pharmaceutica
- NARSAD
- NIMH
- Pfizer Pharmaceuticals
- Stanley Foundation/NAMI
- Wyeth

Consultant
- Abbott Laboratories
- Acadia Pharmaceuticals
- Bristol-Meyers Squibb
- Corcept
- Cypress Biosciences
- Cyberonics
- Eli Lilly
- Forest Laboratories
- GlaxoSmithKline
- Janssen Pharmaceutica
- Otsuka
- Pfizer Pharmaceuticals
- Quintiles
- Wyeth

Speakers Bureau
- Abbott Laboratories
- GlaxoSmithKline
- Janssen Pharmaceutica
- Pfizer Pharmaceuticals

Stockholder
- Corcept
- Cypress Biosciences
- Neurocrine Biosciences
- Acadia Pharmaceuticals

Board of Directors

American Foundation for Suicide Prevention (AFSP)
American Psychiatric Institute for Research and Education (APIRE)
George West Mental Health Foundation
Novadel Pharma
National Foundation for Mental Health (NFMH)

Patents

Methods and devices for transdermal delivery of lithium (US6,375,990 B1)
Methods to estimate serotonin and norepinephrine transporter occupancy after drug treatment using patient or animal serum (provisional filing April 2001)

Equity

Reevax
BMC-JR LLC
CeNeRx

1

INTRODUCTION AND OVERVIEW

Why a book about psychopharmacology for the nonprescribing practitioner? As you read this book's cover, you likely asked that question. After all, if one cannot or does not prescribe medications, what is the use of the information? The point, of course, is that the patient (or client) who is receiving, or better yet, actively participating in treatment needs to be aware of the options, and often desires an educated opinion from the practitioner (s)he is seeing for treatment. Though there may be the temptation to split diseases into those with biological components and those with a psychological basis, the truth is almost always somewhere in the middle. It is the rare patient for whom pharmacotherapy is indicated who would not also benefit from psychotherapy, be it cognitive-behavioral, psychodynamic, interpersonal, supportive, or whatever meets the need of that individual. On the other hand, the person who presents to a psychotherapist may have questions about whether or not medications are indicated, the therapist might think that an evaluation for pharmacotherapy is warranted, treatment may not be going as expected, or there may be medical issues that arise. Any number of questions might prompt the consideration of a pharmacotherapy consultation, and nonprescribing practitioners should be aware of these issues to ensure that patients receive optimal treatment.

Principles of Psychopharmacology for Mental Health Professionals
By Jeffrey E. Kelsey, D. Jeffrey Newport, and Charles B. Nemeroff

The goal of this book is not at all to equip the reader to prescribe psychotropic medications, but rather to convey clinically relevant information to those individuals who deliver a very powerful treatment, namely, psychotherapy, and to ensure that patients are given access to the full array of treatments that are appropriate for them. The information presented in this book is based on the experience of the authors who have taught and collaborated over the years with many therapists, including social workers, psychologists, pastoral counselors, and marriage and family therapists in outpatient and inpatient settings, continuing education courses, and graduate programs. We have also drawn upon the available scientific and clinical literature and, perhaps most importantly, the experiences that our patients have shared with us over the years.

What are the situations in which nonprescribing practitioners need to know about treatments involving medications? These potentially span the entire duration of treatment. The patient who first seeks treatment from a therapist is relying on the therapist to recognize if the disorder is one for which medication is the standard of care (e.g., bipolar disorder or schizophrenia), is an option to be considered in combination with psychotherapy (e.g., many anxiety disorders, depression), or is not indicated (e.g., adjustment disorders, relationship stressors). As treatment duration progresses, the patient with panic disorder who finds the anxiety too high to tolerate exposure therapy may need guidance in deciding if it is time to consider medication treatment. Another example of an appropriately timed referral is the couple in family therapy that is not fully successful because the husband's depression is interfering with the progress of therapy. In addition, the patient who is troubled by bothersome medication side effects, but whose physician has limited appointment times, can often find an effective advocate in the therapist. All of these, and more, are situations for which it is important that mental health professionals be aware of disorders for which medication treatments are and are not available, what the typical course of treatment is, and at least a general familiarity with potential side effects and desired outcome.

The current managed care environment has added a new impetus to the therapist's need to know about psychotropic medicines. More patients today are finding that treatment is taking place in a "split" environment. That is, one person provides psychotherapy, and another provides pharmacotherapy. Done well, "split" therapy can be a win–win situation for all involved; performed poorly, it is the patient who ultimately pays the price. The advantages to "split" therapy are an oftentimes lower overall expense to the patient, perhaps better insurance coverage, and increased access to treatment providers who have expertise in a specific area. The potential downside, which should not be underestimated, includes the complexity of two treatment providers rather than one, the possibility of "split" treatment becoming "fragmented" treatment, the chance that patients with primitive defense mechanisms will split the treatment themselves, the potential for increased resistance, and the limitation of time available with the prescriber. What do patients think about split treatment? Many will find this to be a satisfactory arrangement if the following parameters are clearly defined. Who is in charge of what? Is the frequency and duration of visits with each provider sufficient for the task at hand? And perhaps most importantly, does the patient know that the two providers will communicate back and forth so the patient is not lost between the cracks? These situations of course are descriptive of the ideal collaboration, but the real world arrangement is often not as good. The venue in which patients might be most likely to encounter a less than optimal arrangement is frequently in the delivery of pharmacotherapy. Visits are too short or too infrequent, or the patient may perceive, sometimes correctly, that the prescriber is less concerned about his/her well-being than the therapist. It is essential, therefore, in a dual practitioner treatment paradigm, that the respective roles of each care provider are clearly defined and respected. It invites confusion and ultimately leads to treatment failure if the psychopharmacologist begins to conduct psychotherapy or the psychotherapist makes recommendations concerning specific pharmacotherapies.

Should, Therapists Act as "Gatekeepers"? The term gatekeeper will be familiar to readers who are involved in managed care. In that environment, the gatekeeper is usually a primary care physician who decides if a patient's care can be managed in the primary care setting or if a patient requires the attention of a specialist. There is an analogy in the practice of psychotherapy. Clearly, any patient who first consults a psychotherapist is going to rely on that therapist for treatment recommendations. Perhaps the person is afraid of medications, so (s)he sought psychotherapy first. Furthermore, it is difficult for patients to be fully objective regarding their own care, and few have the training or background to be able to decide independently if medication is indicated. How can therapists know if medications are indicated for a particular patient? They can do so by being aware of the uses *and* limitations of pharmacotherapy. In our experience, not uncommon is the patient who has been in therapy, is referred to a psychopharmacologist like one of us, and tells us that (s)he was relying on the therapist to decide if medication was needed. Yet, patients often do not ask their therapists about medication, because they commonly assume, "If I need to be on medication, surely my therapist will tell me."

How Is a Referral Selected? The first step in making a referral for pharmacotherapy is to recognize that the patient has a disorder that would likely respond to pharmacotherapy. Perhaps the psychotherapy is not proceeding as desired, there is a comorbid condition (psychiatric or medical) requiring treatment, or a second opinion concerning diagnosis and treatment is desired. The following clinical vignette should help to illustrate.

After discussing the therapist's concerns that medications are indicated, and hearing the patient's response, the next step, if the discussion has been productive, is to make the referral. It is helpful for a therapist to pick a few physicians for routine referrals whom (s)he knows share a similar perspective on treatment and with whom (s)he can become increasingly comfortable sharing patient care. The prescriber should not be a physician who will devalue the importance of therapy, but rather one who will be supportive of the process. Limiting the number of physicians to whom the therapist refers enhances networking relationships as more than one shared patient can often be discussed during a single telephone call or hallway encounter. Selecting more than one physician for referrals, however, provides better flexibility for scheduling and matching up prescribers with patients more appropriately.

Clinical Vignette

Deborah is a 35-year-old married female who has had two prior episodes of depression. Both previous episodes were treated by her primary care physician with antidepressants, but Deborah discontinued treatment after 4–5 months because she did not like the side effects of drowsiness and weight gain. A friend of hers had seen a psychotherapist, and when Deborah became depressed again, she decided to try this approach instead of medication. She was in psychotherapy but experiencing only a limited response. She continued to have depressive symptoms of depressed mood, increased sleep, increased appetite, anhedonia (an inability to experience pleasure), and poor concentration. Her therapist suggested a consultation with a psychiatrist who she knows, but Deborah was reluctant based on her previous experience and a belief of "what's the use of taking more drugs if it's just going to come back again anyway?" How do we respond to Deborah? To what extent is she voicing the negative cognitions of her depressed mood as opposed to genuine concerns about side effects that were uncomfortable enough to lead her to stop treatment prematurely in the past? One approach, and this would come best from the therapist who has been working with the patient and has established a rapport, would be to say, "I know you're discouraged. We both thought you would be doing better by now. The symptoms that you have though, the sadness, sleeping and eating more, trouble concentrating, and not enjoying things the way you used to, are all symptoms of major depressive disorder. Major depression is very common and usually responds well to antidepressants. I know you had problems in the past with side effects, but this time I would like you to see a psychiatrist with whom I work to see if (s)he might be able to come up with a treatment that works and that you can tolerate. The other concern I have is that with this being your third episode of depression, there is an 85–95% chance that you will have yet another episode in the future. I would really like to see you get the improvement that you deserve, and as some of these symptoms improve, I believe the therapy will be more helpful to you." This approach addresses a number of useful points. There is empathy for the patient, the depression is framed as a medical disorder with specific medical treatments to address the self-blame or guilt that many patients will have, the high probability of recurrent episodes is pointed out, and a realistic optimism derived from a familiarity with the available treatment options is communicated to the patient.

Should patients be referred to psychiatrists or primary care physicians? Our bias is that the referral should almost always be to a psychiatrist. The patient is already seeing a specialist, the therapist, for psychotherapy and deserves the advantage of seeing a specialist for pharmacotherapy. This is not to suggest that certain primary care physicians, physician assistants, or nurse practitioners are not skilled pharmacotherapists. In fact, nonpsychiatric physicians prescribe the majority of psychotropic medications, particularly antidepressants and antianxiety medicines, in this country. However, problems can arise when the prescriber is a primary care provider if the disease turns out to be more refractory to treatment than was initially appreciated. That said, the psychotherapist should also appreciate that there are differences between psychiatrists in the way they practice pharmacotherapy. There has been an unfortunate trend over the last few years for some psychiatrists to gravitate to the concept of the 10-minute medication check, often performed in conjunction with a visit with a social worker or nurse immediately prior to the physician appointment. This may work for some patients, but it is far from optimal. We prefer the enhanced quality of care that can be provided when greater physician–patient contact time allows for a more comprehensive assessment.

How can good pharmacotherapists be found? First, check with experienced and respected colleagues, take note of which pharmacotherapists are referring patients to you, attend local educational meetings with psychiatrists, or, if there is a medical school nearby, attend the psychiatry department's grand rounds. Local patient advocacy and support groups, such as the Depression and Bipolar Support Alliance (DBSA), the National Alliance for the Mentally Ill (NAMI), the American Foundation for Suicide Prevention (AFSP), and the Anxiety Disorders Association of America (ADAA), are valuable sources of information from the patient's perspective.

What is the current status of pharmacotherapy? The last 10–15 years have been exciting times in the field of pharmacotherapy of mental disorders. For example, when we compare the state of affairs in the mid- to late 1970s, we find that major depressive disorders could only be treated with tricyclic antidepressants, monoamine oxidase inhibitors, or electroconvulsive therapy. All were, and still are, effective but often difficult to tolerate over the long haul. At that time, psychotic disorders were treated with what are now termed the "typical" antipsychotics but were then called "major tranquilizers." These medications, including Haldol (haloperidol), Thorazine (chlorpromazine), Navane (thiothixene), and related compounds, were effective for the "positive" symptoms of psychosis (e.g., hallucinations, delusions) but were less than satisfying for the "negative" symptoms of schizophrenia such as apathy or withdrawal. Moreover, they were plagued by a myriad of uncomfortable side effects that rendered adherence an ongoing problem. Bipolar disorder, then termed manic-depression, could be treated with lithium, but lithium therapy is often unsatisfactory for patients with mixed states or rapid cycling. Anxiety disorders were treated, if even diagnosed, with benzodiazepines or barbiturates, though some pioneers in the field were just beginning to use antidepressant drugs, now a mainstay of treatment for these diseases. Fast forward to the 21st century, and there have been numerous innovations for psychiatric pharmacotherapy. There are several newer antidepressants with more favorable side effect and safety profiles, a burgeoning number of antiepileptic drugs being used for bipolar disorder, and a new generation of "atypical" antipsychotics with improved treatment adherence because they are easier for patients to tolerate. Everyone involved in the treatment of psychiatric disorders must know about current treatments. Otherwise, when the patient asks his/her therapist about medication treatment, providing outdated information may become an obstacle that prevents the individual from seeking effective treatment.

Clinical Vignette

Carol is a 45-year-old woman who has been suffering from an episode of major depressive disorder for 6 months. She has been working hard in psychotherapy but continues to show signs and symptoms of depression such as increased sleep, increased appetite, decreased energy, feelings of guilt, and depressed mood. Her therapist suggests a referral for a medication evaluation. Carol's reply consists partly of the following concern: "My mother gained 40 pounds when she took an antidepressant 20 years ago, and I'm not going to do that." It would be helpful to point out to Carol that her mother probably took a tricyclic antidepressant or a monoamine oxidase inhibitor. Although both are effective medications, they have a number of unpleasant side effects including an often-significant amount of weight gain. Many of the newer antidepressants are relatively neutral in regard to weight gain, and Carol should bring up this concern with the physician, or if she prefers, the therapist could mention that in the referral. A therapist without such information about medication effects can be at a decided disadvantage when trying to encourage a patient to seek optimal care.

When is medication indicated in the treatment of psychiatric illness? There is no short answer to this question. At one end of the continuum, patients with schizophrenia and other psychotic disorders, bipolar disorder, and severe major depressive disorder should always be considered candidates for pharmacotherapy, and neglecting to use medication, or at least discuss the use of medication with these patients, fails to adhere to the current standard of mental health care. Less severe depressive disorders, many anxiety disorders, and binge eating disorders can respond to psychotherapy and/or pharmacotherapy, and different therapies can target distinct symptom complexes in these situations. Finally, at the opposite end of the spectrum, adjustment disorders, specific phobias, or grief reactions should generally be treated with psychotherapy alone.

Why read this book? The purpose of this book is to invite "nonprescribing" practitioners to increase their knowledge of available medication therapies, to understand when they are appropriate to use, and perhaps equally important, to recognize when they are not indicated. This knowledge provides a foundation for therapists to discuss the use of psychiatric medicines with both their patients and the prescribing physicians to whom they make referrals. Again, we want to emphasize that the information in this book is not intended, and is by no means sufficient, to teach someone how to prescribe these medications, but rather to provide a sense of familiarity so that psychiatric medications are not a complete unknown. In the end, the goal is for the patient to be more informed about treatment options so that (s)he is better equipped to determine if treatment is proceeding as it should.

Finally, we would like to add a note about terminology. The terms "patient" and "client" will be used interchangeably, recognizing that different disciplines have their preferred ways of referring to those who come to us seeking help.

ADDITIONAL READING

Beitman BD, Blinder BJ, Thase ME, Riba M, Safer DL. *Integrating Psychotherapy and Pharmacotherapy: Dissolving the Mind–Brain Barrier.* New York: WW Norton, 2003.

Blackman JS. Dynamic supervision concerning a patient's request for medication. *Psychoanal Q* 2003; 72(2): 469–475.

Gabbard GO, Kay J. The fate of integrated treatment: Whatever happened to the biopsychosocial psychiatrist? *Am J Psychiatry* 2001; 158(12): 1956–1963.

Lebovitz PS. Integrating psychoanalysis and psychopharmacology: a review of the literature of combined treatment for affective disorders. *J Am Acad Psychoanal Dyn Psychiatry* 2004; 32: 585–596.

Longhofer J, Floersch J, Jenkins JH. The social grid of community medication management. *Am J Orthopsychiatry* 2003; 73(1): 24–34.

Nathan PE, Gorman JM (eds). *A Guide to Treatments That Work, 2nd Edition.* London: Oxford University Press, 2002.

Patterson J, Peek CJ, Heinrich RL, Bischoff RJ, Scherger J. *Mental Health Professionals in Medical Settings: A Primer.* New York: WW Norton, 2002.

Pilgrim D. The biopsychosocial model in Anglo-American psychiatry: Past, present and future? *J Ment Health* 2002; 11(6): 585–594.

Pillay SS, Ghaemi SN. The psychology of polypharmacy. In Ghaemi SN (ed), *Polypharmacy in Psychiatry.* New York: Marcel Dekker, pp 299–310.

Roose SP, Johannet CM. Medication and psychoanalysis: treatments in conflict. *Psychoanal Inq* 1998; 18(5): 606–620.

Rubin J. Countertransference factors in the psychology of psychopharmacology. *J Am Acad Psychoanal* 2001; 29(4): 565–573.

Sammons MT, Schmidt NB. *Combined Treatments for Mental Disorders: A Guide to Psychological and Pharmacological Interventions.* Washington DC: American Psychological Association, 2001.

2

BASICS OF PSYCHOPHARMACOLOGY

2.1 INTRODUCTION

2.1.1 Learning the Language of Pharmacology

One of the difficulties in learning about any medical field is becoming familiar with the technical jargon. Psychiatry is no different. Doctors like to use as few words as possible but be as specific as they can possibly be. We accomplish this by taking simple root words and adding one or more prefixes and suffixes to derive the specific meaning that we want to convey. The result is that we can say a lot with a few words, though at times it may sound as if we say little with a large number of words. The lengthy words that sometimes arise when several scientific prefixes and suffixes are added to a root word can be very imposing to those who are not initiated into "doctor-speak."

Let us share an example. The body's hormone system is called the endocrine system. Endocrine comes from a Greek prefix that means "within" (*endo-*) and a Greek root word that means "separate" (*krinein*). This makes sense when you realize that hormones are substances that carry instructions between *separate* organs *within* your body. By adding the suffix *-ologist* (which means one who studies) to

Principles of Psychopharmacology for Mental Health Professionals
By Jeffrey E. Kelsey, D. Jeffrey Newport, and Charles B. Nemeroff

endocrine, we get the term endocrinologist. An endocrinologist is simply a doctor who studies and treats illnesses of the hormone system. But the hormone system does not work alone; it functions in concert with other body systems such as the nervous system. By adding the prefix *neuro-* (which means nerve), we arrive at the term neuroendocrinologist. A neuroendocrinologist is a doctor who studies the interaction between the nervous system and the hormone system. When the hormone and nervous systems interact, this has an impact on the way we think and behave. In other words, it affects our mind. By adding the prefix *psycho-* (which means mind), we have the term psychoneuroendocrinologist. A psychoneuroendocrinologist is one who studies how the mind is affected by the interaction between the hormone system and the nervous system.

As you can see, by stringing several simple words together, we can construct complex medical terms that can convey large amounts of information. We will try to avoid using too many of these technical terms as we set off on our journey into the study of (*-ology*) how medications (*pharmaco-*) affect the mind (*psycho-*). In a word, let's take a look at psychopharmacology.

2.1.2 Overview

Before we introduce you to the many psychiatric illnesses and the medications used to treat these illnesses, you first need a general understanding of just how these medications work. In this chapter, we will introduce you to these concepts.

First, you will learn about the human nervous system and how it works when it is healthy. This will include an introduction to the structure (anatomy) of the nervous system and the function (physiology) of the nervous system. Next, we'll describe the things that can go wrong. We'll look at how the system breaks down and malfunctions. Then we'll show you how these breakdowns can result in psychiatric illness. Finally, we'll introduce you to the medications used to treat psychiatric illness. You will learn where these medications work and our best guess of how they work. The presumed mechanism of action of many medications is just that, presumed. In contrast to antibiotics, in which we know quite a lot about the ways that they kill bacteria or stop them from reproducing and how these mechanisms ultimately effect a cure for an infectious disease, less is known about how psychotropic medicines work. Oh, we pretty well understand what psychotropic medicines do when they reach the nerve cell. For example, most of the antidepressants used today block the reuptake of serotonin at the nerve cell, but we're still not sure why blocking serotonin reuptake gradually improves mood in someone with depression. This will lead to a "tour," if you will, of what happens to a medication from the time the pill is swallowed, until it exerts its therapeutic effect.

2.2 NORMAL HUMAN NERVOUS SYSTEM

There are two parts to this story: function and structure. The study of the body's structure is called anatomy, and so, we'll be discussing neuroanatomy (the structure of the nervous system). The study of the body's function is called physiology, and so, we'll also be discussing neurophysiology (the function of the nervous system).

As architects teach us, form follows function. The layout of a building is dictated in large part by its intended use. A hospital, an airport terminal, a restaurant, a home, and a factory are each designed to serve a specific purpose. If the building's design does not facilitate its purpose, then it will soon be abandoned.

Similarly, the structure of the nervous system is interwoven with its function. At all levels, from the microscopic highly branched nerve cell to the multiple connections between large brain regions that are visible to the naked eye, the structure of the nervous system is obviously designed to serve its chief purpose: communication. As a result, it is difficult to talk about structure separately from function. Nevertheless, a divided, stepwise approach may help make these complicated matters easier for you to understand.

2.2.1 Neuroanatomy: Structure of the Nervous System

Central Nervous System (CNS). The human nervous system is an integrated communication network that sends and receives information throughout the body. This network is divided into two main divisions: central nervous system (CNS) and peripheral nervous system (PNS). The CNS is the command center of this network and is made up of the brain and spinal cord. The PNS is the interface of the nervous system with the rest of the body and the external environment. It is comprised of nerve fibers and small clusters of nerve cells known as ganglia.

Neurologists treat nervous system diseases that mainly cause physical symptoms. Therefore, they are concerned with both the CNS and the PNS. Mental health professionals, on the other hand, treat diseases that produce emotional, thought, and behavioral symptoms. As a result, we are more concerned with the CNS and, in particular, the brain.

The Brain. The brain is the most magnificent of the body's organs. But then, as mental health professionals, we may all be a little biased. As you study the brain, you learn very quickly that it is highly organized. If you cut the brain like a loaf of bread, which we can now do visually with computed tomography (CT) and magnetic resonance imaging (MRI) scans, there are many structures that are easy to see. We'll spare you all the details regarding these many brain regions.

Over the years, we have learned a great deal about the functions of each of these structures. This knowledge has come about in several ways. First, we can look at the effect of disease or injury in a particular part of the brain. For example, if a stroke causes paralysis, then we can assume that the injured part of the brain was responsible for movement of the paralyzed body parts. Likewise, if an injury results in certain personality changes, then we can assume that the injured part of the brain contributed to those behavioral alterations. One of the best-known examples is the effect of a stroke upon mood. It is well known that a stroke to the left frontal area of the brain dramatically increases the likelihood of depression. On the other hand, a stroke to the right frontal area increases the likelihood of developing a manic episode. Clearly then, the frontal lobes of the brain contribute to our mood state. As an aside, depression following a stroke occurs in 25–45% of patients. It can be easy to explain the vulnerability to depression after a stroke in terms of disability, loss of independence, or a reminder of our mortality. Such explanations are sometimes used to rationalize that medically ill patients have a "right" to be depressed and therefore don't need antidepressant treatment. However, depression following a stroke, just like depression that may accompany a heart attack or cancer, should be treated aggressively, and the option of medications should be considered. In fact, it is often depressive episodes that occur in response to a stressor such as medical illness that call for consideration of antidepressant therapy. The patient who becomes depressed after a stroke or a heart attack is less likely to be successful in occupational therapy, physical therapy, or making life-style modifications, such as dietary changes or smoking cessation, that are important in reducing the risk of another event.

We are now learning even more about the brain through the use of imaging technology. MRI provides unbelievably detailed pictures of the brain's structure. Computer programs now allow us to use the MRI "slices" to construct three-dimensional views of the brain. The latest developments are the so-called functional brain imaging studies. These include positron emission tomography (PET) and functional MRI (fMRI). With these tools, we can actually see what areas of the brain "light up" or become more or less active during certain activities or certain emotional states. These tools are also providing us a closer look at the brain's circuitry (i.e., the connections between brain structures).

Glial Cells. The tissue of the nervous system is made up of two cell types: nerve cells and glial cells. Glial cells provide a supporting role in the network. They afford protection and provide nutrition to the nerve cells. They also insulate nerve fibers to speed the transmission of information. Although glial cells perform only a supportive role, they are crucial to nervous system functioning. When disease affects the glial cells, severe illness often results. You need only consider multiple sclerosis (MS) or amyotrophic lateral sclerosis (Lou Gehrig disease) to realize the devastating consequences of diseases that attack glial cells.

Nerve Cells. A nerve cell is also known as a neuron. It serves as the basic functional unit of the system. There are approximately 10 billion neurons in the human nervous system. In many ways, the neuron is just like any typical cell. It has a cell membrane and a nucleus. Its cytoplasm contains the usual organelles that you learned about in high school biology: endoplasmic reticulum, mitochondria, storage vesicles, and the Golgi apparatus.

But the structure of the neuron leaves it well adapted to its purpose, namely, communication. Neurons provide the linkages to communicate from the outside environment to ourselves and again to the outside environment if we wish. The neural pathways can be simple, such as the two cell pathways that are activated when a kneecap is struck with a reflex hammer and the leg kicks out, or as complicated as the pathways (as yet poorly defined) that are active in the generation of emotional states.

A neuron is made up of three parts: axon, cell body, and dendrites. The cell body contains the nucleus, and therefore the genetic material, DNA, and much of the "machinery" that allows the cell to function, to synthesize neurotransmitter molecules to communicate with other cells, and to maintain the day-to-day housekeeping chores of the cell. The dendrites, in general, transmit information to the cell body. As such, dendrites are the "eyes" and "ears" of the neuron. The axon, in contrast, sends information downstream to neighboring cells via hundreds, even thousands, of axon terminals.

Plasticity. There is another feature of the neuron that is different from other cells in the human body. Neurons are generally not thought to be capable of dividing to make new neurons, though recent exciting research suggests that nerve cell division (i.e., neurogenesis) does occur on a regular basis in at least some regions (e.g., the hippocampus) of the brain. In general, however, when a nerve cell dies, it is never replaced. This is why people seldom recover from paralysis after a severe spinal cord injury. It is also why the accumulated death of many neurons results in dementias like Alzheimer's disease. Fortunately, the CNS enjoys a tremendous "plasticity." In other words, the brain learns which nerve cell connections to strengthen, and which to weaken. This modifying of connections is the neural substrate for learning and requires the synthesis of proteins. In a classic series of experiments, Bernard Agranoff and colleagues examined the role of protein synthesis on learning. Briefly, they taught goldfish how to swim through a maze. When protein synthesis was blocked, learning did not take place, whereas when protein synthesis was undisturbed, learning did take place. Such observations offer the tantalizing possibility that psychotherapy and pharmacotherapy may achieve their therapeutic benefit by producing similar or complementary changes in the brain. This plasticity is somewhat analogous to what happens when a houseplant is placed next to a window, and a few days later, the leaves have turned to face the light. In a similar fashion, nerve cells are constantly adapting. It happens so gradually that you can't really see it. But the dendrite and axon branches are continuously removing old connections and establishing new connections with neighboring cells. This "pruning" begins before birth and continues throughout life.

It is the process of pruning followed by the growth of new branches that explains why people paralyzed by a stroke or spinal cord injury may experience gradual improvement over several months time. The establishment of new neuron-to-neuron connections to replace those that were destroyed when the injury occurred sometimes allows the communication circuit to be repaired. In addition, there are certain times in life that are preprogrammed for a flurry of pruning activity. One such time is adolescence and early adulthood, which has led some researchers to conclude that problems in the pruning process might trigger the emergence of schizophrenia. We'll tell you more about that later.

2.2.2 Neurophysiology: Function of the Nervous System

In neurophysiology, we encounter another of those medical terms that is a string of prefixes added to a simple root term. The parts of this word (*neuro* + *physio* + *ology*) literally mean "nervous system + function + study." So neurophysiology is simply the study of how the nervous system works.

When we talk about the function of the nervous system, there are two major levels to the discussion. First, what is the purpose of the nervous system? In other words, why do we need it? What does it accomplish? Second, how does the nervous system work? What are its means of accomplishing its tasks?

Purpose of the Nervous System. Overall, in the most simplistic analysis, the nervous system performs three tasks: sensation, processing, and execution. These are the tasks of any information management system. In this respect, your nervous system serves purposes similar to a computer network. In your nervous system, each of these three tasks can occur voluntarily within your full awareness or involuntarily outside your consciousness.

Sensation provides the input to the system. The sources of sensory information can be outside your body through one of the five primary senses: sight, sound, taste, smell, and touch. The source of information can also be inside your body. The nervous system receives and monitors information such as your blood pressure, blood sugar, and blood oxygen level.

Processing is what the nervous system does with the information once it is received. Sometimes this processing occurs without your conscious participation. For example, you don't usually make conscious efforts to control your blood pressure (although with biofeedback training you can exert some level of control). This type of information is processed in "primitive" regions of your brain and don't require your conscious participation. Thought and emotion are also processing functions of the nervous system. This type of processing occurs at the highest level of the system, the brain's cerebrum. At this level, information is largely processed consciously. But this is not entirely true. Freud emphasized long ago that much of what we consider mental life transpires outside our awareness in the dynamic unconscious, a concept now demonstrable with sophisticated functional brain imaging techniques. Through these various levels of processing, you come to understand (or misunderstand) and plan responses to the information your brain is receiving.

Once the information is processed and you (consciously or unconsciously) have decided what it means, your nervous system coordinates a response. This is the task of *execution*. The loop from sensation to processing to execution can occur at many levels. The simplest level is the reflex arc. As noted earlier, when your family doctor strikes your knee with a rubber hammer, the nerves at your knee sense the impact and transmit that information. This information is intercepted and processed well before it ever reaches your consciousness. A reflex center interprets the sensation as a possible threat and automatically executes a command to straighten your knee. The result is a reflex action that protects your leg from injury by kicking away the perceived threat. This sensation to processing to execution loop is completed without any involvement of your brain.

This same loop occurs at all levels of interaction and can become exceedingly complex. You may have attended a professional convention or class reunion recently during which you encountered an old friend whom you had not seen for some time. You caught sight of your friend, and that visual sensory information was transmitted to your brain. This image was processed by your brain, and you recognized that what you were seeing was your old friend and that your friend was coming toward you smiling. Your nervous system quickly executed the command to smile in return. Meanwhile, processing (at a more conscious level) continued as you tried to decide how best to respond. Should you shake hands with your old friend or is a hug more appropriate? Instantaneously, cultural rules, the intimacy of your friendship, and the situation of the encounter were all being considered as you processed this information. You decided upon a handshake, and a command to extend your right hand was executed. But more sensory input was received at that point. You noticed that your friend's arms were outstretched as if to embrace you. Your brain rapidly processed this new information, and a command was executed to extend your arms and embrace your old friend.

As you can see, this loop of sensation to processing to execution can be quite simple or very complex. In social encounters, a host of modifying interactions often comes into play. But in the final analysis, the purpose of the nervous system is quite simple. It is to integrate information and coordinate your responses as you communicate with your environment.

Mechanisms of the Nervous System. We've talked about what the nervous system does. Now let's take a look at how it does it. It does so by transmitting signals known as nerve impulses. The nerve cell is well suited to this task. It is a highly excitable cell. When a nerve cell is stimulated by incoming signals to its dendrites, it responds by opening channels (pores) in its cell membrane. When these channels open, charged particles called ions flood into the nerve cell. Called depolarization, this influx of ions causes a dramatic shift in the balance of electrical charges inside and outside the nerve cell. If the depolarization of the nerve cell reaches a certain threshold, the cell "fires" an impulse, known as an action potential.

Once an action potential is fired, it begins to spread. Remember, a neuron is an excitable cell. Like fans doing "The Wave" at a football game, the excitement of the action potential begins to travel the length of the nerve cell. The action potential travels up the dendrite toward the cell body, opening more channels and allowing more ions to flood into the cell as it goes.

The cell body gathers the incoming action potentials from the dendrites and sends along a single action potential to the axon. The action potential travels the length of the axon until reaching the axon terminals. At this point, the nerve cell must pass the impulse to its neighboring cells. This communication from one neuron to another is accomplished by neurotransmission.

Neurotransmission. This is the most important part of nervous system function for us to understand, both because it serves as the cornerstone of nerve cell signaling, and because it is the process that is modulated by psychotropic medications and thus helps to explain both the therapeutic benefits and the side effects that they produce. Psychiatric medicines have little or no direct effect on the action potential traveling down the length of the excited nerve cell. Instead, they act to enhance or interfere with the talk, or neurotransmission, between nerve cells.

Over 100 years ago, a debate was raging between the two most famous neuroscientists in the world concerning the nature of the nervous system. Golgi believed that all neurons were connected in a "nerve net" or "syncytium" whereas Ramon y Cajal believed that neurons were separated from each other by tiny spaces called synapses. Cajal proved to be correct, and it was later learned that neurons communicate across the synapse by releasing chemical substances known as neurotransmitters or by releasing electrical charges. Because chemical neurotransmission is much more common than electrical transmission, especially in the brain, and it is chemical neurotransmission that is modulated by psychiatric medicines, our discussion will focus on the chemotransmitter process. In simplest terms, the process of chemical neurotransmission occurs in three steps: neurotransmitter production, neurotransmitter release, and neurotransmitter action on specific receptors.

Neurotransmitter Production. Neurotransmitters are relatively simple chemicals, and our bodies make most of the ones that we use. The nerve cell receives precursor substances such as amino acids from proteins in the diet and chemically processes these precursors to form neurotransmitter chemicals. The neurotransmitter is then stored in small sacs inside the neuron called storage vesicles. These storage vesicles reside inside the axon terminals.

Neurotransmitter Release. When the nerve cell is stimulated, an action potential is generated that travels the length of the cell from dendrite to cell body to axon. Once the action potential reaches the axon terminal, it causes the storage vesicles

Clinical Vignette

Patients often ask, "How does this medication work?" We've found the following answer helpful to most patients who are trying, for example, to understand what an antidepressant does. Cells in the brain need to communicate with each other, and they do so by releasing chemicals called neurotransmitters. Examples of neurotransmitter chemicals include serotonin, norepinephrine, and acetylcholine. When cell A wants to talk to cell B, cell A releases the brain chemical, and it drifts across a very narrow gap to cell B, where the chemical binds to a protein called a receptor. This turns the signal on in cell B. Of course, there must also be a way to turn the signal off. When the brain chemical drifts away from the receptor, this turns off the signal in cell B. The cell that released the chemical, cell A, will often take it back up to recycle it. This recycling process is called reuptake, and it saves energy, because it is easier to reuse a molecule of a brain chemical than it is to make a new one. Many antidepressants slow down the reuptake of the brain chemical A so that it stays in the tiny space between the cells for a longer period of time, where it can keep binding to receptors and thus keep turning on the signal in cell B.

to dump their supply of neurotransmitter into the synapse that separates the nerve cell from its neighbors.

Neurotransmitter/Receptor Binding. At this point, the neurotransmitter chemical is free in the synapse (extracellular fluid) and drifts (diffuses) in all directions. Some of the neurotransmitter molecules float across the synapse and bind to receptors on the surface of the adjacent nerve cell. Each neurotransmitter has its own unique three-dimensional shape and binds with certain receptors but not others. The binding between a neurotransmitter and a receptor is similar to fitting a key into a lock. When the neurotransmitter binds the receptor, the signal has been passed to the neighboring nerve cell. This is the process of neurotransmission.

In many cases, the neurotransmitter sends an excitatory signal to its neighbor. In other words, it tells the neighboring nerve cell to wake up and get busy. As a result, an action potential (i.e., nerve impulse) is more likely to be fired in that neuron. Other neurotransmitters act as inhibitory messengers that reduce the possibility that the neighboring cell will fire an action potential. In other words, an inhibitory neurotransmitter tells the neighboring neuron to take a break and get some rest. This actually makes it more difficult (at least for a while) to create an action potential in the neighboring cell. The excitable neighbor is therefore calmed down by the inhibitory neurotransmitter. When the neurotransmitter binds to a receptor on the cell membrane surface of the adjacent nerve cell, a second messenger often carries its signal inside the neighboring nerve cell. This concludes the process called signal transduction. What happens after the second messenger system inside the nerve cell has been activated is now the subject of much research. Although they are poorly understood, the work of these second messengers may eventually help explain the delayed effects of many psychiatric medications.

Stopping Neurotransmission. Turning off the neurotransmitter signal once it has been released into the synapse is critical to successful communication between nerve cells. This is of paramount importance because unbridled stimulation can be harmful to nerve cells. For example, one of the problems in the minutes and hours following a stroke is that nerve cells near the stroke area can literally be stimulated to death. In fact, some of the new medications used to minimize damage to the brain after a stroke act by literally calming the cells in the brain. Thus, signal termination is a critically important aspect of neurotransmission.

As we noted earlier, when the neurotransmitter is released from the axon terminal into the synapse, it is free to diffuse across the synapse to bind the receptors on the neighboring nerve cell. However, other fates may await the neurotransmitter once it's released into the synapse. In general, these other processes act to terminate neurotransmission by preventing the neurotransmitter from reaching the receptor on the adjacent nerve cell. There are, in fact, five distinct mechanisms for terminating the neurotransmitter signal once it has been released into the synapse.

1. *Diffusion.* Instead of drifting to the opposite side of the synapse, the neurotransmitter molecule can also drift outside the synapse altogether. In this free

extracellular space outside the synapse, there are usually no receptors to which neurotransmitter can bind. It simply floats in this space outside the cells (extracellular space), which is continuous with the cerebrospinal fluid (CSF) that bathes the brain, until it is eventually recycled or degraded.

2. *Deactivation in the Synapse.* There are enzymes in the synapse, for example, catechol *O*-methyltransferase (COMT), that deactivate the neurotransmitter by cutting atoms from the ends of the neurotransmitter molecule. This is like rubbing a metal file against your house key. When you've changed the shape of the key's teeth, it no longer fits the lock. Likewise, when the enzymes remove enough of the neurotransmitter's structure, it no longer fits its receptor. At that point, the neurotransmitter is deactivated.
3. *Negative Feedback.* Some of the neurotransmitter diffuses back to the surface of the nerve cell that released it. There are also receptors that fit the neurotransmitter here. When a neurotransmitter binds a receptor (called an autoreceptor) at the axon terminal of the nerve cell that released it, it tells the nerve cell that there's plenty of neurotransmitter already in the synapse. So don't release anymore! This process is called negative feedback and is analogous to the way a thermostat works in your home to control room temperature.
4. *Reuptake.* The nerve cell that released the neurotransmitter also has what are called reuptake sites on its surface. These reuptake sites are actually transporter proteins that are specific to each type of neurotransmitter. They act like miniature vacuum cleaners to retrieve the neurotransmitter from the synapse. The neurotransmitter is removed from the synapse at the reuptake site and returned to the inside of the nerve cell's axon terminal. Although the reuptake process recycles the neurotransmitter molecules for future use, the process does, in fact, serve to terminate the current neurotransmitter signal.
5. *Deactivation Inside the Axon Terminal.* After the neurotransmitter molecule is returned to the axon terminal via reuptake, it is briefly free, and unprotected, inside the cytoplasm of the nerve cell. It is quickly gathered and stored in storage vesicles again, where it is protected and held for future use, but during the brief interval during which the neurotransmitter is free inside the neuron's cytoplasm, it is vulnerable to deactivation by enzymes. Although the enzymes inside the nerve cell (e.g., monoamine oxidase (MAO)), are distinct from those that operate in the synapse, they act in a similar fashion. The enzymes cut off, or cleave, atoms from the neurotransmitter molecule until they change its shape so that it no longer fits its receptor.

Brain Circuitry. When we started this discussion of neurophysiology, we told you that it's hard to talk about nervous system structure without also talking about nervous system function and vice versa. Nowhere is this clearer than when we talk about brain circuitry.

Mention of circuitry naturally engenders comparisons of the brain to a computer. In fact, there are a number of parallels between the structure and function of the nervous system and the structure and function of a computer system. Both receive input, both process this input, and both produce an output. However, computer circuitry is much simpler than the circuitry of the brain in two important ways.

First, computer circuits are hard-wired at the factory. A computer's circuitry never changes. In contrast, as we noted previously, brain circuitry is constantly adapting through a process of pruning and reestablishing connections. This pruning affords the nervous system a plasticity that enables it to adapt continually to the demands of an ever-changing environment.

Second, computer circuits have only two conditions: OFF and ON. Conversely, a single circuit in the nervous system can have a variety of graded responses. Although there are several explanations for this graduated circuit activation, a principal basis is that more than one neurotransmitter can be utilized in a single circuit. Most circuits have a single primary neurotransmitter. There are over 100 neurotransmitter substances that have been identified, and more are yet to be discovered, but the most common primary neurotransmitters that you'll read about are serotonin, dopamine, norepinephrine, acetylcholine, glutamate, and GABA, as well as a novel class of neurotransmitters called neuropeptides. In a given neural pathway, the secondary neurotransmitters typically act as cotransmitters that modulate the signal of the circuit's primary neurotransmitter.

The importance of brain circuitry is that it reminds us that these chemical neurotransmitters are not released willy-nilly throughout the brain. This is why the term "chemical imbalance" is so unsatisfactory. The brain is not a large water bottle into which these chemicals are poured and maintained in some precise balance. For that reason, there is no simple test to check a neurotransmitter level like the dipstick on your car's oil reservoir. Instead, your brain is a delicate instrument with predefined but ever-adapting pathways of communication.

Each of these pathways (or circuits) serves a particular purpose and works in concert with other circuits. Technology has only recently allowed us a glimpse of these circuits in action. Thus, we are just beginning to map out the pathways and functions of the myriad brain circuits involved in the regulation of thought and emotion. As you'll see later, however, understanding brain circuitry can help us to anticipate what the beneficial effects and side effects of a medication may be.

2.3 PATHOPHYSIOLOGY: STUDY OF WHAT GOES WRONG

By now, you know that the nervous system is a communications network that serves to control your body. You also know that nerve impulses are the vehicle that carries information around this network. In addition, you know that chemical neurotransmission is the means by which these signals are passed from one neuron to another. Finally, you know that neurotransmitters, receptors, and enzymes are the key components that make all of these things happen.

We have long suspected that abnormalities in the receptors and enzymes that interact with a neurotransmitter are one of the major underlying causes of many major mental illnesses. As you will learn later, medications that act on these receptors, reuptake sites, or enzymes relieve the symptoms of many psychiatric illnesses. This would seem to validate our prior suspicions. Nevertheless, it has been very difficult to demonstrate these suspected abnormalities.

Part of the reason may be the relatively crude nature of the tools we have had until recently to study brain function. However, this is clearly beginning to change. Genetic research and functional brain imaging, which actually takes pictures of the brain "in action," may ultimately give us a glimpse of brain receptor and enzyme activity that was unthinkable just a few years ago.

2.3.1 What Goes Wrong

Despite these limitations, there are several models of what goes wrong in the brain when mental illness strikes. It is helpful to review these ideas.

1. *Too Little Neurotransmission.* In some cases, disease appears to damage or cause the death of nerve cells, a process called neurodegeneration. These diseases cause problems by stopping normal neurotransmission altogether. One example of this disease process is Alzheimer's disease, the major cause of dementia in the elderly. In this common and devastating illness, acetylcholine-containing nerve cells, and others, die prematurely.
2. *Too Much Neurotransmission.* Other mental illnesses result from too much neurotransmission (i.e., overactivity) of certain brain circuits. One example may be psychosis, for example, hallucinations and delusions that have been hypothesized to result from excessive transmission of the neurotransmitter dopamine in certain pathways. In some cases, the transmission becomes so excessive that it kills the nerve cell, a phenomenon called excitotoxicity. This process is believed to occur in some patients with epilepsy and in those with Huntington's disease.
3. *Faulty Wiring and/or Developmental Delay.* Remember that neurotransmission moves through brain circuits. Some mental illnesses may be caused by misconnections in the circuitry that can result in the brain's equivalent of "crosstalk" that occurs when telephone lines are crossed. Examples of this problem are the so-called neurodevelopmental disorders such as autism, certain forms of mental retardation, and possibly schizophrenia.
4. *Poor Timing of Neurotransmission.* The activity of some brain circuits, like the secretion of certain hormones, varies at certain times of the day. Called circadian rhythms, the timing of these rhythms may be disrupted in some illnesses. Examples include sleep disorders such as insomnia and narcolepsy, as well as other conditions such as nighttime binge-eating disorder.
5. *Imbalanced Neurotransmission.* Most brain regions are innervated by axonal projections secreting multiple neurotransmitters. When the system is healthy, the activity of the two (or more) neurotransmitters is held in a delicate balance. Some illnesses result from an imbalance in transmission of multiple neuro-

transmitters. Examples of this problem include the abnormal movements seen in Parkinson's disease and Huntington's disease. Treatment with certain antipsychotic medications may also produce abnormal movements by causing imbalanced neurotransmission in this same circuit.

2.3.2 Why It Goes Wrong

If it has been difficult to prove that abnormalities of neurotransmission cause certain mental illnesses, you can imagine how difficult it is to show what causes such abnormalities to occur in the first place. However, we have made some progress in this area.

Genetic Factors. Some mental illnesses are well known to run in families, which of course raises the question of genetic inheritance. For many major mental disorders including bipolar disorder and schizophrenia, twin studies have been particularly revealing. For example, if an identical twin has schizophrenia, the chance that the other identical twin also develops schizophrenia is 50%. This is known as the concordance rate for the illness. Studies with identical twins adopted into different families confirm that there is a genetic contribution to certain mental illnesses such as bipolar disorder, schizophrenia, and depression. Many medical illnesses such as cystic fibrosis, hemophilia, and sickle cell disease are the direct result of a single abnormal gene. Except for Huntington's disease, major psychiatric illnesses cannot be explained in this simple fashion.

Nevertheless, there is strong evidence that some mental illnesses are partly inherited. One prevailing theory is the "two hit hypothesis." The first of these two hits is a genetic trait that leaves one vulnerable to the illness. The second hit is some stressful life event or environmental insult (e.g., infection or toxic exposure) that triggers the onset of the illness in the vulnerable individual.

Brain Deterioration (Neurodegeneration). Other mental illnesses are called neurodegenerative because they result from the death of nerve cells in the brain. Neurodegenerative illnesses steadily worsen over time as more and more nerve cells progressively die. These illnesses are most common in the elderly, and the best-known examples are Alzheimer's disease and Parkinson's disease, though others including Huntington's disease and Pick's disease have been described. However, neurodegenerative diseases can strike at any time. For example, Tay–Sachs disease is a relatively rare inherited neurodegenerative disease that most commonly affects Jews of eastern European descent (Ashkenazi Jews). The illness strikes during infancy and quickly leads to death. There are also neurodegenerative disorders of the spinal cord such as amyotrophic lateral sclerosis (ALS) that result in progressive paralysis and ultimately death.

Abnormal Brain Development. In a certain sense, neurodegenerative disorders reside at the opposite end of the spectrum from the so-called neurodevelopmental diseases. These result from abnormal development of brain circuitry. The causes of such disorders are varied and include chromosomal or other genetic abnormalities, nutritional deficiencies, prenatal infections, or toxin exposures.

For obvious reasons, neurodevelopmental illnesses usually appear at birth or in early childhood. It is during these early years that the connections that form brain circuitry are established. Some of the best-known examples of neurodevelopmental illnesses include cerebral palsy, phenylketonuria, and the autistic disorders.

Schizophrenia raises interesting questions in this regard. It becomes apparent in late adolescence or early adulthood, not in childhood. In many, if not most, cases, schizophrenia is manifested by a premorbid period of recognizable prodromal symptoms followed by a progressively worsening downhill course after the first signs of the illness become evident. For these reasons, it was long assumed that schizophrenia is a neurodegenerative disorder like dementia. In fact, schizophrenia was once called dementia praecox, which literally means "premature dementia." However, many researchers now believe that schizophrenia is, in fact, a neurodevelopmental illness, and one of developmental arrest of certain brain cells.

But how does a neurodevelopmental disorder fail to emerge until adulthood? This is certainly seen in other genetically transmitted diseases including certain forms of diabetes and Huntington's disease. The answer to this question remains obscure but may lie in the plasticity of brain circuitry because, as noted earlier, nerve cell connections are continually being pruned away and reestablished. One particularly busy period of nerve cell pruning is late adolescence and early adulthood. It is believed that problems arising during this pruning may play a pivotal role in the emergence of schizophrenia.

2.4 PHARMACOLOGY

2.4.1 Introduction

Pharmacology is the study of the use of medications. There are two subplots to this evolving story: pharmacodynamics and pharmacokinetics. Here we go with the doctor-speak again. In layperson's terms, pharmacodynamics is the effect of the medication on the body, whereas pharmacokinetics is the effect of the body on the medication. An example might be instructive. Benzodiazepines, such as alprazolam (Xanax) or clonazepam (Klonopin), are commonly used to treat anxiety disorders. The *pharmacodynamic* effects include the therapeutic goal of decreased anxiety, as well as potential side effects of sedation or slowed reaction times. The *pharmacokinetic* effect is the metabolism of the drug by the body, primarily the liver. When more than one type of medication is ingested, there can be both pharmacodynamic and pharmacokinetic interactions between them. Returning to the anxiety disorders example, if a patient who is taking a benzodiazepine to treat panic disorder is also taking an over-the-counter decongestant such as pseudoephedrine for seasonal allergies, the pharmacodynamic effects of the two medicines might cancel out one another. Specifically, the anxiety being alleviated by the benzodiazepine might be increased by the pseudoephedrine.

Only when we look at both pharmacodynamics and pharmacokinetics can we predict the net effect that a medication will have. Appreciating these basic aspects of pharmacology helps us not only to anticipate what symptoms or illnesses a medication is likely to treat but also to recognize the side effects and potential interactions the medication is likely to have.

2.4.2 Pharmacokinetics

Before a medication can be of any help, it has to get to where it can act to produce its beneficial effects. For psychiatric medications, the action is, of course, in the brain. The problem is that it is relatively difficult for medications to get there. This is no accident. Our bodies are designed to protect our most vital organs. Our rib cage surrounds our heart and lungs. The skull encloses the brain, and the brain is also protected by the so-called blood–brain barrier from invaders that enter the bloodstream. In this section, we will describe the steps your medication takes to get to your brain and the hurdles it encounters along the way.

Medication Transportation System. If the brain, the spinal cord, and the nerves make up the body's communication system, then the heart, blood vessels, and blood are the body's transportation system. Blood carries oxygen and nutrients to the organs and then returns the wastes for disposal. Medications use this same internal highway system to travel throughout the body.

There are three steps that a medication takes during its travel through the body. First, the medication must somehow travel from outside the body and enter the bloodstream. Second, the medication is escorted while it is circulating in the bloodstream. Third, the medication must exit the bloodstream. We'll now describe each of these three steps in a little more detail.

1. *Entering the Bloodstream.* The way that a medication enters the bloodstream depends largely on how it is taken. There are many ways of ingesting medication, and those that are frequently used for psychiatric medications (or mind-altering illicit drugs) are shown in Table 2.1. The route of administration dictates how much of the medication reaches the bloodstream and how quickly it gets there.

The most common way to take medications is by mouth (orally). This is the slowest and least efficient way to get medication into your system. When a tablet or capsule is swallowed, much of it either passes through the gastrointestinal tract without ever being absorbed into the bloodstream or is inactivated by the liver before it has a chance to reach the rest of the body (more on this later). The fastest and most efficient means to get medication into the bloodstream is to inject it directly into a vein (intravenously). If oral medication is so much slower and so much less efficient, then why do we usually take our medications by mouth? We do so because it is easier, cheaper, safer, and painless to take medications orally.

There is perhaps no better illustration of the impact of the route of administration than the sad story of cocaine. For centuries, coca leaves were chewed by the indigenous peoples of South America for a boost of energy while working in

TABLE 2.1. Routes of Medication Administration with Subsequent Onset of Action and Clinical Efficiency

Route	How It's Taken	Speed of Onset	Efficiency
Oral	Swallowed and absorbed across intestinal lining	Slow	Low
Subcutaneous	Injected into fat beneath skin	Slow to intermediate	Intermediate
Intramuscular	Injected into muscle	Intermediate	Intermediate
Intranasal	Snorted and absorbed across lining of nasal passages	Rapid	Intermediate
Inhaled	Inhaled and absorbed in lungs	Almost immediate	High
Intravenous	Directly injected into bloodstream	Immediate	High

the fields. Although chewing coca leaves can be habit-forming, it does not appear that this was ever a tremendous social problem. Later, cocaine was refined from coca leaves into a powdered form that can be snorted. In this form, cocaine crosses the lining of the nasal passages to enter the bloodstream and, from there, the brain. Snorting powdered cocaine produces a quicker and more intense "high" than chewing coca leaves. Over time, it became apparent that powdered cocaine is also considerably more addictive than chewing coca leaves. Over 20 years ago, a process called "free-basing" was developed that converts powdered cocaine into a form called crack that can be smoked. When this smoke is inhaled, it crosses the lungs into the bloodstream in a matter of seconds with a rapid influx into the brain. The result is that crack cocaine almost instantaneously produces an extremely intense "high." In general, the addictive potential of a drug frequently parallels the rapidity with which it enters the brain following ingestion. Thus, through refinements that have changed cocaine's route of administration from oral (chewing coca leaves) to intranasal (snorting powdered cocaine) and now to inhalation (smoking crack), human ingenuity has created one of the most dangerously addictive substances in history.

2. *Escort in the Bloodstream.* Once the medication enters the bloodstream, it is quite vulnerable to being metabolized or inactivated. The body has provided an escort service for most substances in the bloodstream. These escorts are called carrier proteins. While a carrier protein is escorting the medication, it is protected from degradation. However, it is also unable to leave the bloodstream while under this protein escort.

Most psychiatric medications are highly protein bound. At any point in time, 80% or more of the molecules of most psychiatric medications circulating in the bloodstream are under escort by a carrier protein. It is only the remaining small fraction that is free to leave the bloodstream to reach the target organ or to be eliminated from the body. Knowing this permits the dose to be adjusted so that the "free fraction" of medication is sufficient to deliver enough of the medication to the site of action, namely, the brain.

However, if an individual is prescribed two or more medications that are each highly bound to the same carrier protein, then they could potentially compete for protein binding. In fact, it is possible to saturate, or fill, the available carrier protein binding sites. When this occurs, the free fraction, that is, the non-protein-bound and biologically active portion, of the medication might be larger than anticipated. This will cause the medication to be more potent at lower doses. If the potential for this type of drug interaction is anticipated in advance, then the doses can be adjusted accordingly. However, if the protein-binding interaction comes as a surprise, complications such as drug toxicity can arise. We'll talk more about this in our discussion of drug–drug interactions later in this chapter.

3. *Exiting the Bloodstream.* Medications, nutrients, and other substances are continuously leaving the bloodstream and entering other tissues or organs. They are free to reenter the bloodstream at any time and often do. The effect of the medication depends on where it exits. If it exits at the liver, the body's version of a waste treatment and chemical detoxification facility, then the medication is likely to be inactivated, that is, metabolized. If it exits at the kidney, then it will likely be excreted in urine. We'll describe this in more detail in the next section.

Of course, our main concern is how the medication leaves the bloodstream to enter the brain. The brain has a special mechanism called the blood–brain barrier that protects it from many harmful substances that may be circulating in the bloodstream. The blood–brain barrier is comprised of several distinct components, both structural (e.g., tight junctions between the cells lining the capillaries in the brain) and biochemical (e.g., enzymes present on the blood vessel walls that inactivate various drugs). It is especially difficult for substances that dissolve in water to pass through the fatty blood–brain barrier. To be able to traverse the blood–brain barrier, nearly all psychiatric medicines are slippery, fat-loving (lipophilic) substances that can readily slide through the barrier and enter the brain. The principal exception is lithium, which dissolves in water but as an atom (rather than a big bulky molecule) is so small that it can nevertheless pass through the barrier. Once a psychiatric medication has passed through the blood–brain barrier, it has reached its intended destination and can now begin to do its work.

Medication Elimination System. Obviously, the medication cannot and should not stay in the body indefinitely. The key organs in the system that deactivate chemicals and eliminate wastes are the liver and kidney.

Liver: Chemical Processing. For protection from dangerous accumulation of various toxins, the body has evolved methods to eliminate foreign substances. Potentially harmful chemicals can originate from myriad sources including foods, liquids, air, and, of course, medications. The liver's role is to inactivate these chemicals and to convert (metabolize) them to water-soluble forms (i.e., forms that dissolve in water rather than fat), which can more easily be filtered and eliminated by the kidneys.

To do this work, liver cells have an abundance of enzymes that inactivate these chemicals either by cutting off (cleaving) pieces of the molecules or modifying the molecules by adding components to them so they can readily be eliminated. When the liver is doing its work, it is said to be metabolizing the drug, and what remains of the molecule after its metabolism is called its metabolite. Sometimes, though not always, the metabolite is as active as the original compound. In certain instances, the parent compound is actually a prodrug that is pharmacologically inactive and is transformed by the liver to the active compound. Although many psychiatric medications have no active metabolites, others have one or even several active metabolites. Considering the number of active metabolites can be particularly important when prescribing medication for elderly patients or those with liver disease. For such patients, medications with no active metabolites can be easier to inactivate and may therefore be less likely to accumulate and cause unpleasant side effects or even dangerous toxic effects.

There is yet another important aspect to the liver's work. When blood leaves the heart to travel to all parts of the body, about 30% passes through the liver before completing its return trip to the heart. It is this small percentage of blood that is subject to chemical processing by the liver during each trip around the body. However, there is a key difference for medication taken by mouth. Because most foreign substances enter the body by absorption across the intestines after being swallowed, the body is designed so that fully 100% of the blood returning from the gastrointestinal tract passes through the liver before making its first trip to the heart. Therefore, 100% of an oral dose of a medication is subject to chemical processing by the liver before it has a chance to get to the brain. This phenomenon is called first pass metabolism, and it helps explain why it often takes a larger oral dose of medication to produce an effect that is comparable to that experienced when the medication is administered by a different route.

Kidneys: Chemical Disposal. The kidneys are the body's filter system. In order to be filtered by the kidneys, a molecule must be relatively small and water soluble. Most psychiatric medications fulfill neither of these requirements. However, after successive metabolic steps that are primarily completed in the liver, the molecules are smaller and/or water soluble so that the kidneys can more readily clear them.

Therefore, care must be taken when administering medication to patients with kidney disease. If the kidneys are slow to remove medication, this can create a backlog in the medication elimination system. The liver may try to compensate by slowing its chemical processing efforts. As a result, levels of the active medication can rise extremely high despite using doses that are typically safe in otherwise healthy patients. Often, the doses of medications should be considerably lower in patients with poorly functioning kidneys.

2.4.3 Pharmacodynamics

If pharmacokinetics tells us what the body does to the medication, then pharmacodynamics tells us what the medication does to the body. We are trying to answer the question, "How does this medication produce its effect?" However, you will soon see that for all of our knowledge about what psychiatric medications do, we often fall short of knowing exactly how they work.

When we talk about what a psychiatric medication does, we are invariably discussing its effect on neurotransmission between nerve cells across the synapse. Psychiatric medications act by modulating chemical neurotransmission in the synapse. However, as you probably know, it often takes several days or weeks for depression or psychosis to respond to treatment. Clearly, psychiatric medications work. Why, however, is there often a delay before they begin to do so?

Initiation and Adaptation. The answer to this question is surprisingly simple. Many psychiatric medicines do not work immediately because they work indirectly. By changing neurotransmission, these medicines set in motion a sequence of events in the brain. As brain neurochemistry gradually changes in response to the sustained alterations in neurotransmission produced by the psychiatric medicine, the therapeutic effects of the medication become evident. Taking the medication initiates the process, but the adaptation made by the brain to the continued presence of the medication is what ultimately determines whether or not there is a response.

These paired processes, known as initiation and adaptation, do not represent a new concept. We've long known that taking a drug one time can have very different effects from taking it repeatedly. Perhaps the most familiar examples are the drugs of abuse. For example, the acute effect of cocaine is to produce an intense but brief euphoria. Cocaine produces this effect by enhancing neurotransmission in dopamine-activated reward circuits in the brain. These "initiating" effects happen very quickly in response to the action of cocaine in the synapse.

Some psychiatric medications also produce a response within minutes of taking a single dose. Their therapeutic benefit can come very quickly. For example, taking a benzodiazepine such as diazepam (Valium) can quickly relieve panic and anxiety. Taking a stimulant can often rapidly relieve the symptoms of attention deficit–hyperactivity disorder (ADHD). When psychiatric medications work this quickly, we assume that the therapeutic benefit is a direct consequence of their "initiating" action in the synapse.

Side effects can also occur quickly after a single dose of a medication. For example, some antidepressants (e.g., selective serotonin reuptake inhibitors) can cause nausea, stomach upset, loose stools, and even diarrhea. Likewise, some antipsychotics (e.g., haloperidol (Haldol)) can cause unpleasant or painful muscle spasms called dystonias. All of these side effects can occur within minutes or hours of taking a single dose of the medication. These side effects are also a result of the direct effects of the medication in the synapse.

However, the long-term effects of habitually taking a medication or a substance of abuse can be quite different. For example, when cocaine is used repeatedly, it produces long-lasting changes in the brain's reward regions that precipitate the behavioral manifestations of addiction such as drug craving and, ironically, the loss of the originally experienced euphoria. This represents the adaptation, or we might argue the maladaptation, of the brain to habitual cocaine use.

Fortunately, some adaptation effects of continued medication use are beneficial. The brain also undergoes adaptive changes when a patient habitually takes an antidepressant. Laboratory animal studies and brain imaging studies have revealed that taking an antidepressant over time leads to changes in the number and distribution of certain nerve cell receptors. It's not entirely clear how this happens, but it does appear that the therapeutic response roughly coincides with the timing of these receptor changes. This explains why taking an antidepressant sporadically when one has a bad day does nothing. An antidepressant must be taken regularly and repeatedly to produce the adaptive changes in the brain that are associated with clinical improvement. This scenario also appears to be true for mood stabilizers used to treat bipolar disorder and antipsychotics used to treat schizophrenia and other psychotic illnesses.

Some medication side effects also occur only after prolonged administration and, as such, are products of the adaptive response to the continued administration of the medication. For example, taking a so-called conventional or typical antipsychotic for a long period of time can cause involuntary movements called tardive dyskinesias. These dyskinesias are believed to occur after chronic administration of the antipsychotic has caused changes in the density and/or sensitivity of dopamine receptors in brain regions that coordinate movement.

Initiation: Action in the Synapse. Psychiatric medications essentially work in one of two ways. They either promote neurotransmission or they hinder it. But there are several mechanisms by which they accomplish these tasks. We'll now describe these processes.

A medication can increase neurotransmission in one of the following ways: (1) blocking enzymes that inactivate neurotransmitter, (2) blocking neurotransmitter reuptake sites, (3) blocking negative feedback receptors, (4) stimulating receptors on the neighboring nerve cell, (5) supplying precursor substances to increase neurotransmitter synthesis, and (6) directly stimulating release of the neurotransmitter. Let's briefly review these mechanisms.

1. *Blocking Enzymes.* Remember that there are enzymes both in the synapse and in the cytoplasm of the nerve cells that metabolize and thereby inactivate neurotransmitter molecules. One way to promote neurotransmission is to increase the supply of available neurotransmitter. Blocking (or inhibiting) the enzymes that destroy neurotransmitter will do just that. Certain antidepressants known as monoamine oxidase inhibitors (MAOIs) and some medications used to treat Alzheimer's disease act in this manner.
2. *Blocking Reuptake.* Certain neurotransmitters can be taken back up by the cells that released them into the synapse. Inhibiting this reuptake facilitates neurotransmission by increasing the concentration of the neurotransmitter that is present in the synapse. Many antidepressants, including tricyclic antidepressants and selective serotonin reuptake inhibitors, act via this mechanism.
3. *Blocking Negative Feedback.* Receptors known as autoreceptors are present on the surface of the axon terminal of the nerve cell that releases a neurotrans-

mitter. When a molecule of the neurotransmitter binds an autoreceptor, it produces a negative feedback effect that causes the nerve cell to decrease further neurotransmitter release. Consequently, blocking the autoreceptor promotes neurotransmission by eliminating this negative feedback mechanism. The antidepressant mirtazapine (Remeron) acts in part by this mechanism.

4. *Stimulating Postsynaptic Receptors.* Neurotransmitters carry their signals by diffusing across the synapse from the axon terminals to receptors on the neighboring, so-called postsynaptic, nerve cell. Some medications stimulate postsynaptic receptors and thereby act by mimicking the action of the neurotransmitter itself.
5. *Neurotransmitter Precursors.* Most neurotransmitters are manufactured by the neurons themselves from a variety of simple building block substances that are commonly obtained from the diet. Another way to promote neurotransmission is to increase the available pool of neurotransmitter by supplementing the supply of a precursor substance. In most instances, this is a very inefficient and largely ineffective approach to treatment. However, L-DOPA, the immediate precursor to the neurotransmitter dopamine, remains an effective treatment for Parkinson's disease.
6. *Stimulating Neurotransmitter Release.* Psychostimulants, such as methylphenidate (Ritalin), can directly trigger the release of certain neurotransmitters (e.g., dopamine and norepinephrine) from the neuron's axon terminal.

Psychiatric medications can also act by decreasing neurotransmission in certain circuits either by directly blocking postsynaptic receptors or by increasing the release of inhibitory neurotransmitter substances. When a medication acts by blocking postsynaptic receptors, no matter how much neurotransmitter is released from the axon terminal, the signal cannot be transduced to the neighboring cell if the postsynaptic receptors are blocked. Medications that act by blocking postsynaptic receptors include nefazodone (Serzone), an antidepressant that acts primarily by blocking a certain class of serotonin receptors, and antipsychotics, which act by blocking one or more classes of dopamine and/or serotonin postsynaptic receptors.

2.4.4 Predicting Medication Effects

Every medication exerts multiple effects. The effect for which it is prescribed is called the therapeutic effect. All other effects are side effects. Which of these effects is the therapeutic one is therefore determined when the decision is made to take the medication.

An example is obviously in order. Medications that block the neurotransmission of histamine (i.e., antihistamines) produce several effects including drowsiness, drying of nasal passages, and weight gain. If the common over-the-counter antihistamine diphenhydramine (Benadryl) is prescribed to help a patient who has insomnia, then drowsiness is the therapeutic effect. Weight gain and dried nasal passages are side effects. If it is prescribed for seasonal allergies, then the drowsiness is a side effect, and drying the nasal passages is the therapeutic effect.

Psychiatric medicines exert multiple effects for two principal reasons. First, they usually interact with more than one receptor type. There are two ways to look at this. You will often hear a medication with multiple receptor interactions called a "dirty drug." This is because the more receptor interactions it has, the more effects, and hence side effects, it produces. As a result, great effort has been made to develop newer medications with fewer receptor interactions and, thus, fewer side effects. This effort has been quite successful with antidepressants, as we have moved from the effective but side effect-laden tricyclic antidepressants to newer antidepressants such as selective serotonin reuptake inhibitors.

But some feel that by reducing the receptor interactions we may produce less effective medications. In this view, medications with multiple receptor interactions are said to have a "rich pharmacology." As we will see in a later chapter, these multiple actions in the synapse appear to be a reason why the newer atypical antipsychotics have certain advantages over the older antipsychotic medicines. How many receptor interactions are sufficient? How many are too many? It depends. Certainly, it does no good to interact with a receptor that produces no benefit, but sometimes interacting with two different receptor types in a synergistic manner can produce even greater benefit.

There is another reason why medications exert multiple effects. For example, an antidepressant that very specifically promotes serotonin neurotransmission and has little or no interaction with other receptor types will still produce multiple effects. How can this be? Remember that in different areas of the brain, a single neurotransmitter can assume very distinct roles. When an individual takes a medication that alters the activity of a particular neurotransmitter, it generally does so throughout the brain. Consequently, the dopamine receptor blocking effect of haloperidol (Haldol) reduces hallucinations and paranoia in one brain region but causes upper extremity stiffness through its action in another brain region.

All of this might initially seem confusing. However, if you understand the effects of promoting or blocking the activity of each neurotransmitter, and you know how a medication affects each neurotransmitter system, then it becomes easier to predict both therapeutic effects and potential side effects of a given medication.

2.4.5 Predicting Drug Interactions

In previous sections, we discussed pharmacokinetics and pharmacodynamics. Remember, these are simply fancy medical terms for what the body does to a medication and what a medication does to the body. These twin pillars of pharmacology form the basis for understanding and being able to predict drug interactions.

Before moving on, you should understand that not all drug interactions are bad. Sometimes we use them to our advantage. For example, it's common practice to combine antibiotics that attack bacteria in different ways when treating serious infections like pneumonia or meningitis. The two antibiotics work together to kill the bacteria more effectively than either could alone. Likewise, psychiatric medications that work in different but complementary ways are sometimes combined to achieve a better treatment response.

So why all the hubbub about drug interactions? This is because drug interactions can also produce harmful effects. And if the prescriber, or the patient, doesn't see them coming, the results can be disastrous. For example, a few years ago, the non-sedating antihistamine astemizole (Seldane) was introduced, essentially revolutionizing the treatment of seasonal allergies. In FDA testing, it proved a safe and effective medication. But later, in routine clinical use, it was not uncommon for patients to take the antibiotic erythromycin together with Seldane. The problem is that erythromycin interferes with the liver's ability to metabolize Seldane. As a result, Seldane accumulates when taken with erythromycin. The danger arises because extremely high levels of Seldane can lead to heartbeat irregularities, that is, cardiotoxicity. Consequently, two "safe" medications, taken together, combine to produce a lethal mixture.

We don't, however, have to proceed blindly when two or more medications are prescribed together. If we understand the pharmacokinetics and pharmacodynamics of each medication, then we can predict with reasonable certainty the likely interactions. Let's take a look at how such interactions can occur.

Pharmacodynamic Interactions. Sometimes medications interact pharmacodynamically. If two medications produce similar side effects, then those effects can be additive. This can be advantageous. For examples, coadministering two antidepressants that relieve depression in different ways can be more effective than either medication alone. However, added effects can be problematic. If two medications that each produce drowsiness are coadministered, then the combination may produce intolerable daytime sedation.

On the other hand, the effects of two medications can counteract one another. The result is usually that both medications are rendered less effective. A common example is the patient with Parkinson's disease. On occasion, the L-DOPA that is the mainstay of treatment causes hallucinations. The treatment for hallucinations is an antipsychotic, which blocks the activity of dopamine. The problem is that using a typical antipsychotic to treat L-DOPA-induced hallucinations will interfere with the therapeutic effect of the L-DOPA, thereby worsening the symptoms of the Parkinson's disease. Fortunately, the advent of the newer atypical antipsychotics has provided a remedy to this particular Catch-22 drug interaction dilemma.

Pharmacokinetic Interactions. Remember that pharmacokinetics is the study of what the body does to the medication. This includes how the body transports, inactivates (i.e., metabolizes), and eliminates the medication. Sometimes, one medication can change the way the body handles another medication. This is known as a pharmacokinetic interaction. There are two types of pharmacokinetic interactions. One type occurs in the medication transportation system, and the other occurs in the medication elimination system.

Medication Transportation Interactions. Recall that carrier proteins in the bloodstream escort medications and that over 80% of the circulating concentration of most psychiatric medicines is bound to serum proteins. When there are not enough protein binding sites to go around, however, the biologically active free fraction of the drug is increased.

Doctors are most often concerned by this competition for protein binding sites when their patients are taking either the blood-thinner warfarin (Coumadin) or the heart medicine digoxin (Digitalis, Lanoxin). Adding highly protein-bound medications, like most psychotropic medicines, can increase the biological activity of warfarin or digoxin, causing dangerous complications and even death, if this is not anticipated and closely monitored.

Medication Elimination System. We've already related the sad story of erythromycin and Seldane. We've also briefly described the liver enzymes that inactivate medications. We can now tell you these two stories are related.

The most important enzymes in the liver for deactivating medications are called the cytochrome P_{450} enzymes. This is actually a family of related enzymes, and pharmacologists are constantly discovering new members of this family.

Sometimes, one medication can inhibit (i.e., slow down) the enzyme that inactivates another medication. This is what happened in the erythromycin and Seldane saga. In this case, the result was devastating. Two things must be true for this to go so wrong. First, the medication that inhibits the enzyme (in this case erythromycin) must do so strongly enough that it causes the medication that is metabolized by the enzyme to accumulate. Medications that weakly inhibit one of these enzymes seldom cause other medications to accumulate to any great extent. Second, the medication that accumulates must exert dangerous toxic effects at higher levels. This was clearly the case for Seldane.

In the aftermath of the erythromycin/Seldane debacle, antidepressant manufacturers began to study the effects of their medication on these liver enzyme families.

Certainly, the potential for drug–drug interactions by this mechanism exists, but it's unclear whether P_{450} interactions warrant all the attention they've received in antidepressant marketing brochures. Nevertheless, when prescribing any medication, it's important to know how it might interact with other medications that the patient is taking. Carelessly prescribing without reviewing the other medications that are being taken is akin to ignoring a ticking time bomb. One may get by without any untoward effects, but sooner or later, it might hurt the patient. To avoid this danger, prescribers must be aware of the effects of all psychiatric medicines on liver isoenzyme activity.

2.5 PUTTING IT ALL TOGETHER

The challenge that arises at this juncture is integrating all of the above information with what we know about the pathophysiology (i.e., cause) of the psychiatric illness and the characteristics of the individual patient to devise a rational approach to

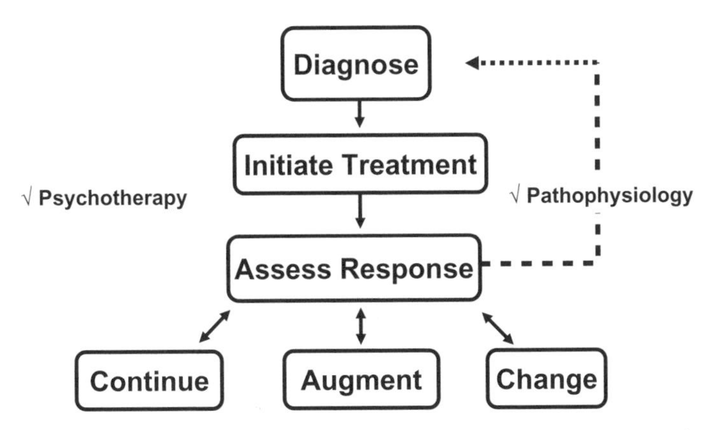

Figure 2.1. An approach to treatment. The first step in initiating treatment is to determine the disorder(s) that is producing distress. Treatment is initiated, and at the appropriate times, a determination of efficacy is made. Depending on this assessment, treatment is continued, something is added, or a change is made. Failure to achieve the desired outcome in a timely fashion should raise issues about (1) the pathophysiology of the disease state and the mechanism of action of the drugs being prescribed, (2) the presence or absence of appropriate psychotherapy, and (3) a determination that the original diagnosis is, in fact, the correct diagnosis.

treatment. A general approach to treatment is shown in Figure 2.1. The diagnosis is made, treatment is initiated, and, at the appropriate time, an assessment of treatment response is made. The timing of assessment can vary widely not only between different illnesses but also within an individual patient at different times. Depending on the results of the assessment, we either continue the treatment, change the treatment, or add to the treatment. Let's review a couple of illustrative examples.

Clinical Vignette

Jim is a 24-year-old male with a 3 year history of bipolar disorder (previously termed manic depression), who had been stable with medication but stopped taking his mood stabilizer 3 weeks ago because he said it made him feel too slowed down. He has had no sleep for the last 48 hours and upon presentation at his therapist's office is disheveled, with pressured speech, grandiosity, and some paranoid ideation. What are the time points for assessment here? First, Jim needs to get some sleep, be less agitated, and not represent a danger to himself or others. Commonly, benzodiazepines such as lorazepam (Ativan) and an antipsychotic would be used. Since sleep deprivation can trigger manic episodes, it is important to reverse his current pattern. So, the first assessment of medication effect is shortly after his admission to the emergency room. The next major assessment time will be days to a week or two to ensure that mood stabilization is taking place. Finally, later on we will want to assess the long-term tolerability of the treatment to maximize the likelihood that Jim remains adherent with treatment in the future.

Clinical Vignette

Sue is 42 years old and experiencing her second episode of major depressive disorder. She has never been on antidepressants before but this time would like to try medication as part of her treatment. The initial assessment period for her will be a few days to a week after starting to make sure that the medication is not producing uncomfortable side effects. After 3–4 weeks, we expect to see some improvement in her mood; if there is no change whatsoever, many physicians would change antidepressants after 4–5 weeks. Finally, when there has ceased to be any further improvement in mood, we want to know, "Is she 'well' or is she only 'better'?" If the answer is that she has only gotten better, but not yet well, then we have more work to do.

Going back to Figure 2.1, if we are stuck in the treatment, we should reconsider the pathophysiology of the disease state, asking ourselves which medications that we are perhaps not exploiting yet act on neurotransmitter systems. If the patient is not yet participating in psychotherapy, we would bring it up again. Finally, if we remain stuck, it is often helpful to take a "blank slate" approach to the treatment, that is, confirm that what we are treating is what the patient really has.

ADDITIONAL READING

Armstrong SC, Cozza KL, Sandson NB. Six patterns of drug–drug interactions. *Psychosomatics* 2003; 44: 255–258.

Black JE. Environment and development of the nervous system. In Gallagher M, Nelson RJ (eds), *Handbook of Psychology: Biological Psychology, Volume 3.* Hoboken, NJ: John Wiley & Sons, 2003, pp 655–668.

Cooper JR, Bloom FE, Roth RH. *The Biochemical Basis of Neuropharmacology, 8th Edition.* London: Oxford University Press, 2003.

Hyman SE, Nestler EJ. Initiation and adaptation: a paradigm for understanding psychotropic drug action. *Am J Psychiatry* 1996; 153: 151–162.

Malhotra AK, Murphy GM, Kennedy JL. Pharmacogenetics of psychotropic drug response. *Am J Psychiatry* 2004; 161: 780–796.

Nemeroff CB. New directions in the development of antidepressants: the interface of neurobiology and psychiatry. *Human Psychopharmacol* 2002; 17(Supplement 1): S13–S16.

Nemeroff CB, DeVane CL, Pollack BG. Newer antidepressants and the cytochrome P450 system. *Am J Psychiatry* 1996; 153: 311–320.

Nemeroff CB, Owens MJ. Contribution of modern neuroscience to developing new treatments for psychiatric disorders. In Weissman M (ed), *Treatment of Depression: Bridging the 21st Century.* Washington DC: American Psychiatric Press, 2001, pp 61–81.

Nemeroff CB, Musselman DL, Nathan KI, et al. Pathophysiological basis of psychiatric disorders: focus on mood disorders and schizophrenia. In Tasman A, Kay J, Lieberman JA (eds), *Psychiatry, Volume 1.* Philadelphia: WB Saunders, 1997, pp 258–311.

Owens MJ, Mulcahey JJ, Stout SC, Plotsky PM. Molecular and neurobiological mechanisms in the treatment of psychiatric disorders. In Tasman A, Kay J, Lieberman JA (eds), *Psychiatry, Volume 1*. Philadelphia: WB Saunders, 1997, pp 210–257.

Preskorn SH. The recommended dosage range: How is it established and why would it ever be exceeded? *J Psychiatr Pract* 2004; 10: 249–254.

Stahl SM. *Essential Psychopharmacology: Neuroscientific Basis and Practical Applications, 2nd Edition*. New York: Cambridge University Press, 2000.

3

MOOD DISORDERS

3.1 INTRODUCTION

The mood disorders were once called affective disorders and are grouped into two main categories: unipolar and bipolar. The unipolar depressive disorders include major depressive disorder and dysthymic disorder; the bipolar disorders include bipolar I, bipolar II, bipolar not otherwise specified, and cyclothymic disorder. Other mood disorders are substance-induced mood disorders and mood disorders due to a general medical condition. In addition, mood disturbance commonly occurs as a symptom in other psychiatric disorders including dementia, post-traumatic stress disorder, substance abuse disorders, and schizophrenia.

The unipolar mood disorders consist solely of episodes of depression. On the other hand, the bipolar mood disorders consist of episodes of both depressed and elevated mood. The periods of elevated mood are characterized by either euphoria or irritability and are called mania or hypomania depending on the level of severity. A schematic of the mood disorders is shown in Figure 3.1. Substance-induced mood disorders and mood disorders due to general medical conditions usually manifest depressed mood; however, manic episodes are occasionally seen as well.

Principles of Psychopharmacology for Mental Health Professionals
By Jeffrey E. Kelsey, D. Jeffrey Newport, and Charles B. Nemeroff

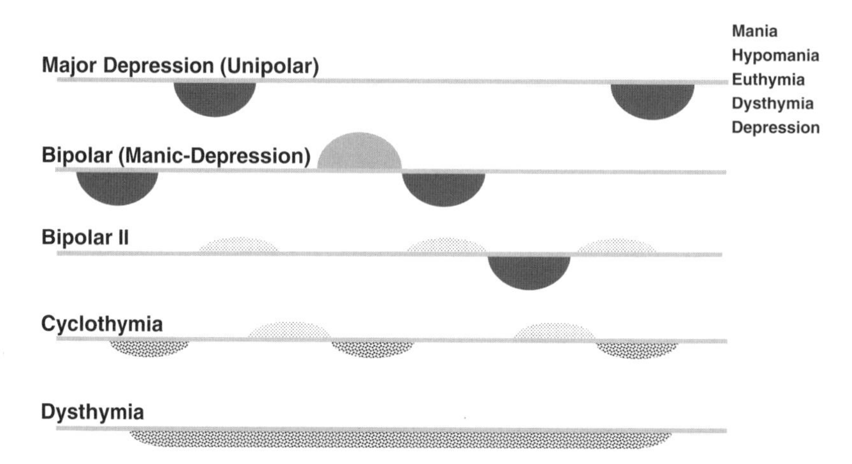

Figure 3.1. Mood Disorders. (From Kelsey, JE and Nemeroff, CB. (1998) Affective Disorders. In SJ Enna and JT Coyle (eds). *Pharmacological Management of Neurological and Psychiatric Disorders.* New York: McGraw-Hill.)

TABLE 3.1. Prevalence of Mood Disorders

Diagnosis	Prevalence
Major Depressive Disorder	Female: 20–25% Male: 7–12%
Dysthymic Disorder	6%
Bipolar I Disorder	0.4–1.6%
Bipolar II Disorder	0.5%
Cyclothymic Disorder	0.4–1.0%

Mood disorders represent a major public health concern around the globe. In the United States alone, the annual cost of major depression is over 40 billion dollars. Less than 30% of the total cost of depression is incurred through direct treatment. The remainder consists of the indirect "hidden" costs of lost productivity due to absenteeism and poor work efficiency, premature death from suicide or medical illness, and the uncounted losses related to a poor quality of life.

These disorders should concern all physicians and mental health professionals for several reasons. First, mood disorders are very common and will be encountered on a daily basis in most clinical settings (see Table 3.1). Second, they disrupt life in numerous ways. During an episode of depression or mania, sleep patterns change, appetite and eating are affected, family life is disrupted, work efficiency suffers, substance abuse rates soar, and physical illness is exacerbated. Thus, comprehensive treatment of mood disorders routinely requires the work of nutritionists, social workers, family therapists, vocational rehabilitation counselors, substance abuse counselors and 12 step groups, primary care physicians, and others.

3.2 MAJOR DEPRESSIVE DISORDER

3.2.1 Brief Description and Diagnostic Criteria

Depression is an imprecisely used term both in public circles and in the mental health community. It may refer to brief feelings of sadness or to a mood disturbance manifesting profound despair that persists over time. In the latter sense, depression represents the key symptoms of a psychiatric mood disorder.

Representative of the unipolar depressive disorders is major depressive disorder (MDD). MDD, or major depression, is a debilitating and potentially life-threatening illness. The ninth leading cause of death in the United States is suicide. Approximately 15% of individuals suffering from major depression or bipolar depression die by suicide. In addition to increasing the risk of suicide, depression also increases the disability and shortens the life expectancy following heart attack, stroke, and the diagnosis of cancer. Depression is a killer but fortunately one that responds well to treatment. Therefore, prompt and accurate diagnosis of major depression is extremely important.

Depressed mood is the hallmark symptom of MDD, but it is neither required nor sufficient for the diagnosis of major depression. In addition to depressed mood, the key symptoms of a major depressive episode include anhedonia, changes in sleep or appetite, psychomotor retardation or agitation, poor concentration or indecisiveness, and recurrent thoughts of death or suicide. The DSM-IV definition of major depression requires that five or more of these symptoms be present for at least 2 weeks in the absence of an identifiable cause such as medication, medical illness, or the death of a loved one. Refer to Table 3.2 for the DSM-IV criteria for MDD.

TABLE 3.2. Diagnostic Criteria for Major Depressive Disorder

A. At least five of the following symptoms are present most of the day nearly every day for 2 weeks and are different from the patient's usual mood. One of the five symptoms must be either depressed mood or anhedonia.
   1. Depressed mood acknowledged by the patient or witnessed by others
   2. Lack of interest or pleasure in usual activities (anhedonia) acknowledged by the patient or witnessed by others
   3. Increased or decreased appetite or body weight
   4. Too much or too little sleep
   5. Fidgetiness or slowed movements that can be seen by others
   6. Feeling tired
   7. Feeling worthless or extremely guilty
   8. Having a hard time concentrating or making simple decisions
   9. Thinking about death or suicide

B. Does not fulfill criteria for a mixed episode (i.e., no evidence of mania).

C. Impairs daily functioning at work or home.

D. Not due to a medication, an illicit drug, or a medical illness.

E. Not better explained by bereavement after the death of a loved one.

Source: Adapted from DSM-IV.

Major depression varies greatly from person to person. Therefore, DSM-IV uses course and descriptive specifiers to further describe the disorder in each individual. The course specifiers quantitatively describe the long-term history of the illness. Patterns of episode recurrence and remission are delineated by these specifiers.

The descriptive specifiers describe the current episode of the illness from a qualitative perspective. The descriptive specifiers of depression include postpartum onset or the presence of catatonic, melancholic, atypical, or psychotic features. *Postpartum onset* applies when the depressive episode begins within 4 weeks after childbirth. It appears that postpartum depression lies between "maternity blues" and postpartum psychosis on a severity spectrum. If untreated, postpartum depression impairs the new mother's ability to bond with her infant and risks potential long-term problems for the child. *Catatonic features* consist of extremes of physical activity from profound immobility to purposeless hyperactivity, a passive resistance to instructions known as negativism, and peculiarities of movement and speech. Depression with *melancholic features* is characterized by anhedonia, an unreactive mood that resists even brief improvement when something pleasurable happens, depression that is worse in the morning, early morning insomnia, loss of appetite, and excessive guilty ruminations. *Atypical features* include increased appetite with craving for calorie-rich foods, excessive sleep, a "heavy" feeling in the extremities termed leaden paralysis, and a heightened sensitivity to rejection by others. Finally, depression with *psychotic features* is characterized by the presence of delusions or hallucinations. The delusions and hallucinations usually contain guilt-ridden or persecutory themes that are consistent with the focus of the mood disturbance and are thus called mood-congruent. Less often, the content of the psychotic symptoms has no apparent connection to the mood disturbance and is labeled mood-incongruent.

3.2.2 Prevalence and Risk Factors

Major depressive disorder is among the most common psychiatric syndromes affecting approximately one in four American women and one in ten American men during their lifetimes. Although the overall prevalence rates have stabilized, the average age of onset for the disorder has decidedly decreased. Numerous risk factors for depression have been identified and are listed in Table 3.3.

TABLE 3.3. Risk Factors for Depression

Female gender
Prior history of depression
Family history of depression
Active substance abuse
Recent stressful life event
Poor social supports
Previous suicide attempt
Postpartum period
Chronic medical illness

The reasons for such high rates of depression in women are unclear. Some have proposed a biological explanation suggesting that hormonal differences place women at greater risk than men; however, studies of the role of female reproductive biology in depression have produced conflicting results. Others claim that cultural factors associated with typical female gender roles predispose women to depression. Some contend that rates of depression in men are underreported due to higher rates of substance abuse that may represent efforts to self-medicate depressive symptoms. All of these factors and perhaps others contribute to the disproportionately higher rate of depression in women.

The higher rate of depression in women is not evenly scattered throughout the life span. Before puberty, the rate of depression in girls and boys is about the same. After menopause, rates of depression among women are also comparable to men. Instead, the rate of depression is highest during the childbearing years from menarche to menopause. Within these reproductive years of a woman's life, the peak rates of depression tend to cluster in early adulthood, in the postpartum, and in the period immediately preceding menopause.

3.2.3 Presentation and Clinical Course

Major depression usually develops over days to weeks following some significantly stressful event. Depressed patients may describe feeling "down" or losing interest in life. Conversely, some patients deny being sad or depressed, but you can often infer depression from the reports of friends and family members or the observation of facial expressions and body language (e.g., downcast eyes, stooped posture, slowed movements, delayed speech, tearfulness, frequent sighing).

Patients with depression usually do not present initially to mental health professionals. Most visit their primary care physicians, complaining not of depressed mood but of other symptoms of depression. Fatigue, insomnia, loss of appetite, loss of interest in sex, muscle tension, body aches, and poor concentration are all commonly reported. These so-called masked presentations of depression may in part explain the documented failure of primary care physicians to diagnose depression reliably. This underscores the importance of considering depression in the differential diagnosis of physical complaints that appear vague or exaggerated.

The long-term course of MDD is highly variable but in approximately half of patients evolves into a chronic, relapsing illness. Untreated, a major depressive episode typically lasts about 6–12 months before resolving spontaneously. The emotional, physical, and social toll exacted during these months of depression can be tremendous. When the illness remits, most patients are able to function at their previous level; however, 20% experience only a partial remission with persistent depressive symptoms that may last months or even years.

There is unfortunately no reliable means to predict which patients suffering from a first episode of depression will have relapses of illness. Of the patients who experience an initial major depressive episode, approximately 50–60% will have a second depressive episode. Of those, 65–75% will experience a third episode of the illness. Once a third episode has occurred, the chances of a fourth are 85–95%. Although the initial episodes of major depression typically follow a stressful life event, a kindling phenomenon has been described in which later episodes arise without precipitating stressors. This suggests that being depressed is somehow bad for the brain, and each episode leaves a person increasingly vulnerable to future episodes of the illness.

3.2.4 Initial Evaluation and Differential Diagnosis

The differential diagnosis of depression is organized along both symptomatic and causative lines. Symptomatically, major depression is differentiated from other disorders by its clinical presentation or its long-term history. This is, of course, the primary means of distinguishing psychiatric disorders in DSM-IV. The symptomatic differential of major depression includes other mood disorders such as dysthymic disorder and bipolar disorder, other disorders that frequently manifest depressed mood including schizoaffective disorder, schizophrenia, dementia, adjustment disorder, and post-traumatic stress disorder, and, finally, other nonpsychiatric conditions that resemble depression such as bereavement and medical illnesses like cancer or AIDS.

The cause of most psychiatric disorders including depression remains unknown; nevertheless, some diagnostic considerations are based on presumed causative factors. In these cases, the distinction from major depression is not based on the symptomatic presentation because there may be no symptomatic difference. The difference lies in the presence of an identifiable biological factor that is presumably causing the depressive syndrome. The causative differential of MDD includes a mood disorder due to a general medical condition in medically ill patients and a substance-induced mood disorder in patients using certain medications or substances of abuse. A comprehensive evaluation of depression must include consideration of potentially treatable causative factors.

Dysthymic Disorder. Dysthymic disorder differs from MDD by being more chronic and less severe. Yet, two issues can cloud the distinction. First, some patients experience "double depression" in which an episode of major depression is superimposed on dysthymia. This can make it difficult to assess treatment response when the baseline mood is dysthymia instead of a normal euthymic mood. Second, a few patients may experience a chronic major depressive episode, which, like dysthymic disorder, lasts 2 years or more. In contrast to dysthymic patients whose insidious onset of symptoms leaves them unable to say exactly when the depression started, most patients with chronic major depression can tell when their depression began.

Bipolar Disorders. You must also distinguish the bipolar disorders from MDD. The distinction is particularly important in young adult patients given that nearly 10% of patients with an initial episode of major depression will go on to develop a bipolar illness. The devastating consequences of untreated mania coupled with the possibility that antidepressants may trigger manic episodes in susceptible individuals adds to the importance of screening for bipolar illness. Although a prior history of full-blown mania seldom escapes detection, you should carefully assess depressed patients looking for any indication of a previous hypomanic episode or a family history of bipolar disorder.

Mood Disorder Due to a General Medical Condition. The diagnosis of depression in medically ill patients is a hotly debated topic. Common symptoms of medical illnesses include fatigue, sleep disturbance, and loss of appetite, each of which resembles the so-called neurovegetative symptoms of depression. Thus, medically ill patients with such symptoms may appear to be depressed when they are not. This debate has centered on whether the physical symptoms of depression should be included when counting symptoms toward the diagnosis of major depression in these patients. For example, should you count weight loss and fatigue as symptoms of major depression in a patient with advanced cancer? Some argue for an inclusive approach in which all the recognized symptoms are counted even if they are conceivably due to a medical illness instead. Others prefer an exclusive approach in which the neurovegetative symptoms are eliminated from consideration when diagnosing depression in medically ill patients. The inclusive approach risks mistakenly diagnosing depression in patients who are not depressed. The exclusive approach risks missing the diagnosis in those who are depressed. Because untreated depression worsens the course of medical illness and interferes with medical treatment, the inclusive approach, which more readily detects depression in medically ill patients, is preferred.

Once it has been decided that a medically ill patient is in fact depressed, you must determine, when possible, if the medical illness is directly causing the depression. MDD is the preferred diagnosis when the depression is triggered indirectly by illness-associated stressors such as unrelenting pain, declining physical health, or the loss of self-sufficiency. On the contrary, depression due to a general medical condition should be diagnosed when it appears that the medical illness precipitated the depression in a direct biological manner.

A number of medical conditions are associated with high rates of depression (see Table 3.4). In some instances, the distinction between MDD and depression due to a general medical condition is largely academic with little bearing on treatment selection. For example, pancreatic cancer may induce depression directly through the release of tumor-secreted substances; however, depression in the pancreatic cancer patient is treated with conventional antidepressant medications. In other cases, the diagnostic distinction bears important treatment implications. One commonly cited example is depression occurring in association with hypothyroidism. Patients with depression and hypothyroidism do not respond to antidepressant treatment alone but require a thyroid hormone supplement.

Substance-Induced Mood Disorder. Many prescription medications and abused substances cause depression (see Table 3.5). This idea is not new. In fact, recognizing that certain medications cause depression has helped us to understand the biology of depression better.

TABLE 3.4. Medical Conditions that May Cause Depression

Classes of Medical Illness	Specific Illnesses
Cancer	Head and neck cancer
	Lung cancer
	Pancreatic cancer
Cardiovascular disease	Cardiomyopathy
	Congestive heart failure
	Myocardial infarction (heart attack)
Endocrine disorders	Adrenal: Addison's disease and Cushing's disease
	Diabetes mellitus
	Parathyroid: hyper-/hypo-
	Reproductive: ovary/testicle failure
	Thyroid: hyper-/hypo-
Infectious diseases	AIDS/HIV
	Hepatitis
	Influenza
	Mononucleosis
	Syphilis
Neurological disorders	Dementia
	Multiple sclerosis
	Parkinson's disease
	Wilson's disease
Nutritional	Folate deficiency
	Iron deficiency
	Vitamin B_1 (thiamine) deficiency
	Vitamin B_2 (riboflavin) deficiency
	Vitamin B_6 (pyridoxine) deficiency
	Vitamin B_{12} (cyanocobalamin) deficiency

Depression caused by a substance is usually indistinguishable from major depression. It's seldom that a substance-induced mood disorder can be diagnosed with absolute certainty. However, when your patient becomes depressed shortly after beginning to use a medication known to cause depression in others, it's reasonable to assume that the substance may be causing your patient's depression.

In the case of prescribed medications, this sometimes leads to difficult decisions. For example, if an anticancer drug is used to treat a life-threatening cancer but that drug is also causing a depression that leads to great suffering and may even shorten life, what should be done? When a substitute for the depression-causing medication is available, this can be tried. However, many times this is not the case. When the depression-causing medication must be continued, then starting an antidepressant may provide some relief.

As for abused substances, the question is usually, "Which came first?" Is the alcoholic depressed because of his drinking or does he drink because he is depressed? The answer is usually "both." The key is that to treat one you must treat the other. Simply giving an antidepressant to a depressed substance abuser accomplishes little.

TABLE 3.5. Drugs[a] that May Cause Depression

Class of Drugs	Specific Drugs
Anticancer	Cycloserine
	Glucocorticoids
	Interferon-α
	L-Asparaginase
	Leuprolide
	Procarbazine
	Tamoxifen
	Vinblastine
	Vincristine
Antihypertensive	Alpha methyldopa
	Clonidine
	Guanethidine
	Propranolol
	Reserpine
Anti-infection	Acyclovir
	Amphotericin B
	Metronidazole
Appetite suppressants	Phenylpropanolamine
Drugs of abuse	Alcohol
	Amphetamines
	Cocaine
	Marijuana
	Opiates (heroin, prescription narcotics)
	PCP (phencyclidine)
	Sedatives
Gastrointestinal	Cimetidine
Hormonal/endocrine	Contraceptives
	Steroids

[a] Prescription and over-the-counter drugs and substances of abuse that can cause depressive symptoms.

Sending that same patient to a drug treatment program with no help for the depression is not much better. A structured "dual diagnosis" program, which treats both the addiction and the depression, has the best chance of helping the patient.

Schizophrenia and Schizoaffective Disorder. Cross sectionally, it is often difficult to distinguish major depression with psychotic features from the schizophrenia spectrum disorders. There are theoretically qualitative differences in the psychosis that may help to make the distinction. Psychosis in the context of a mood disorder tends to be manifested by persecutory and nihilistic themes, but schizophrenia is more often characterized by paranoia and disorganization. However, these characteristics are not totally reliable in a diagnostic assessment. A longitudinal history can clarify the diagnosis, but there are certain circumstances such as the first episode of illness in which a long-term history is not available. Fortunately, the inability to discriminate MDD with psychotic features from schizoaffective disorder or schizophrenia does not interfere with acute treatment. In both cases, treatment must address both mood symptoms and psychotic symptoms. This is accomplished either by giving a combination of an antidepressant and an antipsychotic or by the administration of electroconvulsive therapy (ECT).

Dementia. In the elderly, you may have difficulty distinguishing depression from the early stages of dementia. Depressed patients often report memory problems and may even ask, "Do I have Alzheimer's disease?" It is usually not that their memory itself is impaired. Their forgetfulness is more the result of apathy and poor concentration that leads them to overlook the things going on around them. The result is a false dementia or pseudodementia. On the other hand, patients with true dementia often become depressed as well.

There are a few clues that can help you to distinguish an early dementia from the pseudodementia of depression. True dementia is usually slowly progressive and may not be noticed by family members for months. A pseudodementia usually begins very abruptly so that family members notice almost immediately. Truly demented patients are either unaware of their memory loss or try to hide it. During an interview, demented patients usually try to answer but make many mistakes. Depressed, pseudodemented patients recognize their memory problems. During an interview, they are more likely to answer, "I don't know."

Despite these clues, a definitive diagnosis often cannot be made. In that case, a prudent course is to treat what would be treatable. The initial evaluation should carefully look for treatable medical causes of dementia or depression. These include vitamin B_{12} deficiency and hypothyroidism among others. If no medical causes are found, then treatment for depression should be started. If the patient is depressed and suffering from a pseudodementia, the patient can expect full recovery of memory as the depression resolves. But if the patient has a progressive dementia such as Alzheimer's disease, then treatment for depression has done no harm and may still provide some benefit.

3.2.5 History of Pharmacological Treatment

Biological treatments for depression have emerged through a combination of lucky discovery and systematically targeted research. The result is an antidepressant classification system that is inconsistent and potentially confusing. Some antidepressants are grouped by a similar molecular structure (e.g., tricyclic antidepressants), others are classified by a shared mechanism of action (e.g., selective serotonin reuptake inhibitors, monoamine oxidase inhibitors), and the remaining are lumped into a loosely defined group of so-called atypical antidepressants. The latter group is atypical only in the sense that they do not readily fit into one of the other categories. Table 3.6 presents the traditional antidepressant classification system.

TABLE 3.6. Traditional Antidepressant Classification Scheme[a]

Antidepressant Class	Specific Antidepressants
TCAs/tetracyclics	Amitriptyline
	Amoxapine
	Clomipramine
	Desipramine
	Doxepin
	Maprotiline
	Nortriptyline
	Protriptyline
	Trimipramine
MAOIs	Brofaromine[b]
	Isocarboxizide
	Moclobemide[b]
	Phenelzine
	Tranylcypromine
SSRIs	Citalopram
	Escitalopram
	Fluoxetine
	Fluvoxamine
	Paroxetine
	Sertraline
Atypical antidepressants	Bupropion
	Duloxetine
	Mianserin[b]
	Mirtazapine
	Nefazodone
	Reboxetine[b]
	Trazodone
	Venlafaxine

[a] Listing of antidepressants in traditional groupings. *Abbreviations*: TCAs = tricyclic antidepressants; MAOIs = monoamine oxidase inhibitors; SSRIs = selective serotonin reuptake inhibitors.
[b] Not currently available in the United States.

The traditional scheme is complicated by the fact that some antidepressants exhibit characteristics of more than one class. For example, clomipramine, a tricyclic antidepressant (TCA) with side effects and toxicity similar to other TCAs, works more like the selective serotonin reuptake inhibitors (SSRIs). Similarly, venlafaxine and duloxetine, which are usually grouped with the atypical antidepressants, have a side effect and safety profile comparable to the SSRIs. Although a classification system based on mechanism of action offers some advantage (see Table 3.7), even this scheme is limited by the fact that antidepressants that work in the same way may have widely divergent side effect and safety profiles. In the following discussion, the traditional classification system is adopted. Although fraught with problems and inconsistencies,

TABLE 3.7. Functional Antidepressant Classification Scheme[a]

Functional Antidepressant Class	Specific Antidepressants
MAOIs—irreversible	Isocarboxizide
	Phenelzine
	Tranylcypromine
MAOIs—reversible	Brofaromine[b]
	Moclobemide[b]
NDRI	Bupropion
NRI	Reboxetine[b]
NSRI	Amitriptyline
	Amoxapine
	Desipramine
	Doxepin
	Duloxetine
	Maprotiline
	Nortriptyline
	Protriptyline
	Trimipramine
	Venlafaxine
NSSA	Mianserin[b]
	Mirtazapine
SRI	Citalopram
	Clomipramine
	Fluoxetine
	Fluvoxamine
	Paroxetine
	Sertraline
SRI/serotonin-2 blocker	Nefazodone
	Trazodone

[a] Listing of antidepressants grouped by principal mechanism of action in the synapse. *Abbreviations*: MAOI—irreversible = irreversible monoamine oxidase inhibitor; MAOI—reversible = reversible monoamine oxidase inhibitor; NDRI = norepinephrine/dopamine reuptake inhibitor; NRI = norepinephrine reuptake inhibitor; NSRI = norepinephrine/serotonin reuptake inhibitor; NSSA = norepinephrine/specific serotonin agonist; SRI = serotonin reuptake inhibitor; SRI/serotonin-2 blocker = serotonin reuptake inhibitor and serotonin-2 receptor antagonist.

[b] Not currently available in the United States.

this generally accepted scheme provides continuity with the prevailing psychiatric literature and therefore aids additional study.

Euphorics. In the 19th century, euphoria-inducing substances such as cocaine were recommended for the treatment of melancholia. Although these substances provide transient relief from depression, their use is ultimately self-defeating. The effect of prolonged use is to worsen depression and to risk the development of addiction. Unfortunately, the admitted capacity for alcohol, cocaine, and other abused substances to elevate mood and provide a brief respite from depression all too frequently results in habitual use. The consequence is often a downward spiral into deepening depression complicated by the social, physical, and emotional toll of addiction.

One popular misconception is that modern antidepressants also induce euphoria. This is not true. Antidepressants do not lift the mood of nondepressed individuals. Antidepressants simply relieve depression and hopefully return a person to a normal euthymic mood. The lone exception is the bipolar patient who may have a manic episode triggered by taking an antidepressant without a mood stabilizer. Because antidepressants do not produce pleasurable euphoric feelings in nondepressed people, they are not addictive.

Shock Therapy. The early 20th century saw the development of the first effective biological treatments for depression, the shock therapies. The first shock treatments used injection of horse serum or insulin. A major advance in treatment occurred with the advent of electroconvulsive therapy (ECT) in 1934. Although initially used to treat schizophrenia, ECT was soon found to be highly effective for other psychiatric disorders including depression and mania. ECT remained the primary biological psychiatric treatment until the widespread release of psychiatric medications in the 1950s.

ECT thereafter fell into disrepute partly as a result of indiscriminate application to most any psychiatric symptom and partly as a result of side effects resulting from what are by today's standards extremely high doses of electrical current. This was compounded by unfavorable depictions in the media such as in the popular film *One Flew Over The Cuckoo's Nest.*

Interest in ECT resurfaced in the 1980s with the growing awareness that antidepressants are not always effective. Today, four out of five ECT sessions are used in the treatment of major depression. Although expensive, ECT remains the most effective treatment for depression with response rates of 80–90%, far exceeding that of any antidepressant. ECT should seriously be considered for the treatment of MDD with psychotic features, MDD with catatonic features, mixed bipolar episodes, life-threatening depression, and refractory depression, which is unresponsive to multiple antidepressant trials.

Stimulants. The first stimulant, amphetamine, was introduced in the late 1800s. Over the next 50 years, amphetamines were used to treat a variety of conditions including depression. The stimulants were easier to tolerate than the TCAs and somewhat safer. Unfortunately, they also produced euphoric effects leading to rampart "speed freak" abuse in the 1960s.

In response, the FDA greatly restricted the use of stimulants. They were only approved for ADHD, narcolepsy, and severe obesity. In the 1970s, however, interest in the stimulants as an augmentation to antidepressants began to surface. In particular, stimulants were used to treat depressed patients with severe medical illnesses such as cancer. The stimulants often provide a faster response than antidepressants alone and can be important for medically ill patients who need rapid improvement.

Methylphenidate (Ritalin), dextroamphetamine (Dexedrine), and pemoline (Cylert) are currently available in the United States. Methylphenidate has been the most widely used and is usually the first choice. Pemoline sometimes impairs liver function and is rarely used today due to the potential for toxicity.

In summary, stimulants can still be helpful to augment antidepressants in a medically ill patient. However, you must bear in mind that the stimulants can be abused.

Monoamine Oxidase Inhibitors (MAOIs). The first antidepressant discovered was iproniazid. This medication was developed in the early 1950s as a treatment for tuberculosis but was unexpectedly found to improve mood in depressed patients. It was later found that its antidepressant effect was due to its action on the MAO enzymes. Unfortunately, iproniazid was subsequently found to cause liver damage and was withdrawn from the market.

The MAO enzymes, which come in two types known as MAO-A and MAO-B, perform a scavenger function by metabolizing and thereby eliminating certain molecules from nerve cells. This prevents the accumulation of toxic levels of these substances. In the brain, the MAO-A enzyme metabolizes a variety of substances including norepinephrine and serotonin, and the MAO-B enzyme metabolizes dopamine and several other substances. The effectiveness of MAOIs primarily comes from their ability to inhibit the MAO-A enzyme and thereby boost the availability of norepinephrine and serotonin.

In the United States, there are presently three approved MAOIs: phenelzine (Nardil), tranylcypromine (Parnate), and isocarboxizide (Marplan). These medications are all nonselective, irreversible inhibitors of the MAO enzymes. By nonselective, it is meant that they block the actions of both the MAO-A and MAO-B enzyme subtypes. It is felt that blocking the MAO-B enzyme adds little to the effectiveness of these antidepressants but causes many of the problematic side effects. The MAOIs are irreversible in that they deactivate the enzyme permanently.

The common side effects of MAOIs include dizziness from orthostatic hypotension, drowsiness, insomnia, palpitations, rapid pulse, and sexual dysfunction. In addition, phenelzine appears to cause weight gain and fluid retention.

More concerning are the less common but potentially dangerous interactions of the MAOIs with certain foods and medications. Because the MAOIs permanently disable the MAO enzymes (until the body is able over the course of several weeks to produce a new supply of the enzymes), taking a medication or eating a food that contains one of the substances eliminated by the MAO enzymes can cause toxic accumulation. The result is a so-called hypertensive crisis in which the blood pressure is uncontrollably elevated, risking heart attack, stroke, or death.

One of the substances metabolized by the MAO enzymes is tyramine, which is a naturally occurring component of many foods. Thus, patients taking MAOIs must avoid tyramine-containing foods such as aged cheeses, beer and wine, aged meats, pickled foods, and yeast extracts. These dietary restrictions greatly limit the number of individuals willing to take these otherwise highly effective antidepressants.

Many commonly used medications also contain substances that are eliminated by the MAOIs and must not be taken by these patients. The list of medications to be avoided includes the narcotic pain reliever meperidine (Demerol), and many over-the-counter cold remedies containing dextromethorphan or pseudoephedrine. Finally, patients taking MAOIs must also avoid medications that elevate serotonin levels. This includes certain appetite suppressants and antidepressants including the SSRIs, venlafaxine, duloxetine, mirtazapine, nefazodone, and trazodone. Medications that interact with the MAOIs cannot be taken until at least 2 weeks after the MAOI has been stopped.

In Europe and Canada, reversible MAOIs such as moclobemide are available. Because these medications do not permanently disable the supply of MAO enzymes, the potential for toxic accumulation of substances is greatly reduced. It appears that patients taking these reversible MAOIs may eat tyramine-containing foods without problems. None are currently available in the United States.

Tricyclic Antidepressants (TCAs). Like iproniazid, the first TCA was also developed in the 1950s for another purpose. Imipramine (Tofranil) is structurally similar to the early antipsychotics and was hoped to provide an alternative to chlorpromazine (Thorazine). It proved to be a poor antipsychotic but was surprisingly found to be an effective antidepressant. The tricyclics are so named because a three-ringed structure forms the hub of the molecule.

Long the treatments of choice for depression, the TCAs have in recent years been supplanted by newer agents that are safer and more easily tolerated. Nonetheless, these medications are effective treatments for depression and a variety of other disorders and remain a gold standard for comparative research trials.

TCAs primarily work by blocking the reuptake of norepinephrine, although they block serotonin reuptake as well. The lone exception is clomipramine (Anafranil), which preferentially blocks serotonin reuptake. It is this unique characteristic that makes clomipramine the only TCA that effectively treats obsessive–compulsive disorder (OCD).

In addition to blocking norepinephrine and serotonin reuptake, the TCAs also have numerous other receptor interactions. These multiple actions are a double-edged sword. In a positive light, the TCAs can be said to have a "rich pharmacology," which allows them to be used in many ways. Because of their diverse actions, TCAs can be used to treat such varied problems as migraine headaches, peptic ulcers, insomnia, painful diabetic neuropathy, and diarrhea to name to a few. From a negative perspective, these multiple actions mean that the TCAs can be seen as "dirty drugs" with a long list of side effects (see Table 3.8). The result is that the documented effectiveness of the TCAs in the research setting may be undermined in routine clinical practice by poor adherence due to intolerable side effects. Debate continues, however, as to whether in our efforts to produce safer, more tolerable medications through more specific receptor activity, we have introduced

TABLE 3.8. Tricyclic Antidepressant Side Effects

Antihistaminic	Anti-alpha$_1$ Adrenergic	Anticholinergic	Serotonergic
Sedation Weight gain	Orthostatic hypotension Dizziness	Dry mouth Blurred vision Constipation Memory impairment Difficulty urinating	Anxiety Sexual dysfunction

antidepressants that are less effective than the "dirty" TCAs in treating severely ill or refractory patients.

The common side effects of TCAs frequently limit their usefulness, particularly in older patients. Side effects can be minimized by starting at low doses that are slowly titrated upward or by choosing one of the so-called secondary amine TCAs, nortriptyline and desipramine, with less potent side effects. In addition, it should be remembered that some of the troublesome side effects, such as sedation, tend to disappear over time.

Of greater concern is the safety of the TCAs. Toxic levels of these medications can produce lethal cardiac arrhythmias, seizures, and suppression of breathing. An overdose of a 1–2 week supply of most TCAs is often fatal, a serious consideration when prescribing medication to depressed patients with suicidal thoughts. Children taking imipramine for treatment of ADHD have died from sudden cardiac death; consequently, child psychiatrists seldom use TCAs. Likewise, patients with heart disease or seizure disorders are more likely to have dangerous complications from TCAs and should avoid them.

The TCAs have been presented as a group as if they are uniformly interchangeable. This is not the case. Some TCAs have unique biochemical properties that confer unique clinical characteristics. As previously mentioned, clomipramine is distinct in its selectivity for serotonin reuptake. As a result, clomipramine is more effective in the treatment of anxiety, especially OCD. Amoxapine and maprotiline are actually tetracyclics with a four-ringed structure, but they are discussed here because they resemble TCAs in most clinical respects. Amoxapine is unique in that it is metabolized to the antipsychotic loxapine; therefore, this single medication can be used to treat depression and psychosis. Although this at first seems advantageous, amoxapine is usually not preferred for psychotic depression because this limits the ability to adjust the antipsychotic dose independent of the antidepressant dose. In addition, if amoxapine is continued during long-term treatment, it risks the development of tardive dyskinesia. The other tetracyclic, maprotiline, is associated with greater risk of seizures and is contraindicated in patients with epilepsy.

The true tricyclics are often subdivided into tertiary and secondary amine groups. Structurally, the difference lies in the length of side chains branching off the basic three-ringed hub of the molecule. Clinically, side effects are most common and most severe with the tertiary amine medications such as amitriptyline, imipramine, and doxepin. The secondary amines are generally better tolerated. It should be added that two of the tertiary amine TCAs, amitriptyline and imipramine, are metabolized

TABLE 3.9. Doses and Serum Levels of Tricyclic Antidepressants

Trade Names	Subclass	Starting Dose (mg/day)	Usual Dose (mg/day)	Serum Levels (ng/mL)
Elavil, Endep	Tertiary TCA	25–50	100–300	110–250
Asendin	Tetracyclic	50–100	150–400	200–500
Anafranil	Tertiary TCA	25–50	100–250	80–100
Norpramin	Secondary TCA	25–50	100–300	125–300
Sinequan, Adapin	Tertiary TCA	25–50	100–300	100–200
Tofranil	Tertiary TCA	25–50	100–225	200–350
Ludiomil	Tetracyclic	25–50	100–225	200–300
Pamelor, Aventyl	Secondary TCA	10–25	50–150	50–150
Vivactil	Tertiary TCA	10	15–60	100–200
Surmontil	Tertiary TCA	25–50	100–300	180

to nortriptyline and desipramine before being eliminated. Thus, patients taking amitriptyline or imipramine actually have two active compounds in their systems.

The TCAs are the only antidepressant class in which effectiveness is dependent on serum level. Attainment of the minimal therapeutic level is typically required for effectiveness. Exceeding the maximum treatment level usually provides no additional benefit and risks toxicity. Unique in this regard is nortriptyline, which is the only TCA with a "therapeutic window." This means that beyond the maximum therapeutic level of 150 ng/mL nortriptyline not only risks toxicity but is actually less effective at treating depression. Please refer to Table 3.9 for a summary of dosing guidelines and therapeutic levels.

Despite concerns regarding safety and side effects, TCAs are appropriate for some patients. When starting a TCA, a baseline EKG is required. If the EKG reveals a second-degree or higher heart block, a bundle branch block, or a corrected QT interval exceeding 440 milliseconds, then a TCA should not be started. The initial doses should be low, especially in older patients or those with anxiety who are particularly sensitive to side effects. Over the first 7–14 days, the dose should be increased gradually to the lower end of the expected therapeutic range. After an additional 2–3 weeks, the dose may be increased further if necessary.

During ongoing treatment, serum drug levels and EKGs should be monitored periodically to maximize safety and ensure compliance.

In summary, the TCAs have several advantages. They are less expensive and can be administered once daily. They are backed by nearly 40 years of clinical experience, which has demonstrated their effectiveness for long-term management of depression and for severe cases of illness. Unfortunately, safety and side effect issues limit their usefulness.

Selective Serotonin Reuptake Inhibitors (SSRIs). For 30 years, improvements in antidepressants mainly consisted of further refinements of the TCAs. The dominance of the TCAs for so many years explains why there are so many available, though today many physicians are less familiar with them.

In the 1980s, decades of research began to bear fruit. Pharmaceutical companies were able to design molecules with specific receptor interactions in mind. The driving force behind this effort was the recognition that many of the receptor actions of the TCAs were not helpful and only created unwanted side effects. By designing compounds that did not have so many actions, side effects could be reduced.

In 1983, the first SSRI, fluvoxamine (Luvox), debuted in Switzerland. Five years later, fluoxetine (Prozac) was introduced in the United States. The SSRIs revolutionized the treatment of depression. They improved safety and tolerability, removing much of the stigma of taking an antidepressant. In fact, some think that it has become too easy to take antidepressants and that psychotherapy is being neglected or discouraged.

The selectivity of the SSRIs does not mean that they are totally without side effects. First, serotonin-secreting nerve cells are distributed throughout the brain and control a wide array of nervous system activities. As a result, increasing serotonin not only relieves depression, it can also produce many side effects such as abdominal discomfort, sexual dysfunction, and anxiety. Second, the selectivity of the SSRIs is not absolute but relative. Although the main action of the SSRIs is the same, they do have differences. For patients, this means that the drug interactions and side effects of the SSRIs vary somewhat. It also means that a patient who does not respond to one SSRI may respond to another.

When starting a SSRI, the abrupt increase in serotonin may cause side effects. In the brain, the short-term effects include headache, sleep disturbance, nervousness, anxiety, and tremulousness. The digestive system effects include nausea, loose stools, decreased appetite, and indigestion. Most of these effects are mild and short-lived or can be managed with over-the-counter remedies. Nausea, for example, can be minimized by taking a SSRI after meals. These effects are also commonly seen with venlafaxine and duloxetine, atypical antidepressants that block serotonin reuptake like the SSRIs.

Sexual dysfunction also results from increased serotonin. It can result in delayed orgasm, impotence, or decreased sexual desire. For men with premature ejaculation, the delayed orgasm can be beneficial, but more often this makes it difficult to enjoy sex. Several strategies for managing the sexual side effects have been tried. These include taking medication holidays, reducing the SSRI dose, or adding a second medicine to reverse the side effect. A medication holiday is simply skipping a day's dose when the patient is planning to have sex. Medication holidays are most successful with the short-acting antidepressants paroxetine and venlafaxine and least successful with the extremely long-acting fluoxetine. Taking a medication holiday, of course, requires that sexual activity is planned well in advance and risks inducing a relapse of depression. Lowering the SSRI dose works for some patients but also risks causing a relapse. Medications used to reduce the sexual side effects of SSRIs include buspirone, yohimbine, amantadine, cyproheptadine, or bupropion. If efforts to reduce the SSRI sexual dysfunction are unsuccessful, then switching to another antidepressant may be needed. Bupropion, mirtazapine, and nefazodone are reasonable choices.

Infrequently, SSRIs produce dystonic reactions, which are intense muscle spasms usually of the face and neck. They may cause akathisia, a restless inability to sit still. Dystonic reactions and akathisia are more commonly side effects of the dopamine-blocking antipsychotics. It is believed that SSRIs produce these effects because increasing 5HT activity tends to decrease dopamine. When these side effects occur, the SSRI should be switched to another antidepressant.

Abruptly stopping a SSRI can produce an unpleasant serotonin discontinuation syndrome. This syndrome is not life threatening or otherwise dangerous but can produce symptoms of malaise, nausea, abdominal pain, irritability, anxiety, and shock-like sensations in the arms and legs. It appears to be most common and most severe when stopping the short-acting antidepressants paroxetine and venlafaxine. Conversely, serotonin discontinuation syndrome is least problematic when stopping long-acting fluoxetine. The symptoms of serotonin discontinuation syndrome can be minimized by gradually tapering the dose over several weeks when stopping a SSRI or venlafaxine or duloxetine.

The current SSRIs in the United States include fluoxetine, fluvoxamine, sertraline (Zoloft), paroxetine (Paxil), citalopram (Celexa), and escitalopram (Lexapro). All effectively treat major depression. In addition, one or more of the SSRIs has been shown effective in the treatment of dysthymic disorder, the depressive phase of bipolar disorder, premenstrual dysphoric disorder, panic disorder, social phobia, obsessive–compulsive disorder, bulimia nervosa, and binge-eating disorder.

Fluoxetine (Prozac). The first SSRI introduced in the United States, fluoxetine was for many years the most prescribed antidepressant in the world. It is approved for the treatment of MDD, OCD, and bulimia nervosa. Fluoxetine can be started at 10 or 20 mg in a single dose taken with a meal. Many patients experience a complete recovery at the 20 mg/day dose, but fluoxetine can be increased up to 80 mg/day. The treatment of bulimia nervosa and OCD usually requires these higher doses.

The common side effects are due to increased serotonin and have already been discussed. Some believe that fluoxetine is more activating than the other SSRIs and prefer its use for lethargic patients. Among the SSRIs, fluoxetine is unique for its extremely long half-life. This does not delay it onset of action but does require a longer washout when switching to another antidepressant. The longer action may also be beneficial. Discontinuation symptoms are seldom problematic, and an extended release formulation of fluoxetine is approved for once-a-week dosing.

Fluvoxamine (Luvox). This is actually the oldest of the SSRIs. It is approved in this country for the treatment of OCD but is also an effective treatment for major depression and many other anxiety disorders. It should be started at 50 mg/day, and the effective dose range is from 100 to 300 mg/day. Fluvoxamine is the only SSRI that must be taken twice a day. The common side effects of fluvoxamine are comparable to other SSRIs.

Sertraline (Zoloft). Sertraline was the second SSRI released in the United States and is approved for the treatment of major depression and many anxiety disorders. It should be started at 25–50 mg/day and increased to 100 mg/day over the first 10–14 days. Many patients require doses nearing 150 mg/day for full benefit. The side effects of sertraline are comparable to other SSRIs.

Paroxetine (Paxil). This antidepressant is also approved for the treatment of major depression, and many anxiety disorders. Many patients respond at the typical starting dose of 20 mg/day, making dose titration unnecessary. The effective dosage range is 20–50 mg/day. The side effects are comparable to other SSRIs. Because paroxetine has slightly more anticholinergic effect than other SSRIs, older patients should start at 10 mg and receive no more than 20 mg per day. Paroxetine is also available as a controlled release (CR) formulation that requires 25% dose increase over regular-release paroxetine.

Citalopram (Celexa), Escitalopram (Lexapro). Escitalopram is the enantiomer *S*-citalopram. Citalopram is a 50:50 mixture of *s*- and *r*-citalopram of which the former is the active component. Both are very selective SSRIs. The side effects of citalopram and escitalopram appear to be comparable to other SSRIs.

Atypical Antidepressants. The atypical antidepressants are not a true class in the same sense as SSRIs or TCAs. There is no unifying property to these antidepressants. Each of these antidepressants is actually a class unto itself that is structurally and functionally different from all other antidepressants. The atypical antidepressants include trazodone (Desyrel), bupropion (Wellbutrin), venlafaxine (Effexor), duloxetine (Cymbalta), nefazodone (Serzone), and mirtazapine (Remeron).

Trazodone (Desyrel). Trazodone was the first of the atypical antidepressants and was actually introduced prior to the SSRIs. It does not have the serious cardiac toxicity or anticholinergic side effects of the TCAs and was the most popular antidepressant until the arrival of the SSRIs. It is approved for the treatment of depression and is also commonly used in low doses to treat agitation in demented patients and insomnia.

Trazodone is usually started at 50–100 mg/day given at bedtime. Doses of 400–600 mg/day are required to treat depression. Unfortunately, these higher doses cause extreme sedation and dizziness due to orthostatic hypotension for many patients. As a result, it is nowadays used less often to treat depression. Trazodone is frequently used at lower doses to treat insomnia in depressed patients. One rare but important side effect of trazodone is priapism. Priapism is a severely painful long-lasting penile erection. It is extremely unpleasant and sometimes requires surgical drainage of the blood trapped in the penis. Patients taking trazodone who experience painful or otherwise abnormal erections should seek immediate medical attention. In case you were wondering, trazodone has no place in the treatment of impotence.

Bupropion (Wellbutrin). Bupropion is the only antidepressant that works by blocking the reuptake of norepinephrine and dopamine. It is used to treat depression and attention deficit–hyperactivity disorder (ADHD) and has recently been released under the name Zyban as an aid to smoking cessation. Bupropion does not appear to be effective in the treatment of anxiety disorders. It will however, decrease the anxiety that is often present as a symptom of depression. Bupropion does not cause the sexual side effects seen with the SSRIs/SNRIs or MAOIs and is a reasonable choice for patients bothered by these effects.

The most common side effects of bupropion are decreased appetite and abdominal discomfort. But more serious is the risk of seizure when high doses are taken. For this reason, patients with epilepsy should not take bupropion.

Bupropion is sold in three preparations: immediate-release, sustained-release (SR), and a recently introduced extended-release (XL). The immediate-release form is usually started at 75 mg/day and the effective dose range is 300–450 mg/day in up to three divided doses. In order to minimize seizure risk, no single dose of immediate-release bupropion should exceed 150 mg, and the total daily dose should not exceed 450 mg. The sustained-release formula apparently carries less risk of seizure. It is started at 100–150 mg/day and is usually effective at 300–400 mg/day given in two doses. Up to 200 mg of the sustained-release formulation can be taken at one time with little risk of seizure. The extended-release formula can be administered once daily at doses ranging from 150 to 450 mg/day. When starting bupropion, patients must be warned that if they forget a dose, do not try to catch up by doubling the next dose.

Bupropion has also been used to treat the eating disorders anorexia nervosa and bulimia nervosa. Unfortunately, their electrolyte abnormalities leave patients with eating disorders especially vulnerable to seizures; therefore, bupropion is no longer used to treat them.

Venlafaxine (Effexor, Effexor XR). Venlafaxine works by blocking the reuptake of both serotonin and norepinephrine. Because of this dual action, some believe that venlafaxine may be more effective than the SSRIs when treating severe depression. Its side effects and toxicity are similar to the SSRIs with abdominal discomfort, sexual dysfunction, and anxiety being commonly reported. At higher doses, it may mildly elevate blood pressure; therefore, blood pressure should be checked periodically. When stopping venlafaxine, serotonin discontinuation symptoms may be especially problematic. Therefore, gradually tapering of the dose every 2–4 weeks is recommended.

Like bupropion, venlafaxine comes in immediate-release and extended-release preparations. The immediate-release form is taken twice a day starting at 37.5 to 75 mg/day and increased to 75 mg/day after 1 week. The effective dose range is 75–375 mg/day. The extended release form is started once daily at 37.5 mg/day and is also effective at 75–375 mg/day. The effective dose range is similar to the immediate-release form.

Duloxetine (Cymbalta). Duloxetine, the newest of the antidepressants approved in the United States, like venlafaxine and most TCAs, acts by blocking both serotonin and norepinephrine reuptake. Its side effects and toxicity are similar to venlafaxine and the SSRIs with abdominal discomfort, sexual dysfunction, and anxiety being commonly reported. In adults, duloxetine can be initiated at 30 mg/day administered in a single daily dose. The maximum recommended dose is 60–120 mg/day.

Nefazodone (Serzone). Nefazodone works by weakly blocking serotonin reuptake and by blocking serotonin-2 receptors. The receptor blockade produces more specific serotonin activity and so reduces many serotonin-associated side effects. In particular, nefazodone does not commonly induce anxiety or sexual dysfunction like the SSRIs.

Nefazodone is approved for treatment of major depression and appears particularly effective in treating depressed patients with agitation or anxiety. Its role in treating anxiety disorders is being studied.

Nefazodone is taken twice daily starting at 100 mg/day. This is increased to 200 mg/day in week 2 and 300 mg/day in week 3. The usual effective dosage range is 300–600 mg/day. At these doses, patients sometimes experience drowsiness, gastrointestinal discomfort, and mild visual changes. Recently, life-threatening liver failure has been reported among patients taking nefazodone. Periodic monitoring of liver function is therefore recommended for all patients taking nefazodone.

Mirtazapine (Remeron). Mirtazapine is the newest of the atypical antidepressants. It mainly works by blocking the alpha-2 negative feedback receptor and thus increases norepinephrine and serotonin activity. In addition, mirtazapine blocks serotonin-2 and serotonin-3 receptors to produce a specific serotonin action like nefazodone. Mirtazapine is approved for the treatment of depression. Its use in the anxiety disorders is being studied.

The common side effects of mirtazapine include drowsiness, weight gain, and occasional dizziness from orthostatic hypotension. The drowsiness appears to improve as the dose is increased. On extremely rare occasions, mirtazapine has been associated with agranulocytosis, a dangerous lowering of white blood cell count. Although agranulocytosis is very rare when using mirtazapine, it should not be taken with clozapine or carbamazepine that also cause agranulocytosis.

Mirtazapine is usually started once daily at bedtime at a dose of 7.5–15 mg. The effective dose range is 30–45 mg/day.

Miscellaneous Medications. A variety of other medications have also been used to treat depression. They have mainly been used together with an antidepressant to augment or boost its effectiveness. These augmenting medications include lithium, tri-iodothyronine (T3), buspirone, pindolol, estrogen, and anticonvulsants.

Augmenting antidepressants with lithium has repeatedly been shown to be effective. But lithium is a difficult medication to take. It is very dangerous in overdose and can quickly reach toxic levels due to fluid loss from diarrhea, profuse sweating, or high fevers. Even at treatment levels, lithium can produce unpleasant side effects such as dizziness, frequent urination, and tremors. Despite all its problems, lithium is one of the best medications available to augment antidepressants for severely depressed patients. Please refer to Section 3.4 Bipolar Disorders for more information on lithium.

Triiodothyronine (Cytomel, T3). T3 is also an effective augmenting agent. It is important to use the T3 thyroid hormone instead of thyroxine (T4). T4 is the form most often used to treat hypothyroidism, but T3 crosses from the bloodstream to the brain more easily and thus is better for treating depression. T3 is usually tolerated well and is taken at 25–50 μg/day in split doses. When taking T3, laboratory tests to check thyroid function should be performed periodically.

Buspirone (Buspar). Buspirone is an anxiety-relieving medication that alters serotonin activity. When added to an antidepressant, buspirone may help treat the depression. It will also relieve anxiety and may reverse sexual side effects of a SSRI. Please refer to Chapter 5 Anxiety Disorders for more information regarding buspirone.

Pindolol (Visken). Pindolol is a blood pressure medicine that also alters serotonin activity. Some believe that it helps speed the response to antidepressants, but more study is needed. It is generally well tolerated.

Estrogen (Premarin, Estrace). Estrogen is probably the most intriguing augmentation agent. Estrogen, the primary female sex hormone, was first used with the theory that estrogen deficiency may explain the higher rate of depression in women. In addition, estrogen is known to have some effect on serotonin activity.

For depression, estrogen has mainly been used to treat women during the transition into menopause. Given in normal hormone replacement therapy doses, estrogen does relieve mild depressive symptoms in these women. It may also augment the effect of antidepressants when given to women with major depression, but it does work well alone. Recent safety concerns regarding the long-term use of estrogen have limited its utility.

Anticonvulsants. Finally, several antiseizure medications have been tried. These include valproic acid (Depakote, Depakene), carbamazepine (Tegretol), Lamotrigine (Lamictal), and gabapentin (Neurontin). The anticonvulsants are effective treatments for bipolar disorder. Their use for major depression needs to be studied further. Please refer to Section 3.4 Bipolar Disorders.

Drug Interactions. No modern discussion of the history of antidepressants would be complete without mention of the debate regarding potential drug interactions. As discussed more fully in Chapter 2, medications may interact in several ways, and their interactions may be helpful or harmful. The antidepressant debate has focused on the way these drugs influence the liver's ability to metabolize and thus deactivate other drugs. In particular, it is the impact of antidepressants on the liver's cytochrome P_{450} family of enzymes that has been so extensively discussed.

The cytochrome P_{450} enzyme system first drew widespread attention in the aftermath of the erythromycin/astemizole (Seldane) tragedy. When patients were given both the antibiotic erythromycin and the antihistamine astemizole, some died of sudden heartbeat irregularities (i.e., arrhythmias). It was found that erythromycin inhibits the activity of the cytochrome P_{450} liver enzyme that metabolizes astemizole. Because erythromycin blocked this enzyme, astemizole accumulated to toxic levels and poisoned the heart's electrical conduction system, resulting in the sudden deaths. Because some antidepressants also alter heart conduction in this way, studying the impact of antidepressants on the cytochrome P_{450} enzymes was a logical next step.

The cytochrome P_{450} system is actually a family of related liver enzymes. Each specific enzyme within this family is called an isoenzyme. New isoenzymes within the cytochrome P_{450} system are constantly being discovered. The 1A2, 2C9/2C19, 2D6, and 3A4 isoenzymes are the best understood. Table 3.10 shows the impact of the newer antidepressants on particular cytochrome P_{450} isoenzymes and the drugs that may be affected.

It may be fair to ask, "Is this much ado about nothing?" Although test tube studies have shown that particular drugs interact, it is seldom that this causes problems for patients taking the medications. For example, the antidepressant fluvoxamine inhibits the enzyme that deactivates the antipsychotic haloperidol (Haldol). Does this mean that fluvoxamine and haloperidol cannot be taken together? By no means. Although this would probably raise the blood level of haloperidol somewhat, the main effect if any would be that a smaller dose of haloperidol would be more effective.

Nevertheless, doctors prescribing antidepressants should be aware of possible cytochrome P_{450} drug interactions. This is especially true when one of the drugs is known to be dangerous at toxic levels and when the toxic level is not much higher than the treatment level (see Chapter 2 for a discussion of the therapeutic index). If equally effective alternative medications are available, then drugs with potential interactions should be avoided. However, it sometimes makes sense to prescribe two medications that may interact with one another. When this is done, certain precautionary measures should be taken. Before starting the medications, the symptoms of toxicity should be described to the patient. In addition, the patient should be told in advance what to do if these symptoms occur. Usually, this means going to the nearest emergency room and having the drug levels checked. You should ask your patients about toxic symptoms at each visit, and serum levels should be checked more often.

3.2.6 Current Approach to Treatment

The goals of treatment in depressed patients are to end the current episode and to protect against future episodes of illness. To achieve these goals, the treatment of depression is organized into three distinct phases: acute treatment, continuation treatment, and maintenance treatment. In most patients these goals are accomplished successfully through one or more of the following: psychotherapy, antidepressant medication, and ancillary services such as psychoeducation, support groups, and social services.

TABLE 3.10. Cytochrome P_{450} Interactions of Newer Antidepressants

	Isoenzymes			
Medication	1A2	2C9 / 2C19	2D6	3A4
Citalopram				
Duloxetine			+	
Escitalopram				
Fluoxetine	+	+	++	+
Fluvoxamine	++	++		++
Paroxetine			++	
Sertraline		+	+	+
Bupropion			++	
Mirtazapine				
Nefazodone				++
Trazodone				
Venlafaxine				
Possible interactions with:	Amitriptyline Caffeine Clozapine Estradiol Haloperidol Naproxen Olanzapine Tacrine Tertiary TCAs Theophylline	Diazepam Ibuprofen Omeprazole Phenytoin Tolbutamide Warfarin	Antipsychotics Codeine Dextromethorphan Beta blockers TCAs Type 1C antiarrhythmics	Astemizole Benzodiazepines Carbamazepine Cisapride Clarithromycin Codeine Erythromycin Estrogen Quinidine Phosphodiesterase-5 inhibitors Protease inhibitors TCAs Terfenadine Zolpidem

+ Moderate inhibitor of enzyme.
++ Strong inhibitor of enzyme.

There are several prerequisites to the initiation of treatment for depression. The diagnosis of depression must be firmly established, and any comorbid psychiatric or medical illnesses that may affect the treatment should be identified. Medical causes for the depression must also be ruled out. Finally, the diagnosis, its long-term prognosis, and treatment options should be discussed with the patient. Only then can well-informed treatment begin.

Acute Phase Treatment. The acute phase begins with the decision to treat and ends with remission of the illness. During this phase, depression rating scales can help to establish the severity of the illness and to provide an objective measure of symptomatic improvement. Commonly used scales that your patients can complete in the waiting room include the Beck Depression Inventory (BDI) and the Zung Self-Rating Depression Scale. Scales that you can complete in a timely manner include the Hamilton Depression Rating Scale (Ham-D) and the Montgomery Asberg Depression Rating Scale (MADRS).

The first decision when beginning acute phase treatment is choosing the primary treatment modality: psychotherapy, medication, or both. Several short-term therapies including CBT, IPT, brief psychodynamic therapy, and marital therapy are effective treatments in mild-to-moderate cases of depression without added antidepressant treatment. This is a viable alternative that many patients may prefer.

For moderate-to-severe depression, antidepressants, with or without combined psychotherapy, must be considered. When depression is so severe that hospitalization is warranted or psychotic or catatonic features are present, psychotherapy should be withheld temporarily and medication (or ECT) is required.

Antidepressants have been shown effective in the treatment of major depression with response rates at approximately 60–70%. The only treatment for depression consistently shown to be more effective is ECT with response rates of 80–90%. There is no definitive means of predicting which medication will work best for a given patient; nevertheless, the choice of a medication should not be made capriciously. Several factors can guide medication selection and thereby maximize the likelihood of a successful response.

The first factor consists of historical predictors of treatment response. Patients who have had a good response to a particular medication or who have family members who have had a good response are more likely to respond to that antidepressant. On the other hand, patients who have not responded well or who have had intolerable side effects with a particular medication are likely to do so again. When considering this historical data, be sure that the patients received adequate doses for a sufficient length of time. For example, a patient who tells you that paroxetine does not work for him but goes on to say that he took only 10 mg/day for about 2 weeks has not really told you anything about the effectiveness of paroxetine for his depression. His dose was too low, and he took it for too short a length of time.

The second factor includes symptomatic predictors of treatment response. It has long been recognized that MAOIs, and now SSRIs, are more effective than TCAs in the treatment of atypical depression. In addition, psychotic depression usually does not respond to an antidepressant alone but requires coadministration of an antipsychotic with the antidepressant or a course of ECT.

Third is the presence of other psychiatric or medical disorders. This can help guide antidepressant selection in several ways. In some cases, an antidepressant may be preferred because it can treat both disorders. For example, the extensive evidence that fluoxetine is an effective treatment for bulimia nervosa makes it preferable for patients with depression and bulimia. Similarly, the depressed Parkinson's disease patient whose neurological illness results from a lack of dopamine in a particular area of the brain may have both her depression and her Parkinson's disease improved by bupropion, which increases brain dopamine activity. In other cases, an antidepressant should be avoided if it worsens the other illness or interacts adversely with a medication needed to treat the other illness. For example, TCAs and MAOIs can complicate glucose control in diabetics and should not routinely be used by depressed diabetics. (See Table 3.11.)

The fourth factor influencing medication choice is the safety of the medication. This is especially important given the suicide potential of depressed patients. The newer antidepressants, including the SSRIs and so-called atypical antidepressants, are much safer in overdose than the older TCAs and MAOIs. In the case of the TCAs, ingestion of a 1–2 week supply is lethal 50% of the time.

The fifth factor is the potential for side effects. In general, the newer antidepressants have less cumbersome side effects than the older agents. Your patients should be informed of potential side effects when selecting an antidepressant. By discussing side effects in advance, your patient may help you to decide which side effects would be most distressful to him/her. For example, dizziness may be a problem for an elderly patient at risk for falls, and sexual side effects may be more concerning to others.

The frequency of dosing is another factor that can guide treatment selection. Most antidepressants are administered once or twice daily with the majority given once a day. Some patients may find it easier to comply with once-a-day dosing.

Finally, the expense of treatment can be a decisive factor in treatment selection. Depending on the dose, the cost of the newer antidepressants is $1 to $3 per day. The older TCAs and MAOIs are available in cheaper generic forms. However, these require more stringent medical monitoring and periodic assessment of serum drug levels.

Once an antidepressant is chosen, the side effects can be minimized by starting at a low dose and increasing to the effective dosage range over the first 1–2 weeks. There is wide variability in the timing of treatment response. In most cases, improvement does not begin until the second week of treatment and usually continues for several weeks thereafter.

An adequate trial of an antidepressant requires 4–6 weeks of treatment at a recognized therapeutic dose or serum level. If a patient exhibits no response or an unsatisfactory partial response after an adequate trial, then several options are available. These are discussed in Section 3.2.7 Refractory Depression.

TABLE 3.11. Choosing an Antidepressant for Medically Ill Patients

Organ System	Medical Illness	Antidepressant Recommendation			
		Preferred	Consider	Avoid	Never Use
Cardiovascular	Ischemic heart disease and cardiac arrhythmias	SSRIs	Bupropion Desipramine Duloxetine Nortriptyline Venlafaxine	MAOIs Other TCAs Trazodone	
Endocrine	Diabetes mellitus	SSRIs Duloxetine Venlafaxine	Bupropion Nefazodone	MAOIs Mirtazapine TCAs	
	Hyperthyroidism	SSRIs SNRIs		MAOIs TCAs	
	Hypothyroidism	Thyroid hormone	SSRIs SNRIs	MAOIs TCAs	
Neurological	Dementia	SSRIs	Bupropion Duloxetine Mirtazapine Nefazodone Trazodone Venlafaxine	TCAs	

	Epilepsy	SSRIs	ECT Duloxetine Mirtazapine Nefazodone Venlafaxine	MAOIs TCAs	Bupropion Maprotiline
	Migraine	Mirtazapine Nefazodone	Amitriptyline Doxepin		
	Parkinson's disease	Bupropion Sertraline	ECT MAOIs Other SSRIs TCAs	Amoxapine	
	Stroke	SSRIs	Mirtazapine Nefazodone Venlafaxine	Bupropion MAOIs TCAs	
Ocular (eyes)	Glaucoma	SSRIs	Bupropion Nefazodone	TCAs	
Reproductive	Impotence	Bupropion			
	Inorgasmia	Bupropion Mirtazapine Nefazodone	TCAs	Clomipramine Duloxetine MAOIs SSRIs Venlafaxine	

Continuation Phase Treatment. A relapse is the reemergence of a depressive episode that is still ongoing but has been suppressed by treatment. Although the symptoms of the depressive episode may be in remission, the patient remains at high risk for relapse for the following 4–6 months if treatment is stopped. This suggests that the depression does not fully resolve until nearly 6 months after the observable symptoms have disappeared. This is a vulnerable time as many patients discontinue medications and psychotherapy shortly after their symptoms have subsided. To reduce the likelihood of relapse, treatment should be continued 6–12 months after remission of the acute episode. During this phase, the antidepressant should be continued at the same dose used during the acute phase of treatment. If the decision is made to stop treatment at the conclusion of the continuation phase, then the antidepressant dose should be tapered slowly over 4–12 weeks. Unless dangerous or intolerable symptoms occur, abrupt discontinuation of antidepressants should be avoided as this may precipitate unpleasant discontinuation symptoms and may increase the risk for a recurrence of depression.

Maintenance Phase Treatment. The purpose of this phase of treatment is to provide protection against a recurrence of the illness. In contrast to a relapse, a recurrence is the development of a new episode of depression after the complete resolution of a prior episode. Though theoretically defensible, the distinction between a relapse and recurrence is often vague.

Recommending maintenance therapy requires a careful assessment of the risks of recurrence weighed against the costs and benefits of prolonging treatment. Patients who have had three or more episodes of depression or patients who have had two particularly severe episodes should seriously be considered for long-term maintenance therapy.

As in the continuation phase, the antidepressant that successfully achieved remission should be continued at the same dose during the maintenance phase of treatment. A collaborative decision between patient and physician is crucial to the success of the maintenance phase of treatment. These collaborative assessments should be repeated every 1–2 years and will require exploration of the patient's attitudes toward prolonged treatment.

3.2.7 Refractory Depression

When a patient with depression does not respond to an antidepressant, the first step is to ensure that the patient received an adequate trial. The diagnosis should be reassessed with particular attention given to the possibility of comorbid substance abuse, anxiety, or an undetected medical cause of the depression. In addition, adherence must be assessed thoroughly. If the patient has not been adherent, then the reasons should be explored. Finally, the antidepressant must have been administered at a known effective dose for a reasonable amount of time.

If a patient is truly unresponsive to treatment, then one of two strategies can be implemented: switching or augmentation. Switching entails discontinuing one antidepressant in favor of another. Augmentation involves adding an additional medication to supplement the effect of the antidepressant.

Switching. Switching antidepressants is less costly and simpler and avoids the potential for drug interactions that can occur in an augmentation approach. When a switching strategy is adopted, it is usually best to change to an antidepressant with a different mechanism of action. Theoretically, this provides a greater likelihood of response to the second antidepressant and may help avoid any unpleasant side effects of the first medication.

Switching antidepressants is usually straightforward. Often, the first medication is decreased as the new one is started and gradually increased such that there is an overlap between the two.

When switching between a MAOI and other antidepressants that affects serotonin activity, the first medication must be allowed to "wash out" of the patient's system before the new antidepressant is started. The duration of this washout period is determined by the half-life of the antidepressant that is being discontinued. If a washout is neglected, then a potentially dangerous serotonin syndrome may result.

In addition, whenever an antidepressant that blocks serotonin reuptake is discontinued, an unpleasant but harmless discontinuation syndrome manifested by abdominal discomfort, instability, anxiety, and occasionally painful shock-like sensations in the extremities can arise. The risk appears to be greatest with venlafaxine and paroxetine. Consequently, switching from one of these medications to another that does not block serotonin reuptake requires a gradual taper of the first medication over days to weeks.

Augmentation may be preferable when the patient has already failed trials of several antidepressants or when there has been a partial response to the current antidepressant that would be lost in a switching strategy. In addition, augmentation avoids conveying the demoralizing message to the patient that "we're having to start all over again."

Augmentation. Choosing an augmenting medication is much like choosing an antidepressant. The severity of the depression, the history of prior treatment, and the safety and side effects of the augmenting medication are all important considerations.

If the depression remains very severe, then lithium is a good choice. Although lithium may at times be difficult to tolerate and can be dangerous, it still provides a good possibility of helping a nonresponsive depression.

When the residual depression is mild to moderate, then the risks of using lithium are probably not warranted. A less aggressive approach using a safer but less proven augmenting medication is best. The alternatives include adding T3, buspirone, pindolol, a second antidepressant, a stimulant, estrogen, or an anticonvulsant.

T3 is the best studied of these and is a reasonable alternative, but many prefer adding a second antidepressant in order to recapture some of the "rich pharmacology" of the older antidepressants. Stimulants are highly recommended for medically compromised patients who need a rapid response, and buspirone is probably best for those with an anxious depression. Finally, estrogen may be a good choice for depressed women during the transition into menopause.

Loss of Response. One final dilemma is the recurrence of major depression during maintenance treatment. Nearly one-third of patients who initially respond to an antidepressant will later have a recurrence despite continuing to take the antidepressant.

This can be hard to explain. Potential causes include a worsening of the depression, the development of tolerance to the medication's effect, or the loss of placebo effect. Some believe that in our efforts to find safer and more tolerable medications, we have produced a new generation of antidepressants that are not as effective when used long-term. This harkens back to the "rich pharmacology" versus "dirty drug" debate. Could the older medications with their multiple receptor actions work better long-term? We really don't know.

We also aren't sure what's the best thing to do when a recurrence happens. Alternatives include increasing the dose of the current antidepressant, switching antidepressants, choosing an augmentation strategy, or even attempting a drug holiday to reverse tolerance. Until further research clarifies this phenomenon, the decision to switch treatment, augment treatment, or increase the dose of the current antidepressant must be evaluated on a case-by-case basis.

3.3 DYSTHYMIC DISORDER

3.3.1 Brief Description and Diagnostic Criteria

Dysthymic disorder, also called dysthymia, is by definition a chronic illness that lasts two or more years. It consists of persistently depressed mood that is not as severe as major depression. However, "double depression" can occur in which a major depressive episode is superimposed on a preexisting dysthymia. It is unclear whether double depression is actually two illnesses or a single illness that varies in severity over time. Please refer to Table 3.12 for diagnostic criteria of dysthymic disorder.

3.3.2 Prevalence and Risk Factors

Dysthymia affects 3–6% of Americans in their lifetime. Similar to major depression, women have dysthymic disorder two to three times more often than men. Dysthymia usually begins in childhood or early adulthood.

The risk factors for dysthymia include a family history of depression and the coexistence of a personality disorder. In addition, dysthymic patients often have major depression, anxiety disorders, or substance abuse disorders as well.

3.3.3 Presentation and Clinical Course

Dysthymic patients are less likely to complain of depressed mood than those with major depression. They experience vague feelings of apathy, inadequacy, ruminative

TABLE 3.12. Diagnostic Criteria for Dysthymic Disorder

A. Depressed mood most of the day at least half of the time for 2 years.
B. At least two of the following symptoms are also present during this 2 years:
   1. Increased or decreased appetite
   2. Too much or too little sleep
   3. Feeling tired
   4. Low self-esteem
   5. Having a hard time concentrating or making simple decisions
   6. Feeling hopeless
C. Has not been symptom free for 2 months or more during this 2 years.
D. Did not have a major depressive episode during the first 2 years.
E. Has never experienced a manic, hypomanic, or mixed episode.
F. Not due to a psychotic disorder.
G. Not due to a medication, an illicit drug, or a medical illness.
H. Impairs daily functioning at work or home.

Source: Adapted from DSM-IV.

guilt, and social isolation but, in contrast to the patient with MDD, often come to understand these symptoms as part of their personality. As a result, dysthymic patients can seldom identify when the illness began. They often say, "I've always been depressed."

Untreated, dysthymic disorder is often a persistent, lifelong illness. It leads to significant functional disability, interfering with work productivity and participation in family and social activities. In addition, untreated dysthymic disorder often progresses to chronic or recurrent major depression.

3.3.4 Initial Evaluation and Differential Diagnosis

The assessment of dysthymic disorder is identical to that undertaken for MDD. Causative factors such as medical illnesses, depression-inducing medications, or abused substances must be ruled out. Mild depressive symptoms in the context of other psychiatric disorders must also be ruled out.

The key task is distinguishing dysthymia from major depression. The similarity in symptoms and the potential for double depression can make this difficult. Major depression tends to have an episodic course, more neurovegetative symptoms, and more severe disability. On the other hand, dysthymia is a smoldering, unrelenting mood disturbance.

3.3.5 History of Pharmacological Treatment

For many years, antidepressant medication was infrequently used in the treatment of dysthymic disorder. The reasons are not entirely apparent. One possible explanation is the prevalent view of dysthymic disorder as a "reactive" phenomenon that arises out of psychodynamic conflict in contrast to major depression that is often termed "endogenous," reflecting a presumption that biological factors play a greater role. These conceptions would arguably result in a preference for psychodynamic psychotherapy in treatment of dysthymic disorder and a more ready disposition to prescribe antidepressants for MDD. Another plausible explanation is that the older agents plagued with safety and side effect limitations were not deemed worth the risk of adverse outcome in treating milder forms of depression.

For whatever reason, few controlled trials of antidepressants have been performed in the treatment of dysthymic disorder. The limited evidence available, however, suggests that the same classes of antidepressants that effectively treat major depression also treat dysthymia. Reported side effects are similar with the newer agents tolerated better than TCAs.

3.3.6 Current Approach to Treatment

A trial of antidepressants is highly recommended in the treatment of dysthymic disorder. Although transference attitudes toward medications should always be explored, this may be especially true in treating a dysthymic patient. These patients commonly view their depressive symptoms as an integral part of their personality; therefore, an antidepressant may be seen not as a treatment for an illness but as a confirmation of their defectiveness. In addition, the apathetic and pessimistic outlook of the dysthymic patient occasionally compromises treatment compliance. Because of these transference issues, a psychotherapy that does not ignore but explores the meaning of taking medication is indispensable to successful treatment.

Antidepressants should be titrated to doses equivalent to those used in the treatment of major depression. Titrating to the lower end of the effective dose range should occur within the first 2 weeks. Thereafter, doses can be raised every 2–4 weeks until symptoms improve. Early evidence suggests that dysthymic patients respond more slowly to antidepressants than do patients with major depression. The proper duration of antidepressant treatment for dysthymic disorder is not known. The chronic nature of the disorder perhaps portends that longer term treatment should be anticipated; however, this issue has not been well studied.

3.3.7 Refractory Depression

As in the treatment of major depression, an inability to achieve an adequate response or a loss of response mandates a change in therapy. This may entail a refocus of psychotherapy. Certainly, a medication change should not be made reflexively if it fosters an avoidance of key psychotherapeutic issues. However, medication changes are sometimes warranted.

The options include increasing the dose of the current antidepressant, switching antidepressants, or the addition of an augmenting agent. This decision should account for the current dose of medication, the degree of partial response if any, and the patient's preferences.

3.4 BIPOLAR DISORDERS

3.4.1 Brief Description and Diagnostic Criteria

In the bipolar affective disorders (BPADs), periods of normal mood are interspersed with episodes of mania, hypomania, mixed states, or depression. BPAD differs from MDD in that there is a bidirectional nature to the mood swings and, for many patients, the rate of cycling is more rapid in BPAD than MDD. The phases of BPAD include mania, hypomania, and depression, though mixed states, the simultaneous presentation of symptoms of both mania and depression, are common.

Phases of Bipolar Illness. The depressive phase of bipolar illness is virtually indistinguishable from unipolar MDD and the diagnostic criteria for a major depressive episode (refer to Table 3.2) are used to diagnose bipolar depression as well. The clinical presentation of bipolar depression often resembles atypical depression, which is characterized by severe fatigue and oversleeping.

The elevated phases of BPAD are termed manic or hypomanic episodes. The symptoms of mania and hypomania are qualitatively similar, though they differ, sometimes dramatically, in a quantitative sense. Manic episodes are, by definition, more severe and associated with a greater degree of impairment and/or dysfunction. Symptoms of manic and hypomanic episodes include elevated mood, irritability, rapid thinking, decreased energy, reduced need for sleep, excessive spending, heightened sexuality, and a greater proclivity toward risk-taking behaviors. The impairment seen in manic episodes is usually severe enough to warrant hospitalization, and more than half of patients with acute mania are psychotic. Indeed, severity of symptoms that are sufficient to result in hospitalization distinguishes mania from hypomania. Hypomanic episodes do not produce this same degree of impairment. Patients with hypomania may appear overly confident, more productive and creative with an increased pace of thinking, as well as an overall sense of improved well-being. This symptom profile no doubt accounts for the relatively small number of patients with Bipolar II Disorder (BPAD II), depression interspersed with hypomania, who present for treatment during a hypomanic episode. Typically, it is the disabling and prolonged depressive episodes that bring the patient with BPAD II into treatment. In contrast, the patient with Bipolar I Disorder (BPAD I), depression interspersed with mania, will experience significant distress and dysfunction in either phase of the illness. The DSM-IV diagnostic criteria for the hypomanic and manic episodes that characterize BPAD are listed in Tables 3.13 and 3.14.

It is common for both the depressive and manic phases to occur simultaneously in what is termed a mixed state or dysphoric mania. During these mixed episodes, the patient's mood is characterized by symptoms of both a depression and mania. Mixed episodes often have a poorer outcome than classic euphoric mania and, as a rule, respond better to certain anticonvulsants and atypical antipsychotic drugs than to lithium. As many as 50% of admissions to inpatient psychiatric facilities for the treatment of manic episodes appear to be for mixed manic states. The recognition

TABLE 3.13. Diagnostic Criteria for a Hypomanic Episode

A. At least 4 days of elevated or irritable mood that is different from the patient's usual mood.
B. At least three of the following symptoms (four are required if the mood has only been irritable):
   1. Exaggerated self-esteem
   2. Little need for sleep
   3. Excessively talkative ("hard to get a word in edgewise")
   4. Rapid thinking
   5. Very short attention span
   6. Excessive level of activity or agitation
   7. Excessive pleasure-seeking
C. It impairs daily functioning at work or home.
D. Others notice the change in behavior.
E. It does cause severe impairment that might require a hospital stay.
F. It is not caused by a medical illness, medication, or drug of abuse.

Source: Adapted from DSM-IV.

TABLE 3.14. Diagnostic Criteria for a Manic Episode

A. At least 1 week of elevated or irritable mood that is different from the patient's usual mood. The duration requirement of 1 week is waived if the patient must be hospitalized.
B. Meets the symptoms required for hypomania.
C. It is not a mixed episode (i.e., there is no evidence of depression).
D. Unlike hypomania, the impairment is very severe and may require a hospital stay.
E. It is not caused by a medical illness, medication, or drug of abuse.

Source: Adapted from DSM-IV.

of a mixed episode is important not only for choosing the best treatment, but also due to the importance of discontinuing antidepressant treatment in these patients.

Another BPAD diagnostic modifier is the frequency of mood episodes or "cycling." Patients who experience four or more episodes (depressed, hypomanic, or manic) per year are said to have rapid cycling BPAD. Rapid cycling patients are more likely to be female and, like those with mixed episodes, respond preferentially to certain anticonvulsants and perhaps atypical antipsychotics than to lithium.

Bipolar Syndromes. There are three distinct bipolar syndromes described in DSM-IV: BPAD I, BPAD II, and cyclothymic disorder. The most severe subtype, BPAD I, is comprised of episodes of mania and/or depression. BPAD II, in contrast, is defined by episodes of hypomania and/or depression. BPAD II is arguably the most difficult to distinguish from the mood instability of patients with Cluster B personality disorders. Cyclothymic patients fluctuate between phases of hypomania and those of mild depression reminiscent of dysthymia. Although the symptoms of cyclothymia produce significant morbidity and impairment, the disability falls far short of that associated with either BPAD I or BPAD II. Cyclothymia is perhaps the least understood of the bipolar disorders, precisely because the symptoms are sufficiently mild that patients frequently do not seek treatment. There are virtually no controlled treatment studies of cyclothymia.

3.4.2 Prevalence and Risk Factors

As a group, the lifetime rate of BPAD is approximately 1–1.5%. Some in the field have argued that this is an underestimation and have moreover promulgated the concept of bipolar spectrum disorders from mild to severe that if accepted would surely increase the lifetime prevalence estimates. Prevalence differences based on ethnic group and cultural setting may exist, though no consistent picture has emerged. It is noteworthy, however, that the rate of BPAD is equal between men and women. This contrasts the twofold higher rate of unipolar depression observed in women.

No specific genetic abnormality has yet been identified, but it is clear that BPAD runs in families. Twin and adoption studies have confirmed that this family-based risk is primarily genetic in origin.

Genetic inheritance is likely the single most important risk factor for having BPAD, but what are the risk factors for the onset of an episode? The genetic epidemiology suggests that approximately 50–60% of the risk is derived from genetics, that is, what we inherit from our parents. The balance of the risk is likely attributable to the adverse effects of major life stressors and environmental changes. Over time, the greater the number of episodes in a patient with BPAD, the greater the likelihood, especially if untreated, of additional future episodes. Thus, the prevention of subsequent episodes is one of the many reasons why ongoing maintenance therapy is such a critically important component of treatment.

3.4.3 Presentation and Clinical Course

The term "bipolar affective disorder" is a wonderfully accurate descriptor of the illness, conveying the sense of either mood elevation or lowering. This broad spectrum of mood states is associated with a wide range of clinical presentations. Indeed, many patients with BPAD are initially misdiagnosed as having MDD, which was formerly termed "unipolar depression" to distinguish it from bipolar depression. Episodes of mania or depression are typically the impetus leading a patient to seek treatment or a concerned family member or friend to seek treatment in the patient's behalf. Hypomanic episodes, as mentioned earlier, rarely motivate patients to seek treatment. Instead bipolar depression, typically as severe as the depression seen in MDD and often characterized by the so-called atypical symptoms of increased appetite and sleep, is almost always what leads patients with BPAD II to seek treatment. A complicating factor in making the diagnosis of BPAD in depressed patients is that they often do not recall and/or report periods of hypomania or mania. A patient who is in the depths of depression may find it difficult to remember a time when they were not depressed, much less hypomanic or manic. In these cases, a history obtained from a reliable family member can be invaluable.

Whereas patients with depression commonly seek treatment for themselves, manic patients are usually brought to treatment by someone else, often under some degree of coercion. Despite the havoc that acute mania can wreak upon one's life, the illness so clouds insight and judgment that often the need for treatment is not recognized. Thus, manic patients frequently present for treatment in an emergency room accompanied by a family member, friend, co-worker, or perhaps a police officer.

Acute mania often presents with giddiness, euphoria, anger, or irritability. There will likely be boundless energy, rapid, loud talking, disinhibition, and perhaps a preoccupation with sex or religion.

The course of BPAD can be quite variable. Although BPAD has not traditionally been thought of as a chronic disorder similar to schizophrenia but rather an episodic one, most clinicians have noted a gradually worsening course with more frequent episodes as the illness progresses. This is one psychiatric illness in which treatment not only alleviates the current symptoms but might also improve the long-term course.

3.4.4 Initial Evaluation and Differential Diagnosis

Initially, BPAD is often difficult to diagnose. The symptoms of BPAD resemble elements of depressive disorders, psychotic disorders, and certain personality disorders. In addition, certain medications, substances of abuse, and medical illnesses can produce symptoms that bear a striking resemblance to BPAD. To maximize the likelihood of an accurate diagnosis, the initial evaluation should include not only documentation of the presenting symptoms, but a review of the patient's past psychiatric and medical history, family psychiatric history, and the sequence of symptom emergence during the current episode. The differential diagnosis when evaluating a patient suspected to have BPAD includes MDD, schizophrenia and schizoaffective disorder, brief psychotic disorder, Cluster B personality disorders, attention deficit–hyperactivity disorder, substance-induced (including drugs of abuse as well as certain medications) manic episodes, and manic episodes due to medical conditions such as stroke or certain forms of epilepsy.

Major Depressive Disorder (MDD). The distinction between MDD and BPAD is most problematic during the earliest episodes of illness and at younger ages of presentation. The first episode of bipolar illness is a depressive one in at least one-third of patients with BPAD. The younger the age of onset of an episode of depression, the greater the likelihood that the disease will progress to BPAD.

An episode of bipolar depression is virtually indistinguishable from that of unipolar depression. The key is to gather a careful history of the patient's premorbid functioning, earlier episodes of illness, and family psychiatric illness. This information should be gathered from the patient, as well as family members and friends. Previous episodes of full-blown mania seldom go unreported; however, prior hypomanic episodes are often unrecognized not only by the patient but by friends and family as well. One should inquire about periods of decreased need for sleep (as opposed to insomnia), excessive goal-directed activity (extremely long hours at work), and uncharacteristic excitement or argumentativeness. In addition, any family history of BPAD should be elicited.

The distinction between major depression and bipolar depression is an important one. Treating a depressed bipolar patient with antidepressant monotherapy (i.e., without a concomitant mood stabilizer) can propel such a patient into a manic or hypomanic episode. Although it may not be prudent to initiate a mood stabilizer when the evidence for bipolar illness is equivocal, the clinician should be particularly vigilant for the emergence of manic or hypomanic symptoms when starting antidepressant treatment for the first time in a depressed patient.

Schizophrenia. We are often faced with the challenge of distinguishing bipolar illness from a primary psychotic disorder such as schizophrenia. In particular, the hostility, irritability, paranoia, and excitement that often characterize acute mania cannot reliably be used to distinguish it from the sometimes-agitated psychosis of schizophrenia. Furthermore, the rapid thinking of mania can produce a loosening of associations that is indistinguishable from the thought disorganization that can occur during an acute exacerbation of schizophrenia.

Again, the character of the patient's prior episodes, premorbid functioning, and family history all are helpful. By definition, schizophrenia is marked by a 6-month decline in social and occupational functioning that is seldom seen in bipolar illness. In addition, the delusions and hallucinations of schizophrenia are present during periods of normal mood, whereas bipolar patients only experience psychotic symptoms in the context of severe mood disturbance (i.e., mania or depression).

Finally, the natural course of illness can help to distinguish BPAD from schizophrenia. Many patients with BPAD resume normal functioning between episodes of illness, although those with severe variants of BPAD not uncommonly become chronically ill. Most patients with schizophrenia, in contrast, are unable to achieve their premorbid functional level between exacerbations of illness and many experience a gradually declining course.

Between the mood disorders and schizophrenia lies schizoaffective disorder. Taking both unipolar and bipolar forms, schizoaffective disorder is manifested by periods of mood disturbance accompanied by psychotic symptoms that persist even when the mood disturbance has resolved. Schizoaffective disorder typically produces a greater degree of social dysfunction than bipolar illness but less impairment than schizophrenia.

Brief Psychotic Disorder. This disorder occurs in the immediate aftermath of a markedly stressful event (or series of events). It is marked by emotional turmoil in conjunction with one or more psychotic symptoms such as delusions, hallucinations, disorganization, or catatonia. On presentation, a brief psychotic disorder can be difficult to distinguish from psychotic depression or mania. The presence of a precipitating stressor is not always helpful, because episodes of psychotic mood disorders (especially early in the course of illness) are also commonly triggered by stressful life events. Careful evaluation for symptoms of emerging depression or mania prior to the onset of psychotic symptoms may help clarify the underlying diagnosis.

When brief psychotic disorder is diagnosed, treatment with antipsychotic medication and supportive therapy should be instituted. During treatment, however, the patient should be frequently reassessed for the presence of a mood disorder that was not easily recognizable in the initial agitated and psychotic state.

Borderline Personality Disorder (BPD). The dramatic Cluster B personality disorders should also be considered in the differential diagnosis of bipolar illness. In particular, the affective instability, impulsivity, and attention seeking of BPD resemble certain facets of bipolar illness. The key distinction is that the mood of a patient with BPD is likely to remain reactive to environmental changes, whereas the depressive and manic episodes of BPAD, though frequently environmentally triggered, follow a discrete course that is not as readily responsive to environmental change. Because it is so contingent on contextual stresses, the often severe mood disturbance associated with BPD seldom meets the duration criteria required for BPAD and usually improves rapidly in a structured treatment setting. Furthermore, the patient with BPD seldom experiences the decreased need for sleep, pressured speech, or racing thoughts that so commonly mark episodes of mania and hypomania. It bears noting, however, that BPD and BPAD are not mutually exclusive diagnoses; it is quite possible for a single patient to fulfill the diagnostic criteria for both disorders.

Delirium. Delirium is an abrupt change in mental status often accompanied by agitation and seemingly psychotic symptoms that may resemble mania. Unlike mania, however, delirium is commonly characterized by a fluctuating level of consciousness and disorientation. The chief precipitants of delirium include infections, medications, and metabolic disturbances. Therefore, all patients who present in an acutely agitated state should undergo a comprehensive yet expeditious medical evaluation to rule out potential causes of delirium. This evaluation must include a thorough physical examination and a battery of laboratory tests.

Attention Deficit–Hyperactivity Disorder (ADHD). Only recently has ADHD been added to the differential diagnosis of BPAD. ADHD was long considered a childhood illness that resolved before adulthood. Moreover, the onset of BPAD was long believed to occur exclusively during adulthood. Both of these statements are now known to be untrue. Many of the symptoms of ADHD persist into adulthood. Meanwhile, an increasing number of child psychiatrists and epidemiologists have noted that the onset of BPAD not infrequently occurs in children before they reach puberty.

The common features of ADHD and BPAD include impulsivity and increases in psychomotor activity, but careful assessment can usually distinguish the two diagnoses. The behavioral manifestations of ADHD tend to be continuous, though they are most evident in quiet settings. In contrast, the symptoms of BPAD are episodic and should represent a clear departure from the patient's usual level of activity. In addition, the hyperactivity of ADHD is typically purposeless and nonproductive. This contrasts with the typically goal-directed and often highly productive heightened activity of a hypomanic patient. This distinction should be tempered, however, by the realization that, during manic episodes, the bipolar patient's thoughts and activities often become disorganized and purposeless. Finally, a family history of either ADHD or BPAD can help to clarify the patient's underlying diagnosis.

Substance-Induced Mood Disorder. Numerous case reports exist of abused substances or prescription medications inducing symptoms of mania, though patients with BPAD often abuse illicit substances when they enter a manic phase. Many of the substances reported to induce manic symptoms enhance dopamine activity in the brain. If we recognize that increased dopamine activity improves concentration, leads to feelings of well-being and euphoria, and may even produce hallucinatory experiences, it should not be surprising that these agents might produce mania-like syndromes.

For this reason, the initial evaluation of a patient during an episode of mania or hypomania must include a review of all prescribed medications and illicit substance use, and collection of a urine drug screen. We must bear in mind, however, that many of the newer "designer" drugs such as Ecstasy are not typically detected by most commercial laboratory tests for drugs of abuse.

More controversial is the occurrence of antidepressant-induced mania or hypomania. DSM-IV specifically states that manic or hypomanic episodes triggered by antidepressant treatment should not count toward the diagnosis of BPAD. However, clinicians have traditionally viewed antidepressant-induced switching from depression into mania as an unmasking of a preexisting BPAD that had previously been unrecognized and undiagnosed.

Mood Disorder Due to a General Medical Condition. Commonly called secondary manias, certain medical and neurological illnesses produce symptoms that mimic mania. Often, secondary manias occur when injury or disease interferes with right-sided brain function. As one might anticipate, this is in contrast to the predilection for left-sided brain injury to be associated with depressive symptoms.

Brain injury from trauma, stroke, space-occupying brain tumors, brain infection such as HIV and syphilis, and inflammatory conditions such as lupus and multiple sclerosis can all induce these so-called secondary manias (Table 3.15). For this

TABLE 3.15. Medical Conditions that May Cause Secondary Mania

Neurological	Infection	Metabolic
Head trauma	Encephalitis	Addison's disease
Huntington's disease	HIV/AIDS	Cushing's disease
Multiple sclerosis	Syphilis	Hyperthyroidism
Post-stroke		Postdialysis
Seizure disorders		Vitamin B_{12} deficiency
Tumors		

reason, brain imaging using CT or MRI and laboratory screenings are essential components of the initial evaluation for a manic episode. In cases where secondary mania is highly suspected (e.g., geriatric onset mania), a lumbar puncture (i.e., spinal tap) should also be considered as part of the medical evaluation.

3.4.5 History of Pharmacological Treatment

In contrast to MDD, the bipolar disorders consist of episodes of depression and episodes of hypomania or mania. This poses a problem for treating the depressed phase of this illness, because, as noted earlier, antidepressants can trigger hypomania, mania, or mixed dysphoric mania and can increase the frequency of manic episodes. Therefore, the hallmark of treating BPAD is the use of mood stabilizers, with and without supplemental antidepressant therapy. Please refer to Table 3.16 for a comparison of the traditional mood stabilizers.

Lithium. Discovered in the early 1800s, lithium is a naturally occurring salt that enjoyed a variety of uses in the 19th and early 20th centuries. Popular in medicinal remedies of that era, lithium was touted as a treatment for gout and a host of mental derangements. When its introduction as a salt substitute in the 1940s led to an epidemic of toxicity, the use of lithium was briefly abandoned. However, in the early 1950s, lithium was found to be an effective treatment for acute mania and to provide prophylactic protection against future episodes of bipolar illness.

If we define a mood stabilizer as a medication that is both an effective antimanic and antidepressant, then lithium arguably remains to this day the prototypical mood stabilizer. Lithium not only reduces the symptoms of acute BPAD, it also prevents the recurrence of additional mood episodes. Despite the fact that lithium has revolutionized the treatment of BPAD and remains nearly 50 years after its introduction as the single best treatment for many patients with BPAD, there is still no consensus as to how it works. Lithium exerts effects on several neurotransmitter systems (e.g., serotonin, dopamine, norepinephrine, acetylcholine), on second messenger systems inside the nerve cell, and on nerve cell gene expression. Yet, precisely how these varied effects produce lithium's therapeutic benefit remains unclear.

Lithium remains the treatment of choice for bipolar patients who experience classic euphoric episodes of mania. Current evidence suggests that those with mixed episodes or rapid cycling episodes respond preferably to anticonvulsants or atypical antipsychotic drugs. In addition to its use as a mood stabilizer, lithium is effective in converting unipolar antidepressant nonresponders to responders. Finally, lithium may also be an effective treatment for patients with cluster headaches.

Lithium therapy should be initiated at 300–900 mg/day. The dose should be increased every 3–7 days until a serum level of 0.6–1.2 mEq/L is achieved. Lithium blood levels should be measured approximately 12 hours after the last dose. Therapeutic levels are lower for elderly patients, but young adults often require serum levels of 0.8–1.4 mEq/L or greater for a full therapeutic effect.

TABLE 3.16. Comparison of the Traditional Mood Stabilizers

	Lithium	Valproate	Carbamazepine
Preferred for:	Euphoric mania Bipolar depression	Mixed episode Rapid cycling Poor lithium response Secondary mania	Mixed episode Rapid cycling Poor lithium response
Premedication workup:	Pregnancy test Complete blood count Thyroid function tests BUN/creatinine EKG	Pregnancy test Complete blood count Liver enzymes	Pregnancy test Complete blood count Liver enzymes Reticulocyte count
Starting dose:	600–900 mg/day	500–1000 mg/day Loading: 20 mg/kg	200–400 mg/day
Therapeutic level:	0.6–1.2 mEq/L	60–125 μg/mL	4–12 μg/mL
Minor side effects:	Drowsiness, fatigue Weight gain Nausea, diarrhea Tremor Frequent urination	Drowsiness, fatigue Weight gain Nausea, diarrhea Tremor Hair loss (alopecia)	Drowsiness, fatigue Weight gain Nausea Headache Confusion
Safety and health concerns:	Birth defect Toxicity Hypothyroidism	Birth defect Hepatitis Decreased platelets	Birth defect Hepatitis Agranulocytosis
Drug interactions:	Diuretics[a] NSAIDs (e.g., ibuprofen)[a]	Lamotrigine[b]	Clozapine[c] Contraceptives[d] HIV protease inhibitors[d]

[a] Increased risk of lithium toxicity.
[b] Increased risk of Stevens–Johnson syndrome (rash).
[c] Potential increased risk of agranulocytosis.
[d] Less effective when taken with carbamazepine.

Before starting lithium treatment, a baseline assessment of kidney and thyroid function, a pregnancy test for women of childbearing age, and an electrocardiogram must be obtained. Thyroid and renal function as well as a lithium level should be monitored every 6–12 months after the patient is stabilized. Lithium has a very low therapeutic index, which means that potentially toxic serum levels may be no more than 50% higher than the upper end of the therapeutic range. When starting a patient on lithium, it is important to educate the patient and his/her family of the signs and symptoms of lithium toxicity. These include tremor, nausea, vomiting, confusion, slurred speech, and clumsiness that resembles drunkenness. Advise the patient that if any such symptoms arise, they should immediately visit the nearest emergency room to have their lithium level checked. Lithium toxicity is a medical emergency that can result in coma and even death if untreated.

Lithium toxicity can occur as a result of intentional overdose; therefore, care must be taken when administering lithium to potentially suicidal patients with BPAD. Inadvertent lithium toxicity may also occur. For example, diuretics and nonsteroidal anti-inflammatory drugs such as ibuprofen (Advil, Motrin) slow the excretion of lithium and can lead to accidental toxicity. Consequently, the patient should be advised not to take such commonly available medications while treated with lithium. In addition, dehydration resulting from varied causes such as diarrhea, vomiting, and profuse sweating can lead to accidental lithium toxicity. One should advise the patient who takes lithium to be careful to remain well hydrated at all times and to contact his/her physician if any medical condition arises that may cause rapid fluid losses (e.g., stomach virus, high fevers).

Electroconvulsive Therapy (ECT). Introduced in the mid-1930s, ECT was initially used to treat schizophrenia (for which it is not effective) but was later found to be very effective in the treatment of major depression and mania. It gained widespread use and was the primary biological psychiatric treatment until the introduction of newer psychiatric medications in the 1950s.

In the 1980s, interest in ECT resurfaced. Unlike most of the so-called mood stabilizers, ECT is effective for the treatment of both the manic and depressive episodes of BPAD. In addition, it is often the safest and most effective treatment when treating BPAD during pregnancy. ECT should be given serious consideration for patients with BPAD who are not responding well to conventional medication therapies, whose illness is so severe as to present a life-threatening crisis, or who would be unwise to take one of the primary mood stabilizers due to safety concerns (e.g., first trimester pregnancy).

Typical Antipsychotics. Since their introduction in the 1950s, antipsychotics have played a prominent role in the treatment of bipolar mania. When we recognized that dopamine activity is critical in the brain's reward centers, the notion arose that dopamine hyperactivity may contribute to the euphoria of bipolar mania. Therefore, it was natural to assume that the dopamine-blocking antipsychotics would be effective antimanic medications.

In fact, the typical antipsychotics do have antimanic properties, but the overall results compared to lithium are disappointing. In head-to-head competitive trials against lithium, typical antipsychotics including haloperidol and chlorpromazine were not as effective, and they had unfavorable side effect profiles. Nevertheless, these drugs found a niche in the treatment of BPAD. First, they were helpful and indeed necessary in the treatment of severely ill bipolar patients who had become psychotic. Second, the tranquilizing effects of the antipsychotics begin rapidly within minutes to hours, whereas the calming effect of lithium (and subsequently the anticonvulsants) may require several days. Therefore, antipsychotics were widely used to manage agitation even in nonpsychotic bipolar patients during a manic episode.

Using typical antipsychotics when treating a bipolar patient can be problematic, however. In particular, bipolar patients treated with a typical antipsychotic are at especially high risk for ultimately developing tardive dyskinesia, a disfiguring and potentially irreversible syndrome of involuntary movements triggered by prolonged exposure to the typical antipsychotics. For this reason, the use of the typical antipsychotics has largely been supplanted by first, the benzodiazepines, and more recently, the so-called atypical antipsychotics. Judicious dosing of typical antipsychotics (usually haloperidol) occasionally remains a useful tool when other agents fail, or in certain patient groups where the safety of these medications has been better demonstrated (e.g., pregnancy, severe medical illness).

Benzodiazepines. The benzodiazepines were developed in the 1950s and introduced into the U.S. market in the 1960s. They have found a variety of uses including the treatment of several anxiety disorders, insomnia, seizure disorders, alcohol withdrawal, surgical anesthesia, and others. The benzodiazepines have also been used to calm agitated patients and are therefore useful during the acute treatment phase of bipolar mania.

Benzodiazepines are safe and remarkably well tolerated. The most common side effect is drowsiness. However, elderly patients may experience confusion and a lack of coordination that increases the risk of falls. The benzodiazepines are not without abuse liability and should be used sparingly in patients with a history of a substance use disorder.

Among the benzodiazepines, clonazepam and lorazepam have been most often used in the treatment of mania. Clonazepam is a longer-lasting benzodiazepine with a gradual onset of action over several hours. It is therefore dosed two to three times daily during the management of acute manic episodes in order to provide a general tranquilizing effect. In contrast, lorazepam has a shorter onset and duration of action and has the added advantage of being available in both oral and injectable forms. Lorazepam is typically used on an as-needed basis during acute manic episodes, often in conjunction with clonazepam, to manage breakthrough agitation.

Benzodiazepines also play a critical role in optimizing sleep both during acute manic episodes and during periods of symptomatic quiescence when sleep disturbance can precipitate an episode of illness. Finally, clonazepam has been tested as a prophylactic agent during long-term maintenance therapy, but the results have been disappointing. It appears that clonazepam and the other benzodiazepines do not possess antimanic properties per se but instead offer nonspecific tranquilizing effects that are beneficial during acute episodes of illness. They clearly do not, however, provide reliable prophylaxis against future episodes.

Antidepressants. The use of antidepressants in the treatment of major depressive episodes has already been thoroughly discussed in Section 3.2. Therefore, we will not repeat that discussion here. Antidepressants that are useful for treating unipolar depression are most likely effective for bipolar depression as well, but several issues warrant discussion.

The chief concern when using antidepressants in treating bipolar depression is to avoid switching the patient into a manic episode. Although any antidepressant can theoretically precipitate a manic episode in a susceptible patient, the tricyclic antidepressants (TCAs) are the greatest offenders in this regard. TCAs should, in general, be the antidepressant of last resort when treating bipolar depression. Monoamine oxidase inhibitors (MAOIs) are more effective than TCAs in treating bipolar depression but also quite commonly cause switches into mania, despite coadministration with a mood stabilizer.

It appears that SSRIs and bupropion are less likely than TCAs to induce mania. Venlafaxine, perhaps because of its dual effects on serotonin and norepinephrine like the TCAs, also appears to increase the likelihood of switching into mania. Rarely, if ever, should an antidepressant be used in bipolar patients without concomitant treatment with a mood stabilizer.

Anticonvulsants. In the 1970s, several researchers theorized that the tendency for BPAD to worsen over time with more frequent episodes might indicate the presence of a kindling phenomenon. This model had earlier been validated in certain seizure disorders (i.e., complex partial seizures). Thus, studies of anticonvulsants in the treatment of BPAD were initiated. Although there remains no conclusive evidence that kindling plays a role in the pathophysiology of BPAD, numerous anticonvulsants have been demonstrated effective in the treatment of BPAD.

Valproate (Depakote, Depakene). Valproate is an anticonvulsant that has been demonstrated in multiple controlled clinical trials to be an effective mood stabilizer and, in fact, has obtained FDA approval for the treatment of acute mania. It appears to be particularly effective in bipolar patients who experience mixed episodes or rapid cycling or who have not responded well in the past to lithium.

To be effective, valproate usually requires a serum level of 60–125 μg/mL. Valproate can be given in a "loading dose" of 20 mg/kg in the inpatient setting, but in outpatients it is usually started at 500–1000 mg/day in two divided doses, though many practitioners prescribe valproate as a single bedtime dose, especially with the extended release (ER) formulation. (Which while indicated only for the treatment of migraine headaches and epilepsy, is now commonly used in the treatment of BPAD.) Switching from the regular formulation to the ER formulation typically requires an increase of approximately 25% in the total daily dose due to a reduction in the percentage of the ER formulation that is absorbed. The typical target dose of valproate needed to achieve a therapeutic level is 1000–2500 mg/day.

Before initiating valproate, a patient should undergo liver function tests, a complete blood count with platelets, and a pregnancy test. Long-term therapy requires regular (every 6 months) monitoring of the plasma valproate level, liver enzymes, and blood count. Most patients will experience a mild and transient elevation of liver enzymes (AST and ALT), but up to a two- to threefold elevation is not a sufficient cause for stopping the medication. Liver enzyme elevations beyond this threshold, however, may be an indicator of valproate-induced hepatitis, in which case the drug should be discontinued. Valproate occasionally reduces the platelet count, but this is not generally a concern unless it falls below 100,000.

The most commonly observed side effects of valproate are gastrointestinal complaints, tremor, sedation, and weight gain. Gastrointestinal symptoms such as nausea, vomiting, dyspepsia, indigestion, anorexia, or diarrhea, if present, are often transient. Using the divalproex sodium preparation (Depakote) rather than valproate (Depakene) minimizes the gastrointestinal complaints, and the ER formulation further improves tolerability. Hair loss (alopecia) may also occur, though much less frequently, and oral supplements of selenium and zinc may remedy this problem.

Due to the high rate of serious adverse effects during pregnancy, valproate should be avoided in women of childbearing age. First trimester exposure is associated with an increased risk of neural tube defects (e.g., spina bifida), and later exposure during pregnancy is associated with a risk for mental retardation and developmental delay. To afford a small degree of protection from neural tube defects in the event of unplanned pregnancy, we recommend that all women of childbearing age prescribed valproate should also be prescribed an oral supplement of folic acid (4 mg daily).

Carbamazepine (Tegretol, Equetro). Carbamazepine is another anticonvulsant with documented efficacy in treating BPAD, and was recently FDA approved for this indication. Like valproate, carbamazepine is usually preferred to lithium in cases of mixed mania or rapid cycling.

Carbamazepine therapy is initiated at 200–400 mg/day in two divided doses, and the typical daily dose is often in the 1000–2000 mg/day range. There are no established plasma levels for carbamazepine specifically established for BPAD, so the levels used in monitoring the drug in the treatment of epilepsy (i.e., 4–12 μg/mL) are typically used.

Before beginning treatment with carbamazepine, liver function tests, a complete blood count with platelets and reticulocytes, and a pregnancy test should be performed. Long-term monitoring of carbamazepine therapy includes periodic assessment of liver function tests, complete blood count, reticulocyte count, and carbamazepine levels. These should be performed every 2 months during the first 6 months of treatment and every 6–12 months thereafter.

The most common side effects of carbamazepine include dizziness, drowsiness, weight gain, headache, and fatigue. Many of these side effects can be minimized with a gradual upward titration of the dose. Like valproate, carbamazepine also increases the risk for neural tube defects when administered during the first trimester of pregnancy. Data is conflicting as to whether carbamazepine exposure during later pregnancy increases the risk for mental retardation. Carbamazepine should always be prescribed to women of childbearing age along with 4 mg/day folic acid supplement to provide some degree of protection in case of inadvertent conception.

Rarely, carbamazepine is associated with bone marrow failure, causing a condition known as agranulocytosis or aplastic anemia in which the levels of all circulating blood cells decrease, often dramatically. Although this condition is rare, all patients taking carbamazepine should be cautioned that an unexplained fever or signs of bleeding are early indicators of this condition. If this occurs, the patient should immediately seek a medical evaluation. To avoid potentially fatal agranulocytosis, carbamazepine should be discontinued if the white blood cell count is less than 3000, the hematocrit less than 32, the platelet count less than 100,000, or the reticulocyte index less than 0.3%. Furthermore, carbamazepine should never be coprescribed with the atypical antipsychotic clozapine, which carries a much higher risk for developing agranulocytosis. Carbamazepine can also, on rare occasion, cause a potentially dangerous dermatological condition known as Stevens–Johnson syndrome, and patients should have rash that develops promptly assessed.

Drug–drug interactions are often more problematic with carbamazepine than other mood stabilizers. Carbamazepine increases the activity of certain liver enzymes. Because these enzymes metabolize and eliminate medications and other substances introduced to the body, carbamazepine therapy can decrease the blood level and thereby reduce the effectiveness of itself (a phenomenon called autoinduction) and other medications that are metabolized by these enzymes. It is not unusual to find that the dose of carbamazepine must be increased after several weeks, because it has increased its own elimination. Other medications may likewise be less effective. Of particular concern are the oral contraceptives, Depo-Provera, and protease inhibitors used for the treatment of HIV+ patients. Oral contraceptives often require an increase in dose.

Lamotrigine (Lamictal). Lamotrigine, another anticonvulsant used to treat BPAD, is currently FDA approved for the prevention of both depressive and manic episodes during BPAD maintenance therapy. This represents a shift in the paradigms for BPAD therapy, as medications used to treat acute episodes have also typically been used for antimanic prophylaxis. Lamotrigine is not effective in the acute treatment of mania but has become for many the drug of choice for bipolar depression as well as for prevention of subsequent mood episodes of either polarity.

A concern with the administration of lamotrigine is that it has the potential to induce the Stevens–Johnson syndrome (exfoliative dermatitis). The incidence of a serious rash in clinical trials appears to be about 0.08% with monotherapy and 0.13% with combination therapy. The rash usually resolves when lamotrigine is stopped, but all patients starting lamotrigine should be cautioned to be vigilant for the development of a rash, especially during the first 6 months of treatment.

The risk for rash is increased when lamotrigine is started at a high dose or when the dose is rapidly increased. In addition, administering lamotrigine with valproate (which slows the clearance of lamotrigine) also increases the risk of rash unless the initial dosing is reduced. A typical dosing strategy is 25 mg/day for 2 weeks, then 50 mg/day for 2 weeks, followed by 100 mg/day for a week, and then 200 mg/day. When the patient is also taking valproate, the starting dose of lamotrigine is 25 mg every other day. The usual effective daily dose is 200 mg/day taken in a single dose or 100 mg/day when combined with valproate. Patients taking enzyme-inducing drugs such as carbamazepine often require a dose of at least 400 mg/day. Laboratory monitoring is not required.

Gabapentin (Neurontin). Another anticonvulsant, gabapentin, is unique among psychiatric medications in that, like lithium, it is not metabolized by the liver but excreted unchanged in urine. Gabapentin is not effective as a monotherapy (single-drug) approach in the treatment of BPAD, though it may be helpful as an adjunctive therapy in reducing anxiety and insomnia.

The dose of gabapentin should be started at 600–900 mg/day in two or three doses per day. The usual effective dose is 900–4800 mg/day. Laboratory monitoring is not needed when prescribing gabapentin. It is well tolerated with the most common side effects being drowsiness and headache.

Topiramate (Topomax). Topiramate, yet another anticonvulsant, is also ineffective in the treatment of mania when used alone. It may be helpful as an adjunctive agent, but it does not appear to be effective in the treatment of bipolar depression. Topiramate is distinguished by its minimal impact on weight. Whereas many mood stabilizers are associated with some degree of weight gain, many topiramate-treated patients actually lose weight. Therefore, topiramate has found a niche as a favorite add-on medication for bipolar patients troubled by the weight gain associated with their primary mood stabilizer or atypical antipsychotic agent. Topiramate therapy is initiated at 25–50 mg/day. The usual effective daily dose is 100–200 mg/day, though cognitive dysfunction has been reported in patients at the higher end of the dose range. Laboratory monitoring is not required. Although weight loss may seem to be an attractive effect of topiramate therapy, it should not be considered a first-line substitute for other mood stabilizers that have documented efficacy.

Atypical Antipsychotics. The so-called atypical antipsychotics have revolutionized the treatment of schizophrenia and other psychotic disorders since their introduction in the 1990s. Similarly, they are replacing the older antipsychotics in the treatment of BPAD as well. They offer a similar degree of antimanic efficacy without a lessened long-term risk of tardive dyskinesia. For more information regarding the atypical antipsychotics, please refer to Chapter 4 Schizophrenia.

Clozapine (Clozaril). Clozapine was introduced over 30 years ago but has only been available in the United States since 1990. It remains the medication of choice for treatment-resistant schizophrenia. Since its introduction, it has been used to treat acute mania with excellent results. Furthermore, it avoids the potential for tardive dyskinesia posed by haloperidol and the other typical antipsychotics.

The daily dose of clozapine ranges from as low as 200 mg/day to as high as 900 mg/day, though most patients with mania require lower doses than those with schizophrenia. Due to side effects such as dizziness and sedation, patients must be titrated gradually to the effective dose range.

Clozapine causes virtually no extrapyramidal side effects and can actually relieve tardive dyskinesia. Nevertheless, it is a difficult medication to tolerate. Its common side effects include drowsiness, weight gain, dizziness, constipation, and drooling (sialorrhea). Clozapine also increases the risk that vulnerable individuals may have seizures.

The most talked about and concerning side effect of clozapine is a potentially dangerous reduction in the number of white blood cells. This side effect, called agranulocytosis, occurs in about 1% of patients treated with clozapine. Although we cannot predict in advance who might experience agranulocytosis, we do know that it occurs most often in the first 6 months of treatment. Patients taking clozapine must have a complete blood count performed weekly during the first 6 months of treatment and every 2 weeks thereafter.

Carbamazepine and possibly the antidepressant mirtazapine should not be coadministered with clozapine because these drugs may further increase the risk of agranulocytosis. In addition, the antidepressant bupropion should not be coprescribed with clozapine because it may increase clozapine's seizure risk.

Olanzapine (Zyprexa). Olanzapine has received FDA approval for the treatment of acute mania, long-term maintenance therapy, and bipolar depression in a combination product of olanzapine and fluoxetine. The dose range for olanzapine is 5–30 mg/day. It is usually given once daily at bedtime.

The most common side effects of olanzapine are drowsiness, dizziness, constipation, weight gain, and the expected complications of weight gain including type II diabetes and the metabolic syndrome associated with an increased risk for cardiovascular disease and stroke. Olanzapine does not cause agranulocytosis, nor does it significantly increase the risk of seizure. The risk of developing extrapyramidal symptoms or tardive dyskinesia while taking olanzapine is also very low.

Risperidone (Risperdal). Risperidone is also approved by the FDA for the treatment of acute mania. It acts as an atypical antipsychotic at doses up to 4–6 mg/day. Over this dose, and at lower doses in children and the elderly, risperidone acts more like a typical antipsychotic in that extrapyramidal side effects are common.

Risperidone can be administered once or twice daily in doses ranging from 2 to 6 mg/day. Risperidone is well tolerated with comparatively few mild side effects. It can cause drowsiness, weight gain, dizziness, nausea, indigestion, diarrhea, and sexual dysfunction. Finally, risperidone does not increase the risk for agranulocytosis or seizures.

Quetiapine (Seroquel). Another atypical antipsychotic, quetiapine has also been approved by the FDA for the treatment of acute mania. It is usually administered twice daily at doses of 150–750 mg/day. Like its counterparts, quetiapine is a well-tolerated medication. Its common side effects are drowsiness, dizziness, and headache. It causes less weight gain than olanzapine or clozapine but more than ziprasidone or aripiprazole. Quetiapine also does not cause agranulocytosis nor does it increase the risk of seizures. It can occasionally cause mild changes in liver function tests, but these usually return to normal even if the patient continues taking quetiapine.

Ziprasidone (Geodon). Ziprasidone is indicated for the treatmet of acute mania with typical doses of 40–80 mg twice a day. Ziprasidone is well tolerated, with the most common side effects being sedation, extrapyramidal symptoms, and akathisia. Low magnesium or potassium may cause potentially serious cardiac conduction problems with ziprasidone.

Aripiprazole (Abilify). Aripiprazole is indicated for the treatment of acute mania and for maintenance therapy. It is dosed at 5–30 mg/day. Aripiprazole is well tolerated with the most common side effects being headache, agitation, anxiety, insomnia, and nausea.

Calcium Channel Blockers. The calcium channel blockers work by blocking the influx of calcium, an excitatory ion, into the cell. The first calcium channel blocker, verapamil (Calan), was introduced in the 1960s. Others, including diltiazem, nifedipine, and nimodipine, are now available. The calcium channel blockers have been used to treat a variety of medical conditions including high blood pressure, cardiac pain (angina) and arrhythmias, migraines, seizure disorders, and premature labor.

Studies using calcium channel blockers in the treatment of BPAD began in the late 1970s and early 1980s when it was suspected that abnormalities of calcium activity inside nerve cells might contribute to the brain dysfunction of BPAD. Unfortunately, all of the double-blind placebo controlled studies of calcium channel blockers in the treatment of BPAD have failed to demonstrate their efficacy.

Thyroid Hormone (Thyroxine, Synthroid). The most common use of thyroxine in bipolar patients is the treatment of lithium-induced hypothyroidism. Approximately 5% of patients receiving long-term lithium treatment ultimately develop hypothyroidism. When this occurs, the patient with bipolar disorder may present with symptoms of a depressive episode. Therefore, periodic thyroid axis monitoring, that is, a serum thyroid stimulating hormone (TSH) test, is required for all patients taking lithium and should always be performed when the bipolar patient experiences a depressive episode.

When laboratory testing indicates that a patient with BPAD is clinically hypothyroid, even if lithium is the readily apparent cause, we recommend starting thyroid hormone replacement. Lithium should not be discontinued, particularly if it has otherwise managed the BPAD well. Thyroxine should be started at 50 μg/day. TSH levels can then be checked 6–8 weeks later. The daily dose of thyroxine can be increased in 25 μg increments every 1–2 months until TSH levels have normalized.

Recently, thyroxine has also been suggested to be useful for the management of rapid cycling that has not responded well to conventional mood stabilizers. Thyroxine in this case has been used in so-called hypermetabolic doses even when thyroid function tests are normal. Although limited data suggests that this treatment may be helpful, it carries the risk of inducing bone mineral loss or clinical hyperthyroidism. Consequently, hypermetabolic thyroid supplementation can only be recommended for especially severe, treatment-resistant cases of rapid cycling bipolar illness.

3.4.6 Current Approach to Treatment

As we have noted earlier, BPAD, like MDD, is an episodic illness. Therefore, the treatment goal in treating both mood disorders is to alleviate the current episode and to provide protection from future episodes of illness. Bipolar syndromes by their very nature tend to cloud patient insight. Furthermore, patients with BPAD often experience a "craving" for the euphoria of the hypomanic and manic phases of the illness. Consequently, poor adherence with medication is not an uncommon problem. As a result, psychoeducation and supportive psychotherapy are critical components of a successful comprehensive treatment plan for the bipolar disorders.

Acute Phase Treatment. The treatment of bipolar illness can be organized into two stages: acute treatment and maintenance treatment. The goal of acute phase treatment is to achieve euthymia and thereby bring the current episode of illness to a conclusion. The treatment approaches needed to achieve these ends vary with the nature of the current episode. In other words, episodes of mania, hypomania, and bipolar depression require distinct treatment strategies. But in each case, euthymia is the goal. Bipolar depression is not treated by inducing mania, and mania is not treated by inducing depression. Therefore, one must always be cautious during acute phase treatment to avoid precipitating another episode of illness. Because the strategies employed to treat bipolar mania and hypomania are in many ways distinct from those used to treat bipolar depression, we will discuss these treatment approaches separately.

Manic, Hypomanic, and Mixed Episodes. The first step in managing an acute episode of BPAD is to choose the appropriate venue for treatment. Even when the patient is not overtly suicidal, the agitation, disinhibition, and impulsivity inherent to a severe manic or mixed episode of the disorder commonly require hospitalization. Hypomania, however, can usually be managed outside the hospital with frequent outpatient visits. This is particularly true if the longitudinal course of the patient's illness indicates that the patient is unlikely to progress to a full-blown manic episode.

Three tasks comprise the goals of the acute phase of treatment. First, an appropriate mood stabilizer must be chosen and safely initiated. Second, agitation and psychosis, if present, must be managed while waiting for the mood stabilizer to take effect. Third, the patient's sleep must be optimized.

Choice of a Mood Stabilizer. With the advance of atypical antipsychotics and an ever-expanding list of anticonvulsants, the number of medications reported to treat acute mania and hypomania continues to grow. In fact, all of the atypical antipsychotics, olanzapine, quetiapine, risperidone, ziprasidone, and aripiprazole have FDA approval for the treatment of acute mania. Long-term protection against future episodes of illness has also been demonstrated with several of these agents, which can influence the choice of initial therapy.

Consequently, the choice for a primary mood stabilizer in acute therapy now includes lithium, valproate, carbamazepine, and the atypical antipsychotics. Among these, lithium and valproate remain first-line agents. Valproate and lithium are probably equally effective in the treatment of classic euphoric mania, but valproate and, for that matter, carbamazepine do not appear to provide the same degree of protection from bipolar depression as lithium. As a result, patients taking one of these anticonvulsants may be more likely to require the concurrent use of an antidepressant than those who are taking lithium. This not only necessitates closer monitoring for potential drug interactions, but treating a bipolar patient with an antidepressant, although sometimes necessary, invariably conveys some risk for antidepressant-induced mania. In addition, valproate is considerably more likely than lithium to cause birth defects when administered in early pregnancy and can have adverse effects on cognitive development when prescribed later in pregnancy. When we consider that a substantial proportion of pregnancies in the United States are unplanned, that bipolar patients often exhibit impulsivity and a heightened interest in sex during episodes of illness, which likely further increases their risk of inadvertent conception, and that on average women with unplanned pregnancies don't recognize that they are pregnant until the highest risk period for valproate-associated birth defects has already passed, then we must question the practice of routinely and uncritically using valproate to treat women of childbearing age with BPAD without giving due consideration to the use of lithium.

When selecting a mood stabilizer, four factors can guide selection: (1) the phase of the current episode (i.e., euphoric mania vs. mixed mania), (2) the relative frequency of various episode types in the past as determined by review of the patient's life chart, (3) the patient's past response to particular mood stabilizers, and (4) the response of immediate family members (i.e., parents and siblings) to particular mood stabilizers.

As a rule, we prefer lithium when treating bipolar patients who most often manifest classic euphoric mania. We also prefer lithium for patients whose illness consists of a preponderance of depressive episodes with less frequent manic or hypomanic episodes. We typically initiate lithium at 300–900 mg/day given in a single bedtime dose or two divided doses. The target therapeutic level is 0.8–1.2 mEq/L.

Valproate is preferable when treating patients with frequent mixed episodes, who have a rapid cycling course, or who have a so-called secondary mania arising in the context of medical illness such as multiple sclerosis, AIDS, or a stroke. The target therapeutic level for valproate is 60–125 μg/mL. We prefer using the extended-release (ER) formulation of Depakote that enables us to initiate valproate at 750–1000 mg/day in a single bedtime dose. Once-daily dosing improves adherence and takes advantage of the fact that the sedating effects of a bedtime dose are most pronounced at night when the patient may need help maintaining a restful night's sleep. A loading dose of valproate can be used in young healthy patients who are hospitalized during a severe manic or mixed episode. On day 1 of treatment, 20 mg/kg valproate is administered when loading a patient. This loading procedure may shorten the patient's hospital stay by 1–2 days, but it should probably be avoided when treating elderly or medically ill patients who may not tolerate the large loading dose.

Carbamazepine is also most beneficial for patients with mixed episodes and rapid cycling. However, many patients find the side effects of carbamazepine more troublesome than those of valproate, and because carbamazepine has a penchant for untoward drug–drug interactions, we reserve the use of carbamazepine for those patients who are unable to tolerate valproate, lithium, and the atypical antipsychotic agents. Carbamazepine therapy is initiated at 400 mg/day in two divided doses. The target therapeutic level is 4–12 μg/mL.

Management of Agitation and Psychosis. Like antidepressants, mood stabilizers do not work immediately. It often takes a week or longer for a mood stabilizer to reach a therapeutic level and exert its beneficial treatment effects. Meanwhile, one may have a labile, impulsive, and agitated patient on one's hands. Clearly, rapidly acting tranquilizing medications are needed at this juncture to calm an agitated patient.

The medications used to manage agitation during severe mixed or manic episodes include benzodiazepines and antipsychotics. For restless, agitated bipolar patients who are psychotic or exhibiting grandiosity or paranoia that borders on psychosis, we prefer using an antipsychotic to manage both the psychosis and agitation. For the nonpsychotic bipolar patient, we prefer using benzodiazepines as a first-line medication to manage agitation. Admittedly, both antipsychotics and benzodiazepines in combination are often needed to manage agitation in the most severely ill patients.

When an antipsychotic is needed, we prefer using one of the newer atypical agents: olanzapine, ziprasidone, risperidone, quetiapine, or aripiprazole. Each of these medications reliably reduces agitation and is well tolerated. In particular, they decrease the potential for acute dystonic reactions and tardive dyskinesia caused by the typical antipsychotics. Both ziprasidone and olanzapine are now available in an injectable form that is very rapidly acting and effective in this setting.

Benzodiazepines are preferred by many for the management of agitation in nonpsychotic bipolar patients, though antipsychotics are effective as well. The most widely used benzodiazepines for this purpose are lorazepam and clonazepam. Lorazepam is perhaps the most versatile of the benzodiazepines. It has an intermediate duration of action, does not tend to accumulate and thereby cause confusion or excessive drowsiness, and can be administered by mouth, intramuscular injection, or intravenous injection. Lorazepam should be administered on an as-needed basis several times daily at 0.5–2 mg per dose. The calming effects of lorazepam are usually evident within 20–30 minutes and will last for several hours.

By contrast, clonazepam is an especially long-acting benzodiazepine that is only available in an oral preparation. Clonazepam can be started at 0.5–1 mg/day given in one or two doses per day. Whereas lorazepam provides a relatively quick onset of its tranquilizing effects, clonazepam offers a calming effect that lasts throughout the day.

Optimizing Sleep. Not only is decreased need for sleep a symptom of mania and hypomania, but sleep deprivation in itself serves to further destabilize mood in patients with BPAD. Therefore, one of the initial goals of acute management is to help the patient achieve a good night's rest. Sedating antidepressants, such as trazodone and the TCAs, which are commonly used to treat insomnia, can further elevate the already heightened mood of a bipolar patient. Therefore, they are to be avoided. Hypnotic agents such as zolpidem can be used, but we prefer using bedtime doses of a benzodiazepine or the atypical antipsychotic quetiapine. Because lorazepam and/or clonazepam are often already being used to manage agitation, a bedtime dose of one of these medications is often the most straightforward means to ensure that the patient will sleep.

Depressive Episodes. The emphasis of treatment research in bipolar illness has understandably been on the management of manic and hypomanic phases of these disorders. However, there is clearly room for improvement in the treatment of the depressive phase of BPAD as well. Depression accounts for the majority of BPAD episodes in both men and women, especially the latter. Furthermore, bipolar depression is associated with an increased risk of suicide.

The first step in managing bipolar depression is, of course, to arrive at the correct diagnosis. Producing a life chart that delineates the duration, severity, and frequency of illness episodes is critical to treatment selection. Treatment that focuses on the management of the depressive phase is especially important for patients with three or more depressive episodes, particularly severe depressions, or significant subsyndromal depressive symptoms between episodes.

The next step in the management of the depressed bipolar patient is to evaluate thyroid function. This is especially important for patients treated with lithium in order to rule out lithium-induced hypothyroidism. When this occurs, the addition of thyroid hormone replacement may relieve the depressive symptoms without any additional changes to the bipolar treatment regimen.

The third step in managing bipolar depression is to maximize treatment with the current mood stabilizer. This includes checking a medication level and possibly making a dose adjustment. Patients who are tolerating their mood stabilizer well and whose medication level is in the lower half of the therapeutic range may benefit from an increase in their dose. Among the three classic mood stabilizers (lithium, valproate, carbamazepine), only lithium has well-documented efficacy as an antidepressant. Therefore, depressed patients with BPAD who are being treated with valproate or carbamazepine may benefit from augmentation with lithium or switching to lithium. Lamotrigine is a unique mood stabilizer FDA approved for the prevention of the recurrence of both manic and depressive episodes. It has also been reported to be remarkably effective in the treatment of bipolar depression and warrants consideration as a first-line agent.

If the depressive symptoms do not resolve when treatment with one of the aforementioned mood stabilizers has been maximized, adjunctive therapy with an antidepressant or second mood stabilizer should be considered. SSRIs and bupropion are well tolerated by bipolar patients and appear to hold less potential to induce mania than TCAs. Nevertheless, treatment with any antidepressant should not be started until it has been confirmed that the patient's mood stabilizer is at a therapeutic level. If treatment with two or more of these first-line antidepressants is unsuccessful, a MAOI should be considered.

Finally, when depressive symptoms persist after treatment with both a mood stabilizer and an antidepressant has been maximized, other treatment alternatives remain. These include the use of electroconvulsive therapy (ECT) or the addition of other medications such as atypical antipsychotics, anticonvulsants, or thyroid hormone. ECT has the advantage of being highly effective even in the most severely depressed patients, and it is unlikely to induce mania. Atypical antipsychotics may confer some benefit to depressed patients with BPAD who have not responded to other treatments and are increasingly being added to mood stabilizers prior to trials of antidepressants with often times good results.

Maintenance Phase Treatment. BPAD is a lifelong illness, but the severity and frequency of episodes are highly variable from patient to patient. In addition, episodes of BPAD tend to occur more frequently as the illness progresses. When we consider the kindling models suggesting that each episode of BPAD increases the patient's vulnerability to future episodes, then early and vigorous prophylactic treatment should theoretically improve the long-term course of the disorder. Consequently, appropriate maintenance therapy is critical to the successful treatment of BPAD.

We recommend long-term maintenance treatment in nearly all cases of BPAD. This is especially true after two or more episodes of illness or even a single episode of severe mania. Furthermore, a long family history of BPAD is another indication that maintenance therapy is indicated after even a single episode of illness. However, patients with an apparent secondary mania arising as a consequence of a medical illness or drug treatment may not warrant long-term maintenance therapy if the precipitating factor has been defined and eliminated.

The mainstay of therapy, a mood stabilizer, should be continued at the same dose that was used to achieve remission during acute phase therapy. Ongoing use of the mood stabilizer requires periodic monitoring of medication levels to ensure compliance. In addition to other laboratory evaluations such as complete blood counts, liver, kidney, and thyroid studies are needed to ensure that the mood stabilizer is being well tolerated. Lamotrigine is the only mood stabilizer that does not require periodic laboratory monitoring.

A common issue during maintenance treatment is to determine whether and how long to continue adjuvant treatments that were started during the acute phase of therapy. The particular concern here is the use of antipsychotics. Typical antipsychotics such as haloperidol have long been used during acute episodes of mania to alleviate both psychotic symptoms and agitation. With the exception of the bipolar subtype of schizoaffective disorder, the common dictum was to discontinue the typical antipsychotic not long after the acute episode of illness had resolved. This practice was no doubt due to the realization that bipolar patients are at an especially high risk for developing tardive dyskinesia when typical antipsychotics are administered on a long-term basis. These concerns have largely been obviated by the introduction of atypical antipsychotics. These medications not only serve to calm agitation and relieve psychosis, but increasing evidence suggests that they have mood stabilizing properties as well. Consequently, these medications play a more prominent role in the maintenance therapy of bipolar illness than their predecessors, the typical antipsychotics. However, long-term therapy with certain atypical antipsychotic drugs, most notably olanzapine and clozapine, is associated with a very significant risk of type II diabetes, increased plasma lipids, and the metabolic syndrome.

Sleep is another concern during maintenance therapy. As we noted in the discussion of acute phase treatment, sleep deprivation can destabilize mood and is often the first sign of an impending episode of illness. Therefore, it remains imperative that the patient sleeps well. It is common practice for patients to keep a small supply of a hypnotic agent such as zolpidem or a benzodiazepine to use as needed in the event of sleep disturbance. Furthermore, patients should routinely be advised to notify their physician should they have two or more consecutive nights of poor sleep so that more aggressive measures can be taken to circumvent the possible development of an illness episode.

Managing Breakthrough Illness. Perhaps more than any other psychiatric disorder, BPAD commonly requires that patients take more than one medication to be successfully managed. Episodes of breakthrough mania or breakthrough depression sometimes occur despite therapeutic levels of the primary mood stabilizer. When this occurs, augmentation strategies are frequently required. Our previous discussion of the acute phase management of depression is applicable to the topic of breakthrough depression and therefore will not be repeated here. In this section, we will briefly discuss the management of breakthrough mania.

Obviously, the first step in treating breakthrough mania is to ensure the patient has been adherent with the primary mood stabilizer. Once this has been assured, then the options for managing breakthrough mania include: (1) increasing the dose of the current mood stabilizer, (2) augmenting with one of the other primary mood stabilizers, (3) augmenting with a secondary mood stabilizer such as an anticonvulsant or atypical antipsychotic, or (4) ECT. Should the patient currently be taking an antidepressant, this should be discontinued.

Increasing the dose of the current mood stabilizer deserves consideration when the medication level is at the lower end of the therapeutic range. This has the advantage of keeping the treatment simpler and less costly. However, as the dose is increased, the potential for intolerable side effects or toxicity (especially with lithium) becomes greater.

When increasing the dose of the current mood stabilizer is not an option, then augmentation strategies are needed. If the decision is to use two of the primary mood stabilizers together, our key recommendation is that one of these two mood stabilizers be lithium. If the patient is already taking lithium, then add one of the anticonvulsants. If the patient is already taking one of the anticonvulsants, then add lithium. Coadministration of two of the primary mood stabilizers is typically a very effective treatment alternative; however, it may carry a significant side effect burden and it increases the need for costly laboratory monitoring.

If the breakthrough symptoms are milder, then more tolerable second-line medications may offer a preferable augmentation strategy. These include the anticonvulsants gabapentin and topiramate, though no controlled data of their use in this regard is available. In addition, the atypical antipsychotics olanzapine, risperidone, quetiapine, ziprasidone, and aripiprazole are also available. Lamotrigine is another reasonable alternative, though it must be titrated slowly (especially when coadministered with valproate) to minimize the risk of treatment emergent rash.

ADDITIONAL READING

Arean PA, Cook BL. Psychotherapy and combined psychotherapy/pharmacotherapy for late life depression. *Biol Psychiatry* 2002; 53(2): 293–303.

Bauer MS, Mitchner L. What is a "mood stabilizer"? An evidence-based response. *Am J Psychiatry* 2004; 161: 3–18.

Bodner RA, Lynch T, Lewis L, Kahn D. Serotonin syndrome. *Neurology* 1995; 45: 219–223.

Calabrese JR, Kasper S, Johnson G, et al. International consensus group on bipolar I depression treatment guidelines. *J Clin Psychiatry* 2004; 65(4): 569–579.

Carney S, Cowen P, Geddes G, et al. Efficacy and safety of electroconvulsive therapy in depressive disorders: a systematic review and meta-analysis. *Lancet* 2003; 361(9360): 799–808.

Ertugrul A, Meltzer HY. Antipsychotic drugs in bipolar disorder. *Int J Neuropsychopharmacol* 2003; 6(3): 277–284.

Evins AE. Efficacy of newer anticonvulsant medications in bipolar spectrum mood disorders. *J Clin Psychiatry* 2003; 64(Supplement 8): 9–14.

Fava M, Schmidt ME, Zhang S, et al. Treatment approaches to major depressive disorder relapse. Part 2: Reinitiation of antidepressant treatment. *Psychother Psychosom* 2002; 71(4): 195–199.

Friedman MA, Detweiler-Bedell JB, Leventhal HE, et al. Combined psychotherapy and pharmacotherapy for the treatment of major depressive disorder. *Clin Psychol Sci Pract* 2004; 11(1): 47–68.

Geddes JR, Burgess S, Hawton K, et al. Long-term lithium therapy for bipolar disorder: systematic review and meta-analysis of randomized controlled trials. *Am J Psychiatry* 2004; 161(2): 217–222.

Gijsman HJ, Geddes JR, Rendell JM, et al. Antidepressants for bipolar depression: a systematic review of randomized controlled trials. *Am J Psychiatry* 2004; 161: 1537–1547.

Goodwin FK, Goldstein MA. Optimizing lithium treatment in bipolar disorder: a review of the literature and clinical recommendations. *J Psychiatr Pract* 2003; 9(5): 333–343.

Hirschfeld RMA. The efficacy of atypical antipsychotics in bipolar disorders. *J Clin Psychiatry* 2003; 64(Supplement 8): 15–21.

Iosifescu DV, Nierenberg AA, Alpert JE, et al. The impact of medical comorbidity on acute treatment in major depressive disorder. *Am J Psychiatry* 2003; 160(12): 2122–2127.

Jeste DV, Dolder CR. Treatment of non-schizophrenic disorders: focus on atypical antipsychotics. *J Psychiatr Res* 2004; 38(1): 73–103.

Keck PE, McElroy SL. Bipolar disorder, obesity, and pharmacotherapy-associated weight gain. *J Clin Psychiatry* 2003; 64(12): 1426–1435.

Keck PE, McElroy SL, Richtand N, et al. What makes a drug a primary mood stabilizer? *Mol Psychiatry* 2002; 7(Supplement 1): S8–S14.

Labbate LA, Croft HA, Olehansky MA. Antidepressant-related erectile dysfunction: management via avoidance, switching antidepressants, antidotes, and adaptation. *J Clin Psychiatry* 2003; 64(Supplement 10): 11–19.

Newport DJ, Fisher A, Graybeal S, et al. Psychopharmacology during pregnancy and lactation. In Schatzberg A, Nemeroff CB (eds), *The American Psychiatric Publishing Text-*

book of Psychopharmacology, 3rd Edition. Washington DC: American Psychiatric Publishing, 2004, pp 1109–1146.

Nierenberg AA, Petersen TJ, Alpert JE. Prevention of relapse and recurrence in depression: the role of long-term pharmacotherapy and psychotherapy. *J Clin Psychiatry* 2003; 64(Supplement 15): 13–17.

Sachs GS. Decision tree for the treatment of bipolar disorder. *J Clin Psychiatry* 2003; 64(Supplement 8): 35–40.

Schatzberg AF. Pharmacological principles of antidepressant efficacy. *Hum Psychopharmacol* 2002; 17(Supplement 1): S17–S22.

Scott J, Pope M. Nonadherence with mood stabilizers: prevalence and predictors. *J Clin Psychiatry* 2002; 63(5): 384–390.

Silverstone PH, Silverstone T. A review of acute treatments for bipolar depression. *Int Clin Psychopharmacol* 2004; 19(3): 113–124.

Sloan DME, Kornstein SG. Gender differences in depression and response to antidepressant treatment. *Psychiatr Clin North Am* 2003; 26(3): 581–594.

Suppes T, Dennehy EB. Evidence-based long-term treatment of bipolar II disorder. *J Clin Psychiatry* 2002; 63(Supplement 10): 29–33.

Weller EB, Calvert SM, Weller RA. Bipolar disorder in children and adolescents: diagnosis and treatment. *Curr Opin Psychiatry* 2003; 16(4): 383–388.

Yonkers KA, Wisner KL, Stowe Z, et al. Management of bipolar disorder during pregnancy and the postpartum period. *Am J Psychiatry* 2004; 161(4): 608–620.

4

SCHIZOPHRENIA

4.1 BRIEF DESCRIPTION AND DIAGNOSTIC CRITERIA

Schizophrenia is arguably the most devastating of all mental illnesses. It typically takes a young vibrant person just entering adulthood full of hopes and aspirations and devastates his/her life. Education is interrupted. Career plans change. Family life is disrupted. Often a shell of the former person is all that remains.

Fortunately, new treatments have greatly improved the plight of the patient with schizophrenia. Thanks in large part to the introduction of newer antipsychotic medications, few patients with this disease spend their lives in long-term psychiatric hospitals anymore. However, we have a long way to go. Individuals with schizophrenia are currently a sizeable proportion of both the homeless population and the prison population in the United States. Even with the great advances in schizophrenia treatment in the last 50 years, this illness still takes a tremendous toll on the lives of its sufferers and their families.

The diagnostic criteria for schizophrenia have evolved considerably (Table 4.1). In DSM-IV, there are three symptom domains including symptom characteristics, social/occupational dysfunction due to these symptoms, and symptom duration. In

Principles of Psychopharmacology for Mental Health Professionals
By Jeffrey E. Kelsey, D. Jeffrey Newport, and Charles B. Nemeroff

TABLE 4.1. Diagnostic Criteria for Schizophrenia

To fulfill the diagnosis all five criteria must be met.

A. At least two characteristic symptoms for 1 month:
   1. Delusions (only one of these symptoms is needed if delusions are bizarre)
   2. Hallucinations
   3. Incoherent or disorganized speech
   4. Peculiar or disorganized behavior
   5. Negative symptoms: flat affect, mutism, and lack of motivation
B. Social or employment impairment due to the illness.
C. At least 6 months of some partial signs of the illness.
D. Not due to medical illness, substance abuse, psychotic mood disorder, or schizoaffective disorder.
E. Not autism. Delusions or hallucinations must be present to diagnose schizophrenia in an autistic child or adult.

Source: Adapted from DSM-IV.

addition, DSM-IV lists exclusion criteria for other disorders that in some way resemble schizophrenia.

The characteristic symptoms of schizophrenia have historically been conceptually divided into positive and negative symptoms. At least two of these symptoms must be present for a month during the so-called active phase of illness. One can conceptualize the positive symptoms as the presence of abnormal beliefs or behaviors, whereas, in contrast, negative symptoms are a deficit or absence of normal behaviors.

Positive Symptoms. The positive symptoms of schizophrenia include delusions, hallucinations, disorganized speech, and disorganized or catatonic behavior. Delusions are false beliefs that patients with schizophrenia often hold onto tenaciously. Delusions are often paranoid (e.g., "My neighbor is trying to kill me"), but they may also be grandiose (e.g., "I own the Chrysler Building"), or erotomanic (e.g., "My neighbor is in love with me"). We can also describe delusions as bizarre (logically impossible) or nonbizarre (theoretically possible but untrue). When bizarre delusions are present (e.g., "The fillings in my teeth are transmitters planted by the KGB"), then only one characteristic symptom is required.

Hallucinations are false perceptions of one of the five primary senses (sight, hearing, touch, taste, smell). In schizophrenia, hallucinations are usually auditory of one or more voices. When these take the form of two voices carrying on a conversation or a voice making a running commentary on the patient's behavior, they are especially suggestive of schizophrenia.

The other positive symptoms include various degrees of disorganization in speech or behavior. Disorganized speech can be as mild as beating around the bush (circumstantiality) to total incoherence (word salad). Those with schizophrenia also frequently make up words (neologisms) or speak with singsong rhyming (clanging) or parrot words (echolalia). Disorganized behavior may include odd posturing or repetitive purposeless activity.

Negative Symptoms. Although the odd nature of positive symptoms draws the most attention, the negative symptoms are perhaps the most disabling. These hinder a schizophrenia patient's desire and ability to maintain relationships or hold employment. The negative symptoms include poor motivation (avolition), a bland expressionless face (flattened affect), minimal speech (alogia), and social withdrawal.

Other Symptoms. Although they are not reflected in the DSM-IV criteria, it now appears that mood and cognitive symptoms also hinder the patient with schizophrenia. Depressed mood, often short of the duration or severity needed to diagnose major depression or schizoaffective disorder, is an all too common problem. Because the negative symptoms of the illness and certain antipsychotic side effects resemble depression, this was long overlooked. Indeed, depressed mood may in part explain the extremely high rates of attempted and successful suicides by those with schizophrenia.

Finally, patients with schizophrenia also experience a variety of intellectual or cognitive problems. This includes poor memory, poor attention, and learning difficulties.

Subtypes of Schizophrenia. Schizophrenia is divided into five subtypes based on the most prominent symptoms (Table 4.2). In some cases, the subtype has a bearing on the long-term prognosis of the illness. *Paranoid type* schizophrenia probably has the best prognosis and tends to begin at a later age. On the other hand, *disorganized type* schizophrenia tends to start early and carry a poor prognosis. *Catatonic type* schizophrenia has the most striking presentation with bizarre behaviors including mutism, statue-like posturing, purposeless agitation, mimicking speech, and odd gestures. This form of schizophrenia is much less common today than it was in the pre-antipsychotic drug era. *Undifferentiated type* schizophrenia

TABLE 4.2. Schizophrenia Subtypes

Subtype	Prominent Symptoms	Less Prominent Symptoms
Paranoid	Delusions Hallucination	Disorganized thoughts Disorganized behavior Mutism, catatonia Flat affect
Disorganized	Disorganized thoughts Disorganized behavior	Paranoia Mutism, catatonia
Catatonic	Mutism Negativism	
Undifferentiated	Variable	Variable
Residual	Negative symptoms Mild positive symptoms	Delusions Hallucinations Gross disorganization

simply does not fulfill the specific characteristics of one of the other types. The final type, *residual* schizophrenia, very much resembles the prodromal phase of the illness. It is limited to negative symptoms and mild forms of the positive symptoms.

4.2 PREVALENCE AND RISK FACTORS

For decades, the lifetime incidence of schizophrenia has been reported at about 1%. This figure has remained remarkably constant despite the inherent difficulties in diagnosing schizophrenia. The rates of schizophrenia are approximately the same in all cultures worldwide.

The risk factors for schizophrenia have been studied intensely. Together with bipolar disorder, schizophrenia has long been believed to be a principally "biological" illness. Of course, the artificial wall between biological and psychological roots of psychiatric disease is beginning to crumble. Nevertheless, there is considerable evidence that biological factors laid down even before birth considerably increase the risk for developing schizophrenia.

From the biological studies we have learned that schizophrenia runs in families. Studies of twins and adopted siblings have repeatedly shown that this is mainly due to genetic inheritance. However, this is not the entire story. Some patients with schizophrenia have no family history of the disease. Viral infections during pregnancy may also increase the risk for developing schizophrenia. We believe this because schizophrenia appears to be more common among those born during flu outbreaks and those born during the winter months.

Demographic risk factors have also been studied. They reveal first that gender is not a risk factor. There is no difference in the rates between men and women. However, the illness tends to appear earlier in men (early 20s) than women (late 20s). Race is also not a risk factor. It was once believed that schizophrenia was more common in poor families. We now know this not to be true. It appears that poverty is a result of schizophrenia not a risk factor for it.

4.3 PRESENTATION AND CLINICAL COURSE

The "first break" of schizophrenia usually occurs in the late teens or twenties. This is one of the most heartbreaking aspects of the disease. It so often strikes down bright young people just as they are entering adulthood. This age range, however, is not as fixed as we once believed it to be. Schizophrenia may begin as early as childhood or as late as the 60s or 70s.

Leading up to the first break, most individuals with schizophrenia go through a prodromal phase of illness. This prodrome is a departure from the patient's usual behavior, but patients seldom seek treatment during this phase. The prodromal symptoms are usually limited to negative symptoms of apathy or social isolation or to lesser variants of the positive symptoms taking the form of eccentric beliefs or a strange preoccupation with odd mystical practices. Families often explain these away as "just a phase" and understandably so. If the patient is brought for an evaluation at this point, he/she is more likely to be diagnosed with depression than with a psychotic disorder.

The initial presentation is usually in the context of a crisis that has triggered the acute phase of the illness or a crisis that has arisen as a consequence of the illness. At this point the behavior has become so bizarre or the social deterioration so pronounced that it could no longer go unnoticed.

Because patients with schizophrenia often have little insight into their illness, they are usually brought to clinical attention by a family member, a friend, or, in unfortunate cases, the police. They may have suddenly failed school, been fired from a job, been arrested for trespass (commission of violent offenses is rare in schizophrenia), and been reclusive in their room for days or roaming the house at all hours of the night.

By the time the "first psychotic break" patient is seen, his/her behavior and thoughts are invariably strange. Sometimes the patient may be docile and adherent with the evaluation, but at other times agitated or prone to combativeness. Remember, this is a patient who does not think anything is wrong. Being forced to consult a mental health professional may confirm fears of a conspiracy. This patient may be frightened by this interaction. This is why it is so important for mental health professionals to be aware of both their own and the new patient's fearfulness during a first interview and to ensure a safe environment for all concerned.

Our understanding of the clinical cause of schizophrenia has evolved considerably in the last 20 years. Until the 1980s, Emil Kraepelin's notion that schizophrenia is a neurodegenerative disease basically went unquestioned. What we now call schizophrenia, Kraepelin called *dementia praecox*, literally precocious dementia. He believed that the illness followed a progressive downhill course and culminated in dementia. It later became clear that not all schizophrenia patients follow this deteriorating course, but the neurodegenerative concept of the illness continued for years to hold sway.

In the 1980s, it was first suggested that schizophrenia might in fact be a neurodevelopmental disease. The theory suggested that, like Huntington's disease, a severe and disabling movement disorder, the seeds of the disease are planted before birth but lie dormant for years. The disease later emerges during preprogrammed periods of pruning the communication points (synapses) between nerve cells. In recent years, the neurodevelopmental hypothesis of schizophrenia has gained considerable favor. One consequence of this shift in thinking is that it has opened the door to look again at the long-term course of schizophrenia.

It now appears that the course of schizophrenia generally follows three distinct stages: deteriorating, stable, and improving. The deteriorating form of the illness follows Kraepelin's model with a progressive decline in function, and it is these patients who often require frequent or constant hospitalization. The impairment remains severe in the stable form but does not further worsen. Finally, a significant number of patients with schizophrenia experience distinct improvement. At this improving stage, they are unlikely to be hospitalized and have better social function.

In DSM-IV parlance, schizophrenia patients at this stage would most likely be diagnosed with residual type schizophrenia.

4.4 INITIAL EVALUATION AND DIFFERENTIAL DIAGNOSIS

There are many illnesses that in one respect or another closely resemble schizophrenia. Therefore, it takes considerable skill to diagnosis this disorder reliably. It is so difficult to diagnose accurately at a single time point that a patient with psychotic symptoms may over time have his/her diagnosis changed to and from schizophrenia repeatedly.

The evaluation of a psychotic patient should include a careful history, a thorough mental status examination, a complete physical examination, and a laboratory evaluation. When collecting the history, it is easy to become fascinated with the acute positive symptoms. There is, however, a risk in forgetting to ask about prodromal symptoms such as social withdrawal and apathy. It is of paramount importance to collect a longitudinal history, not only from the patient but from a close friend or family member as well. Friends or family can usually give you a clearer picture of how the patient is performing at work or school and whether the patient had recently become reclusive and withdrawn from usual social activities with friends. It is also particularly important to collect a family history of psychiatric illness. Remember, schizophrenia has a largely genetic influence for risk, so there is often some indication that it runs in the patient's family. The importance of obtaining a longitudinal history versus a simple cross-sectional history is critical. Patients in acute manic episodes can present in a manner that is virtually indistinguishable from those with schizophrenia when only the acute cross-sectional presentation and mental status examination are considered. The approach to treatment and prognosis are, of course, quite different between the two, reinforcing the importance of an accurate diagnosis.

The mental status examination remains an essential part of the evaluation. Often patients with schizophrenia will appear unkempt or otherwise oddly dressed. Sometimes they will be friendly and affable, but when they are paranoid, they can be angry and hostile. Patients may have odd stereotypical movements that can become extreme in catatonic states. The patient with schizophrenia is usually quite alert and well oriented to his/her surroundings. This observation helps to distinguish the psychosis of schizophrenia from that of a delirium due to a medical illness or substance use.

The term "thought disorder" is often used to describe schizophrenia. This is because the flow of thought often becomes disrupted in some way. This can take a variety of forms from poverty of thought and thought blocking to tangentiality and loose associations. The worst-case scenario is "word salad" in which speech becomes totally incomprehensible. Let us offer one tip here. If you find yourself repeatedly becoming lost or confused when interviewing a patient, it's probably not you. It's likely due to some defect in the patient's thought processes.

Finally, hallucinations (usually auditory) and delusions are a common feature of schizophrenia. But please remember, not everyone who hears voices has schizophrenia.

A physical examination is another critical part of the initial assessment. This is not so much because particular physical findings will clue one in to the presence of schizophrenia. Although there are certain neurological "soft signs" reported to be associated with schizophrenia, physical findings instead can lead away from the diagnosis. In particular, abnormal vital signs may indicate that a medical illness or drug ingestion is causing the mental disturbance. A thorough neurological examination is probably the most important part of the physical exam as it can detect telltale signs of undiagnosed brain disease (i.e., infection or tumor).

Finally, a laboratory evaluation completes the initial evaluation. This includes a battery of blood tests to rule out infection, metabolic abnormality, or hormonal disturbance. It must also include a drug screen. Unfortunately, most drug screens do not detect the "designer drugs" like Ecstasy that are an ever-increasing cause of acute psychosis. The initial evaluation should always include a CT or MRI brain scan, preferably the latter.

We also recommend that all female patients receive a pregnancy test. This is not because pregnancy in any way increases the risk for psychotic illness though the postpartum period does. However, knowing whether the patient is pregnant can guide subsequent medication choices. If there is any evidence to suggest a neurological illness, a delirium, or a seizure disorder, then an electroencephalogram (EEG) or a lumbar puncture (LP) should be performed.

Having performed this thorough evaluation, the clinician should be in a good position to differentiate schizophrenia from other disorders described below. But sometimes, time is the only way to be relatively certain about the diagnosis, with a reasonable degree of certainty. By time, we mean following the patient longitudinally for several months or years to "allow the disease to declare itself diagnostically." However, we also mean going backward in time by reviewing old records if the patient has had similar episodes in the past. Now let's closely examine the differential diagnoses for schizophrenia.

Schizophreniform Disorder. This diagnosis differs from schizophrenia only in that the total duration of symptoms is less than 6 months. Many patients originally diagnosed with schizophreniform disorder will ultimately go on to fulfill full diagnostic criteria for schizophrenia. Those who develop marked positive symptoms of psychosis within the first month of illness, who are particularly confused during the acute episode, who had normal social functioning up until the onset of illness, or who do not exhibit the flattened affect so prominent in schizophrenia are said in DSM-IV to have "good prognostic features." In other words, they are less likely to be rediagnosed later with schizophrenia.

During its earliest stages, schizophrenia is notoriously difficult to diagnose reliably. Once diagnosed (even incorrectly), it is a label that tends to stick. Because the diagnosis of schizophrenia is associated with such significant social, medical, and legal baggage, schizophreniform disorder also exists as a diagnostic entity to avoid prematurely diagnosing schizophrenia.

Brief Psychotic Disorder. This diagnosis also differs from schizophrenia by virtue of the duration of symptoms. The symptoms must last less than 1 month, and the patient must return to his/her previous level of social functioning when the illness subsides. Formerly called brief reactive psychosis, an episode of this illness usually arises in reaction to some markedly stressful event, though this is not always the case.

Delusional Disorder. Patients with delusional disorder share the presence of delusions with schizophrenia patients. However, the delusions are not bizarre as they often are in schizophrenia. Patients with delusional disorder often function fairly well in society. They can usually hold employment and typically remain active members of their families. Delusional disorder patients do not have the negative symptoms of schizophrenia, do not experience hallucinations, and do not suffer from the gross social impairment of schizophrenia. They may, however, have circumscribed social problems that are directly related to the content of their delusions. The delusions often are believable or at least somewhat plausible.

Substance-Induced Psychotic Disorder. Nearly every psychiatrist has had the experience of admitting to a psychiatric hospital a paranoid, disorganized young adult whom they were convinced was in the throes of a "first break" of schizophrenia only to see that patient dramatically "clear" within 24–48 hours. This has become all the more familiar with the rising popularity of PCP and "designer drugs" (Table 4.3).

In addition to the acute ingestion of these hallucinogenic drugs, the chronic use of alcohol, amphetamines, or cocaine can lead to paranoia that in many respects resembles the psychosis of schizophrenia. In these cases, the psychotic symptoms may persist long after the substance use has been stopped.

It is important to collect a careful history of drug use both from the patient and from close friends or family. In addition, urine drug screens should always be performed whenever a patient presents with new-onset psychosis.

TABLE 4.3. Substances that Can Produce Psychotic Symptoms[a]

Alcohol	Amphetamines	Bromocriptine
Bupropion	Cannabis	Cocaine
L-DOPA	LSD	Methamphetamine (speed)
Peyote	Phencyclidine (PCP)	Steroids
Stimulants (methylphenidate, dextroamphetamine)		

[a] This is a partial listing of substances that may mimic symptoms of schizophrenia. Psychosis may occur during intoxication, withdrawal, and occasionally as prolonged sequelae long after substance use has ceased. Rarely will substance ingestion produce all five criteria for schizophrenia as outlined in Table 4.1.

TABLE 4.4. Medical Illnesses that Can Produce Psychotic Illness[a]

Brain infection
Brain tumor
Cushing's disease
Hyperthyroidism
Syphilis
Vitamin B_{12} deficiency
Seizures

[a] In addition to this partial listing, a wide assortment of medical illnesses can produce a state of delirium, which though distinct from psychotic illnesses often does manifest certain psychotic symptoms like hallucinations and paranoia.

Psychotic Disorder Due to General Medical Condition. Certain medical illnesses occasionally present with symptoms of paranoid delusions or hallucinations that resemble schizophrenia (Table 4.4). When these illnesses are successfully treated, full resolution of the psychotic symptoms invariably occurs. All patients presenting with new-onset psychosis should undergo a thorough medical evaluation including a physical exam, family and personal medical history, and laboratory studies including electrolytes, thyroid function tests, syphilis screen, vitamin B_{12} and folate levels, and a CT or MRI brain scan. A lumbar puncture (spinal tap) and electroencephalogram are sometimes also warranted.

Delirium. Closely related to the previous disorders is delirium, which includes both psychosis and a fluctuating level of consciousness. The fluctuating sensorium is the key to distinguishing delirium from other causes of psychosis. Medical illnesses or drugs cause delirium; it is a medical emergency that requires prompt medical treatment.

Mood Disorder with Psychotic Features. One subtype of major depression and many episodes of mania are associated with psychotic symptoms. Like schizophrenia, the most prominent psychotic symptoms of psychotic depression or mania are delusions and auditory hallucinations. Unless a longitudinal history is available, it is often difficult to distinguish schizophrenia from a psychotic mood disorder.

Some qualitative features might suggest a diagnosis of schizophrenia, as opposed to a psychotic depression or a psychotic mania, but these are not wholly reliable. For example, bizarre, mood incongruent delusions are particularly suggestive of schizophrenia but can occasionally be seen in manic states as well. Negative symptoms are also suggestive of schizophrenia, but the vegetative symptoms of depression very much resemble the negative symptoms of schizophrenia.

The key to distinguishing schizophrenia from a psychotic mood disorder is to obtain a history of the patient prior to the acute episode of psychosis. This includes both the past history from medical and psychiatric records and collateral history provided by friends and family. In the case of schizophrenia, the history is usually one of a gradual decline in functioning marked by withdrawal from friends, work, and school, worsening performance at school, and increasingly odd, eccentric behavior. Ultimately, it may require following the patient into the future after the acute flareup of illness has subsided to clarify the underlying diagnosis.

Obsessive-Compulsive Disorder (OCD). In theory, distinguishing the obsessions and compulsive rituals of OCD from the delusions and behavioral peculiarities of schizophrenia should be straightforward. Usually, the OCD patient is aware of the excessive nature of his/her obsessions and wishes to be rid of them. The delusional patient with schizophrenia is unaware that these false beliefs are not based in reality and clings to them tenaciously. However, a few OCD patients lose the insight that their obsessions are excessive. At this point, the distinction between obsession and delusion often becomes blurred.

There are some clues that should steer one toward a diagnosis of schizophrenia. First, hallucinations are a common symptom of schizophrenia; they are not associated with OCD, though very strong obsessions are sometimes described as being like voices in the person's head. Second, even severe cases of OCD do not exhibit the disorganized thinking (e.g., loose associations) of schizophrenia. Finally, the odd rituals of the OCD are purposeful; they are intended to alleviate the anxiety created by the obsession. The odd posturing of schizophrenia is generally purposeless.

Autism (Pervasive Development Disorder). The association between schizophrenia and autism is of particular historic significance. Bleuler, who coined the term schizophrenia, included autism as one of his "four As" among the symptoms of schizophrenia, the others being affect, ambivalence, and association. By autism, Bleuler meant the indifference to and separation from normal social interaction that is characteristic of schizophrenia.

The relationship between autism and schizophrenia is still recognized in the latest edition of the DSM. In DSM-IV, the diagnosis of schizophrenia can only be made in someone previously diagnosed with autism when hallucinations or delusions are a prominent feature of the illness.

Cluster A Personality Disorders (Schizotypal PD, Schizoid PD, Paranoid PD). These are the "odd and eccentric" personality disorders. They all share certain features in common with schizophrenia, but schizotypal PD in particular appears to be most closely related to schizophrenia. The schizophrenia-like symptoms of these personality disorders (e.g., magical thinking, paranoia, social withdrawal) are less severe and generally don't impair social or employment function as severely as schizophrenia.

Schizoaffective Disorder. Some psychiatrists consider this a wastebasket diagnosis when one cannot make a decision between schizophrenia and bipolar disorder. We believe this is an unfair criticism. In fact, this diagnosis gives recognition to the fact that there is indeed a continuum between mood disturbance and psychosis and that some patients fluctuate from one end of the spectrum to the other.

The schizoaffective diagnosis is warranted when the patient at times fulfills criteria for schizophrenia while no mood disturbance is evident but at other times also fulfills criteria for a major depressive episode or a manic episode.

4.5 HISTORY OF TREATMENT

Antiquity. The treatment of what we now call schizophrenia probably dates back to prehistoric times. In early cultures, "madness" was usually believed to result from some malevolent external force that invaded the person and took possession of the individual. Treatment efforts would then be directed at enticing or driving out these evil spirits. This would explain the rise of shamanistic exorcisms that existed in a variety of cultures and remain prevalent today. In addition, it may be that trepanation (removing a piece of the skull) practiced by Stone Age peoples may have been the first psychosurgery used to allow the evil sprits an avenue of escape.

Opiates. The first modern attempts to treat schizophrenia with medication included the use of narcotic analgesics such as tincture of opium and paregoric in the late 1800s and early 1900s. These drugs had a calming effect and made management of agitated patients easier in crowded institutions. However, they did not truly relieve the psychosis and certainly did nothing to return these patients to any semblance of a normal life.

Shock Therapy. Insulin coma treatments were used in the early 1900s but offered no tangible improvement. Electroconvulsive therapy (ECT) arose in the 1930s and 1940s and was the first treatment to provide some relief from psychosis. However, its effects are only temporary and it proved too costly for continuous use. ECT continues to have some use for life-threatening catatonia, but it is mainly used to treat refractory depression or bipolar disorder.

Psychosurgery. Frontal lobotomy, and later leukotomy, became popular in state institutions in the 1930s. Like opiates, it calmed agitated, violent patients. It did not relieve psychosis and thankfully was abandoned in the late 1940s.

Reserpine. The first steps toward a true antipsychotic medication began to unfold in the early 1950s. The herb *Rauwolfia serpentina* had for centuries been used to treat "insanity" and a variety of medical illnesses, especially hypertension, and in the 1950s its active ingredient reserpine was isolated. Reserpine was found to improve psychotic symptoms in many patients, but only a few improved enough to leave the hospital. In addition, it produced many troublesome side effects including low blood pressure, nasal congestion, drowsiness, increased salivation, and what we now call extrapyramidal effects. Fortunately, a better alternative, chlorpromazine (see below) was being developed at about the same time. For this reason, reserpine was never widely used to treat schizophrenia. Reserpine was presumed to act by depleting dopamine in the brain and was one of the major pieces of evidence of the "dopamine hypothesis" of schizophrenia.

Chlorpromazine (Thorazine). The first of the modern antipsychotics was developed in the early 1950s, not as an antipsychotic but as an antihistamine that could be used during surgery to minimize the amount of anesthesia needed. It was hoped that this would lessen the danger of shock (dangerously low blood pressure) during surgery. It was actually quite successful, but it was soon found to have other benefits. Of key importance, it could relieve the positive symptoms of schizophrenia. In the years to follow, this led to the production of other similar antipsychotics collectively known as the typical antipsychotics.

Dopamine Pathways. Before we describe the "typical" antipsychotics in any detail, we should digress briefly to talk about the role of dopamine in the brain and how these medications affect it. First, there are four key pathways of dopamine activity in the brain, and each pathway has a particular significance:

- Mesolimbic
- Mesocortical
- Tuberoinfundibular (hypothalamic)
- Nigrostriatal

In admittedly oversimplified terms, it is believed that hyperactivity of dopamine neurons in the mesolimbic pathway contribute to the positive symptoms of schizophrenia. All the typical antipsychotics are believed to work by reducing the activity of the mesolimbic dopamine pathway. More specifically, they do this by blocking dopamine receptors on the nerve cells. Over a period of 1–3 weeks, the dopamine-blocking effect of the typical antipsychotic begins to relieve the positive symptoms of schizophrenia.

In contrast, it is often hypothesized that the negative symptoms of schizophrenia are a result of decreased activity of the mesocortical dopamine pathway. Unfortunately, dopamine blocking by typical antipsychotics in the mesocortical pathway does not improve the negative symptoms, and may even worsen them.

The tuberoinfundibular dopamine pathway modulates secretion of the hormone prolactin. Dopamine released from this circuit naturally acts to decrease prolactin secretion; therefore, the dopamine-blocking effects of the typical antipsychotics increase prolactin secretion. This can be a source of problematic side effects. Marked elevations of prolactin in women can cause amenorrhea (i.e., cessation of menstrual cycling) or galactorrhea (i.e., spontaneous milk secretion from the breasts). In men, high prolactin can produce gynecomastia (i.e., increase in breast size). These severe effects of elevated prolactin are now largely avoided because we no longer use the very high doses of antipsychotics that were used 10–20 years ago. However, elevated prolactin secretion remains a problem with some antipsychotic drugs. Even moderate increases in prolactin levels can interfere with sexual function in both men and women. It appears that even with today's more moderate dosing of the typical antipsychotics, patients sometimes struggle with sexual dysfunction and this may be a key reason for patient nonadherence.

The nigrostriatal pathway participates in the production of smooth physical motion. It is not the brain area that works to initiate movement, which is in the cerebral cortex (pyramidal tract); it is the region that helps one to have fluid motion (extrapyramidal tract). Although many neurotransmitters are found in this latter system, two neurotransmitters—dopamine and acetylcholine—are predominantly involved in this pathway. The brain normally maintains a relatively stable ratio of dopamine and acetylcholine in the pathway. However, when something happens to upset this ratio, problems arise.

Let us use Parkinson's disease (PD) and Huntington's disease (HD) as examples to explain how this system functions. In PD patients, the dopamine/acetylcholine ratio in the nigrostriatal pathway decreases due to the death of dopamine-containing nerve cells. This results in the common physical symptoms of PD: expressionless face, stiffness, stooped posture, shuffling gait, and a resting tremor. In contrast, HD produces excessive dopamine activity in the nigrostriatal pathway, increasing the dopamine/acetylcholine ratio. This results in some of the physical symptoms of HD, namely, involuntary movements known as dyskinesias. This commonly takes the form of lip-smacking, grimacing, or peculiar movements of the hands, legs, or trunk.

As you might anticipate, dopamine receptor-blocking antipsychotics lower the functional dopamine/acetylcholine ratio in the nigrostriatal pathway. As a result, the antipsychotics have the same effect in this pathway as idiopathic PD. This is how antipsychotics produce their so-called extrapyramidal side effects (EPS). EPS can take the form of parkinsonism (e.g., rigidity, tremor) or acute dystonic reactions.

Strategies to treat EPS focus primarily on attempting to reinstate the balance of dopamine/acetylcholine activity in the nigrostriatal pathway. Giving a dopamine receptor agonist or a dopamine precursor can increase dopamine activity, but this carries the risk of exacerbating the patient's psychotic symptoms. Decreasing the dose of the antipsychotic will also decrease the magnitude of dopamine receptor blockade and thus indirectly increase dopaminergic activity, but again, at the risk of increasing psychotic symptoms. However, many patients were often treated with higher than necessary doses of antipsychotics so that a dose reduction was helpful. With the "typical" antipsychotics this was often a successful maneuver to treat akathisia (a restless inability to sit still), which was sometimes mistaken as a worsening of psychosis. The other side of the ratio, cholinergic activity, is also amenable to intervention. If the goal is to reinstate the ratio of dopaminergic to cholinergic activity, and blocking DA receptors decreases net dopaminergic activity, then another strategy is to reduce cholinergic activity. Thus, anticholinergic drugs such as diphenhydramine (Benadryl), benztropine (Cogentin), or trihexyphenidyl (Artane) can usefully serve this purpose. Another strategy with older style antipsychotics was to switch to a less potent agent. High potency antipsychotics such as haloperidol

(Haldol) or fluphenazine (Prolixin) are potent dopamine receptor antagonists with little inherent anticholinergic effect. In contrast, the lower potency antipsychotics such as chlorpromazine (Thorazine) are less potent dopamine receptor antagonists but possess inherently more anticholinergic activity. The lower potency agents are less likely to produce EPS than the higher potency agents but can be associated with anticholinergic side effects such as dry mouth, blurred vision (from pupil dilatation), rapid heart rate, urinary hesitancy, and constipation. Another not uncommon side effect of treatment with the typical antipsychotics, akathisia is often listed among the extrapyramidal side effects. The problem is that akathisia does not respond to anticholinergic medications. However, it does improve when a norepinephrine receptor blocker, propranolol (Inderal), is added. We do not fully understand this, but there may be another as yet unidentified pathway in which the ratio of dopamine/norepinephrine activity is involved.

The occurrence of tardive dyskinesia after treatment with conventional antipsychotics for a long term raises some interesting questions. Remember, dyskinesias are a symptom of HD and other neurological disorders in which there is too much dopamine flowing through the nigrostriatal pathway. How can a dopamine-blocking medication produce symptoms similar to HD?

Tardive dyskinesia (TD) is most likely to occur when a patient takes *high* doses of a *high* potency antipsychotic for a *long* time, though there are reports of TD following relatively brief exposures. It is thought that the chronic blockade of the D_2 dopamine receptor subtype leads to a state of "supersensitivity" of the receptors. Keep in mind that much of the energy the brain consumes is directed at maintaining homeostasis, or keeping the milieu essentially as close to unchanged as possible. Therefore, when dopamine receptors are being blocked by antipsychotics, there is a compensatory upregulation or increase in the number of the receptors so that together they are more sensitive to dopamine binding. This tends to amplify the dopamine signal more than usual, and, therefore, some of the information from the dopamine pathways can still be transmitted. This occasional "leak" of dopamine to a supersensitive receptor is one theory of the etiology of TD. Stopping the antipsychotic usually worsens the TD, as least temporarily, and some patients will have symptoms of TD when their antipsychotics are rapidly decreased. This withdrawal dyskinesia fortunately is relatively short-lived in most patients. In contrast, TD tends to be a chronic condition, though with months to years perhaps as many as half of patients with TD will improve and experience relief of these debilitating symptoms. In severe cases of TD, the involuntary muscle movements can impair swallowing or even breathing. When TD has progressed to that stage, often increasing the antipsychotic dose produces the only relief, though the improvement is usually only short term.

Typical Antipsychotics. The earliest antipsychotics were all structurally similar and belonged to the phenothiazine class. However, over the years, many medications with many different structures have been found to work in essentially the same manner.

As a group, these medications have been known by several names. They have been called *major tranquilizers*. This is not altogether inaccurate; these medications do calm or "tranquilize." Physicians still use this name sometimes, especially when they're reluctant to use the word "psychotic" in a discussion with a new patient or his/her family. These medications have also been called *neuroleptic*, literally meaning "seize the nerve cell," in the original Greek. This term is derived from the potential for the medications to cause extrapyramidal side effects. Finally, and most accurately we contend, these medications are called *antipsychotics*.

The typical antipsychotics vary widely in their potency. This serves as the basis for dividing them into three groups: low, medium, and high potency. When we talk about potency, we are talking about the dose of the medications required to block the dopamine receptor. In terms of relative strength, it is helpful to think in terms of powers of 10. Medium potency antipsychotics are about ten times more potent than the low potency antipsychotics. The high potency medications are about ten times more potent than the medium potency medications. These are, of course, rough estimates, but they serve as a helpful guideline. Refer to Table 4.5 for a summary of the antipsychotics in each potency group.

These medications cannot be dosed solely based on their dopamine receptor blocking potency, because they also have effects on other receptors that must be factored into their dosing (see Table 4.6). For example, it is not unusual to begin treatment of a psychotic patient with a 5 mg dose of haloperidol. In terms of dopamine receptor blocking potency, 5 mg of haloperidol is more or less equivalent to 500 mg of chlorpromazine. If a patient were immediately treated with 500 mg of chlorpromazine, however, he/she would likely have side effect problems such as dizziness and excessive sedation. This is because the medications with the lowest dopamine receptor blocking potency are the most potent at other receptor systems responsible for these side effects. (See Table 4.7) The evolution of antipsychotics from low to medium to high potency has been driven not only by the desire to find

TABLE 4.5. Typical Antipsychotics and Their Dosing Ranges

Potency	Generic Name	Trade Name	Daily Dosage	Depot Dose
Low	Chlorpromazine	Thorazine	200–1000 mg	—
	Thioridazine	Mellaril	50–300 mg	—
	Mesoridazine	Serentil	150–600 mg	—
Medium	Loxapine	Loxitane	25–100 mg	—
	Molindone	Moban	50–225 mg	—
	Perphenazine	Trilafon	8–64 mg	—
	Thiothixene	Navane	5–30 mg	—
	Trifluoperazine	Stelazine	50–225 mg	—
High	Pimozide	Orap	2–6 mg	—
	Fluphenazine	Prolixin	2–20 mg	6.25–50 mg/2 wks
	Haloperidol	Haldol	2–20 mg	50–200 mg/month

TABLE 4.6. Antipsychotic Receptor Actions and Effects[a]

Receptor Action	Effects
Dopamine blocking (mesolimbic)	Decreased positive symptoms
Dopamine blocking (mesocortical)	Worsened negative symptoms
Dopamine blocking (tuberoinfundibular)	Amenorrhea (menstrual cycling stops)
	Galactorrhea (milk formation in breasts)
	Gynecomastia (breast formation in men)
	Sexual dysfunction
Dopamine blocking (nigrostriatal)	Parkinsonism
	Acute dystonic reactions
	Tardive dyskinesia
	Akathisia(?)
Histamine blocking	Drowsiness
	Weight gain
Acetylcholine blocking	Dry mouth
	Blurred vision
	Constipation
	Confusion/poor memory
	Reduced parkinsonism/dystonic reactions
Norepinephrine α-1 blocking	Dizziness
	Increased risk of falls

[a] Not every person will experience side effects equally.

TABLE 4.7. Atypical Antipsychotics and Their Dosing Ranges

Generic Name	Trade Name	Daily Dosage	Depot Dose
Aripiprazole	Abilify	5–30 mg	—
Clozapine	Clozaril	100–900 mg	—
Olanzapine	Zyprexa, Zydis	5–30 mg	—
Quetiapine	Seroquel	150–750 mg	—
Risperidone	Risperdal	2–6 mg	25–50 mg/2 weeks
Ziprasidone	Geodon	80–160 mg	—

more effective antipsychotics but also by the desire to eliminate these troublesome antihistamine, anticholinergic, and anti-α-1 adrenergic side effects. This has in fact been quite successful. The high potency antipsychotics have few of these latter side effects. The cost of this, of course, is that they are more prone to side effects (e.g., EPS and endocrine) caused by dopamine receptor blocking in the nigrostriatal and tuberoinfundibular pathways.

The net result is that low potency antipsychotics cause more histamine-blocking, acetylcholine-blocking, and α-1 adrenergic blocking side effects. The high potency antipsychotics are more likely to produce dopamine-blocking side effects. Now, let's take a brief look at each of the specific medications.

Chlorpromazine (Thorazine). The first of the modern antipsychotics, chlorpromazine has in recent years been more widely used in Europe than the United States. In addition to treating psychosis, chlorpromazine is sometimes used to treat insomnia. Due to its overall side effect burden and potential risk of TD, we prefer not to use chlorpromazine to treat insomnia unless the patient also has a psychotic disorder.

It is available in both oral and injectable forms and has a calming effect on agitated patients. Chlorpromazine should typically be started at doses no higher than 100 mg/day and increased stepwise. Otherwise, dizziness due to orthostatic hypotension is quite a problem.

Thioridazine (Mellaril). The potency and effects of thioridazine are very similar to chlorpromazine. It should also be started at a relatively low dose and increased stepwise to help patients become adjusted to its effects.

There are three additional side effects that are relatively specific to thioridazine. It occasionally causes retrograde ejaculation in men, an unpleasant experience in which semen flows in the wrong direction during orgasm. Of greater concern is the fact that at doses above 800 mg/day, thioridazine can cause a retina-damaging condition known as pigmentary retinopathy (retinitis pigmentosa) that results in blindness. For this reason, the daily dose of thioridazine should never exceed 800 mg. Finally, thioridazine has an adverse effect on the electrical conduction of the heart, specifically increasing the QT interval on electrocardiograms (EKGs). This EKG change is associated with an increased risk of serious cardiac side effects.

Mesoridazine (Serentil). This antipsychotic has effects similar to its other low potency counterparts. It should also be started at a low dose and gradually increased.

Loxapine (Loxitane). Loxapine is a medium potency antipsychotic, and it has several interesting features. First, it is chemically very similar to clozapine, the first of the atypical antipsychotics. In the test tube, loxapine actually behaves more like an atypical antipsychotic (more on that later), but when patients are treated with it, loxapine acts more like a traditional typical antipsychotic. A second point of interest is that loxapine is actually the major active metabolite of the antidepressant amoxapine (Ascendin). As a result, one can use a single medication (amoxapine) to treat both depression and psychosis. In practice, however, the use of what is essentially a fixed dose combination medication should be avoided. Using amoxapine does not allow separate adjustment of the antipsychotic and antidepressant, and most importantly, amoxapine is the only antidepressant associated with the risk of TD.

As a medium potency antipsychotic, its dose and side effects are intermediate. Sometimes, it may be better to use a medium potency antipsychotic for patients who are especially sensitive to the EPS of high potency antipsychotics. Young, well-muscled males are particularly prone to EPS and so loxapine may be a good choice for those individuals.

Molindone (Moban). Molindone is another of the medium potency antipsychotics. There are two features that set it apart. First, it is less prone to causing weight gain than other antipsychotics. As a result, it is sometimes preferred for obese schizophrenia patients. Second, although typical antipsychotics do not necessarily cause seizures, they may make them more likely to occur in people who are already prone to seizures. There is some evidence to suggest that molindone may be the least likely antipsychotic to increase the vulnerability to seizures. For this reason, molindone is frequently used to treat patients with schizophrenia who also have epilepsy.

Perphenazine (Trilafon). Perphenazine has a potency and side effect profile similar to other medium potency antipsychotics.

Thiothixene (Navane). Thiothixene is sometimes grouped with the medium potency and at other times with the high potency antipsychotics. Its potency is actually about halfway between these two groups. Thiothixene is available in both oral and injectable forms. It should be initiated at doses of about 5 mg/day and can be increased as needed.

Trifluoperazine (Stelazine). Trifluoperazine is very similar to thiothixene. It comes in both oral and injectable forms. Its dose range is the same as thiothixene.

Pimozide (Orap). Pimozide is probably the most potent of all antipsychotics, but it is seldom used to treat schizophrenia. Instead, pimozide is most often used to treat Tourette's syndrome. There is actually no reason why pimozide can't be used to treat psychosis and no reason why other antipsychotics are not effective in Tourette's syndrome. Pimozide was simply used first in controlled clinical trials to treat Tourette's syndrome, and the physicians who routinely treat that illness became accustomed to using it. Pimozide is only available in an oral form. The lack of an injectable form to treat agitated patients as well as the lack of availability of data from controlled trials in schizophrenia patients likely explains why it has not been used very often in the treatment of schizophrenia.

Fluphenazine (Prolixin). Fluphenazine is another high potency antipsychotic. It is widely used to treat psychosis and comes in oral, injectable, and long-acting injectable (depot) forms. Its side effect profile is typical of the other high potency antipsychotics.

Fluphenazine should be initiated at 5 mg/day to treat schizophrenia and increased as needed. The depot form is administered every 2 weeks in doses from 6.25 to 50 mg per dose. The depot form is generally believed to cause less EPS; however, some physicians have raised the concern that depot fluphenazine may be prone to "dose dumping." Dose dumping means that a significant portion of the depot dose might be prematurely released into the bloodstream.

Haloperidol (Haldol). There are a handful of medications that for various reasons have had a significant cultural impact; that is, they are popular among patients and physicians. Among antidepressants, it is obviously Prozac. Among benzodiazepines, it was Valium, which 25 years ago was often called "mother's little helper." Among antipsychotics, it is likely Haldol. Part of the reason may be haloperidol's versatility. It has many uses other than the treatment of schizophrenia. It is by far the most widely prescribed antipsychotic in the United States.

In addition to treating schizophrenia, haloperidol is the antipsychotic with the most proven safety record in medically ill patients. For this reason, haloperidol is the treatment of choice for delirium (in low doses). It has also been used to treat hyperemesis gravidarum (persistent vomiting during pregnancy). Haloperidol is the treatment most often used for both the abnormal movements and agitation of Huntington's disease. In addition, haloperidol has been widely used to treat agitation in dementia though it has given way to mood stabilizers and atypical antipsychotics. Together with pimozide, haloperidol is one of the two most often used treatments for Tourette's syndrome.

Like fluphenazine, haloperidol is available in oral, injectable, and depot forms. In schizophrenia, haloperidol is begun at doses of 5 mg daily and increased as needed. Lower doses are used for most other indications. The depot form of haloperidol is initiated by administration of a 50 mg test dose. Depot haloperidol is given monthly at about 20 times the daily dose of the oral form. The maximum depot dose is 200 mg per month. "Dose dumping" does not seem to be a problem with depot haloperidol.

Lithium (Eskalith, Lithobid). Before the recent proliferation of atypical antipsychotics, lithium was tried as an alternative for schizophrenia. By and large, this represented another effort to circumvent the risk of tardive dyskinesia. It is not effective either as monotherapy or as combination therapy with antipsychotics in schizophrenia.

Atypical Antipsychotics. In the 1980s and early 1990s, the SSRIs began a revolution in the treatment of depression. Tried-and-true but side effect laden tricyclic antidepressants fell into disfavor as newer and safer medications became available. A similar revolution is taking place in the treatment of psychosis. A new generation of antipsychotics that have fewer of the more disturbing side effects and may well be more effective are now available.

The seeds of this transformation were sown some years ago. The first so-called atypical antipsychotic, clozapine (Clozaril), was devised in the 1960s. Clozapine was used widely in Europe until a series of deaths from a toxic hematological (blood) side effect called agranulocytosis occurred in the mid-1970s. Clozapine resurfaced in the 1980s and was approved for use (under strict guidelines) in the United States in 1990. Since that time, several other atypical antipsychotics have been approved, and others loom on the horizon.

Before we discuss specific medications, there are two questions that demand attention. First, just what is an "atypical" antipsychotic? Second, how does an atypical antipsychotic work? Several proposed definitions of atypicality have been tossed about. They include:

- Less prone to causing EPS or tardive dyskinesia
- Better treatment for negative symptoms
- More effective than conventional antipsychotics
- Some different mechanism of action on nerve cell receptors

Most people settle on the first definition, that is, they are less prone to causing EPS, when they refer to an atypical antipsychotic. We generally agree, but this is not a perfect definition because, for example, low potency typical antipsychotics such as thioridazine are less likely than high potency typical antipsychotics to cause EPS. Of course, the reason that the low potency antipsychotics cause less EPS is because their acetylcholine-blocking effects tend to offset their dopamine-blocking effects in the nigrostriatal pathway. However, they do possess the same dopamine-blocking effects as the high potency drugs, and they still carry a significant long-term risk of tardive dyskinesia.

Therefore, we believe that this alone is not a sufficient definition for atypicality. We prefer to define atypical antipsychotics as those that are less prone to causing EPS because they work differently than the typical antipsychotics. This, of course, raises the question of just how these medications work. Using clozapine as the starting point to answer this question has proved difficult. Why? The problem is that clozapine interacts with so many different types of nerve cell receptors that it becomes hard to tell which of these actions makes the difference.

At present, there are several theories that have gained favor. First, it appears that some of the atypical antipsychotics act by blocking a different type of dopamine receptor than the typical antipsychotics. The typical medications work by blocking dopamine type 2 (D_2) receptors while some of the atypicals seem to work by blocking dopamine type 4 (D_4) receptors. Why does this matter? Well, it seems that there are fewer D_4 receptors in the nigrostriatal pathway but many in the mesolimbic pathway. Therefore, blocking the D_4 receptor preferentially reduces dopamine activity in the area where it causes the psychosis (i.e., the mesolimbic pathway) but has minimal effect where lowering dopamine would cause EPS (i.e., the nigrostriatal pathway). This dopamine receptor theory is far from proved and other dopamine receptors may play a role in atypicality.

The second theory is that some atypicals work by balancing dopamine blockade with serotonin receptor blockade. We know that one of the roles of serotonin is to attenuate (or lessen) dopamine activity. Blocking serotonin action therefore may release just enough dopamine activity in the nigrostriatal pathway to avoid EPS without interfering with the antipsychotic effects in the mesolimbic area.

There are, of course, several other theories as to how the atypical antipsychotics work. These focus on other neurotransmitters, including the neuropeptide neurotensin and the amino acid glutamate, and on a variety of other complex receptor activities. In the final analysis, we are still not sure just what makes the atypical antipsychotics work so well, but we are glad that they do.

Clozapine (Clozaril). Clozapine has been available in other parts of the world for about 30 years. The FDA has only approved it since 1990. Clozapine is clearly the most effective antipsychotic. It is as effective in reducing the positive symptoms of schizophrenia as the typical antipsychotics, like haloperidol, but also relieves many of the negative symptoms. In so doing, clozapine more than any of its predecessors opened the door for many patients with schizophrenia to be gainfully employed and to become vital contributors to society. Clozapine occupies a smaller percentage of D_2 receptors, approximately 70% as compared to the typical antipsychotics that occupy >90%.

In the treatment of schizophrenia, the daily dose of clozapine ranges from 200 mg/day to as high as 900 mg/day. Most patients respond best in the 500–700 mg/day dose range.

In addition to being effective in the treatment of schizophrenia, clozapine also is effective in the treatment of the manic phase of bipolar disorder. Although not a first-line treatment for mania, clozapine is useful for patients who are not responding well to more traditional treatments. Finally, clozapine is the one antipsychotic proven to help treatment-resistant schizophrenia. Fully one-third of patients who do not respond to other antipsychotics will respond to clozapine.

Clozapine causes virtually no extrapyramidal side effects and can actually relieve the symptoms of tardive dyskinesia. Nevertheless, it is a difficult medication to tolerate. The most talked about and concerning side effect is a potentially dangerous lowering of a certain class of infection-fighting white blood cells. This side effect, called agranulocytosis, occurs in about 1% of patients who take clozapine. Although we cannot predict in advance who might experience agranulocytosis, we do know that it occurs most often in the first 6 months of treatment.

If a patient continues taking clozapine when the white blood cell count has fallen, then the immune system can fail, ultimately leading to death. Fortunately, the condition reverses when clozapine is discontinued. Because of this potential danger, the FDA has approved clozapine under the strictest of guidelines. Any patient who takes clozapine must have a blood sample obtained weekly for the first 6 months of treatment, and thereafter, the monitoring can be decreased to every 2 weeks. If the white blood cell count drops at any time below a predetermined safety level, then the patient must stop taking clozapine immediately and be monitored carefully until the cell counts return to normal. In addition to the required weekly monitoring, patients need to be vigilant for the physical signs and symptoms of agranulocytosis, namely, signs of possible infection such as sore throat or fever. Should these occur, he/she should immediately report to the nearest emergency room for a complete blood cell (CBC) count.

Another serious side effect of clozapine is a risk of seizures. This mainly occurs at higher doses of the drug, and having a seizure is not necessarily a sufficient reason to stop clozapine permanently. If the clozapine has been especially helpful, an anticonvulsant can be added to protect against further seizures. Valproate (Depakote) may be best in this regard because it not only provides protection from seizures but also may help to relieve some of the symptoms of schizophrenia. Recently, it has become clear that two atypical antipsychotic drugs, clozapine and olanzapine, are associated with an increased risk for the development of type II diabetes.

More common than seizures or agranulocytosis are a host of other nagging side effects of clozapine. These include drowsiness, weight gain, drooling, dizziness, dry mouth, constipation, and blurred vision. In addition, patients taking clozapine can occasionally have harmless but frighteningly high fevers during the first few months of treatment. These can be treated with over-the-counter fever medications, but the patient should first have a CBC count checked just in case the fever is due to an infection resulting from agranulocytosis.

Care should be taken when prescribing other medications with clozapine. The mood stabilizer carbamazepine (Tegretol) and perhaps the antidepressant mirtazapine (Remeron) should not be taken with clozapine because they might further increase the risk of agranulocytosis. Likewise, the antidepressant bupropion (Wellbutrin, Zyban) should not be taken with clozapine because it may add to the seizure risk.

Clozapine can certainly be a difficult and expensive medication to take. However, for the treatment-resistant patient with schizophrenia, clozapine is often well worth the trouble.

Risperidone (Risperdal). Risperidone was the second atypical antipsychotic released in the United States. It is actually quite different from clozapine, and, in general, members of the class of "atypical" antipsychotics are often not all that similar among themselves. Risperidone blocks D_2 receptors as do haloperidol and fluphenazine, but it probably blocks a lower percentage of D_2 receptors, more like clozapine than haloperidol. In addition to blocking dopamine D_2 receptors, risperidone also blocks serotonin type 2 receptors.

In reality, risperidone acts as an atypical antipsychotic at doses up to 4–6 mg/day. At higher doses, risperidone begins to act more like a typical antipsychotic, and EPS can become a problem. The dose at which this occurs for individual patients is quite variable. In elderly patients, even low doses can cause EPS. Whether this risk for EPS translates into a risk for TD after long-term use remains unknown. There is now considerable evidence that risperidone is also effective in treating mania and in augmenting antidepressants in particularly low doses.

Risperidone treats schizophrenia at doses from 2 to 6 mg/day. Doses as high as 16 mg/day have been used, but as noted before, EPS becomes more frequent at these higher doses. It was initially recommended that risperidone therapy be initiated with divided daily doses because it is a relatively short-acting medication. However, with the discovery that risperidone has a longer-acting active metabolite, the current recommendation is that it be given once a day at bedtime. Risperidone has comparatively few side effects that are generally mild and disappear after chronic treatment. It can cause drowsiness, slight weight gain, dizziness, nausea, indigestion, diarrhea, and sexual dysfunction. As mentioned previously, EPS is usually not a significant problem when risperidone is taken in the recommended doses. Risperidone does not cause agranulocytosis. An exciting development is the recent introduction of a depot injection form of risperidone (*Risperdal Consta*), the first atypical antipsychotic approved in depot form by the FDA. Depot risperidone is administered every 2 weeks in 25 mg, 37.5 mg, or 50 mg doses. It should find widespread use in nonadherent patients and largely replace depot haloperidol.

Olanzapine (Zyprexa). The olanzapine molecule is structurally very similar to clozapine and therefore exerts very similar effects on brain receptors. The dose range of olanzapine for treating schizophrenia is from 5 to 30 mg/day. Like clozapine, olanzapine appears to treat both positive and negative symptoms. It is also approved for the treatment of the manic phase of bipolar disorder. It has also been shown to augment the antidepressant effects of fluoxetine in refractory patients.

The most common side effects of olanzapine are drowsiness, potentially considerable weight gain, dizziness, and constipation. Olanzapine does not cause agranulocytosis nor does it significantly increase the risk of seizure. The risk of developing EPS while taking olanzapine is also very low. A concern with olanzapine, like clozapine, is the increased risk of developing type II diabetes in patients receiving long-term treatment. There have also been reports of patients developing diabetic ketoacidosis, a potentially life-threatening illness, while on olanzapine therapy, even in the absence of weight gain.

An intramuscular injection form of olanzapine, administered at doses from 2.5 to 10 mg, is now available for the management of acute agitation in the inpatient setting. This injectable olanzapine has no role in outpatient care; however, a depot formulation of olanzapine is expected in the near future.

Quetiapine (Seroquel). Quetiapine is the fourth of the atypical antipsychotics introduced in the United States. It is effective in both positive and negative symptoms of schizophrenia within a dose range of 150 to 750 mg/day in two divided doses.

Quetiapine is also a reasonably well-tolerated medication. Common side effects are drowsiness, dizziness, and headache. It causes neither weight gain nor agranulocytosis and incurs no increase in the risk of seizures. It can produce mild changes in blood tests of liver function, but these tests usually return to normal even if the patient continues taking quetiapine.

Ziprasidone (Geodon). Ziprasidone, like risperidone, blocks serotonin type-2 and D_2 receptors. Ziprasidone is effective in treating psychosis at doses from 80 to 160 mg/day. It is effective in treating both positive and negative symptoms, and new data suggests efficacy in the treatment of mania. Interestingly, ziprasidone also has high affinity for both norepinephrine and serotonin transporter sites, which suggests that it might be an effective antidepressant at higher doses.

Ziprasidone is well tolerated. Its common side effects are drowsiness, nausea, and constipation. Though there were initial concerns about untoward cardiological side effects similar to those produced by thioridazine and the tricyclic antidepressants, ziprasidone appears to be safe though it should probably not be used in patients with preexisting heart disease.

Injectable ziprasidone, administered in intramuscular doses of 10–20 mg, is now available for managing agitation in the inpatient setting, though it has no routine use in the outpatient setting. A depot formulation of ziprasidone is expected to be approved soon.

Aripiprazole (Abilify). Aripiprazole, the newest of the so-called atypical antipsychotics to be introduced in the United States, has a unique mechanism of action. It is a "partial agonist" at dopamine receptors. This means it stimulates dopamine receptors, but it does so in a much weaker fashion than does dopamine itself. The result, at least in theory, is that the partial dopamine agonist, aripiprazole, strikes a balance by slowing down dopamine activity in brain areas where there's too much but stimulating dopamine activity in brain areas where there's too little. Because some evidence indicates that the positive symptoms of schizophrenia result from too much dopamine activity in the mesolimbic circuit and the negative symptoms result from too little dopamine activity in the mesocortical circuit, a partial dopamine agonist like aripiprazole represents an ingenious approach to addressing both the positive and negative symptoms of the illness.

Daily doses of aripiprazole range from 5 to 30 mg. Aripiprazole is very well tolerated. Common side effects include headache, insomnia, nausea, dizziness, and constipation.

4.6 CURRENT APPROACH TO TREATMENT

In the era of modern psychiatry, the treatment of schizophrenia has undergone two revolutions. The first revolution began in the 1950s with the debut of the typical antipsychotics, the first proven effective treatments for psychosis. These medications enabled patients who in years past would have been relegated to long-term hospitalization to return to the community.

The second revolution began in the past 10 years with the arrival of the atypical antipsychotics. Although the atypicals are no panacea for schizophrenia, they represent an advance in at least three areas. First, they lessen the burden of antipsychotic side effects and therefore frequently increase adherence dramatically. Second, the atypicals may treat all of the schizophrenia symptom clusters (positive, negative, mood, cognitive), whereas the typical antipsychotics chiefly treat the positive symptoms. Third, atypical antipsychotics sometimes benefit patients whose schizophrenia is unresponsive to typical antipsychotics.

When approaching the treatment of schizophrenia, it is best to view the illness in one of four distinct phases: prodromal phase, acute phase, maintenance phase, and residual phase. Let us take a look at the treatment options at each of these phases of the illness.

4.6.1 Prodromal Phase

This is the first phase of illness occurring before the start of overt psychotic symptoms. During this phase, patients so seldom come to clinical attention that we know very little about the appropriateness of various treatment options. It may be that early intervention can alter the course and lessen the ultimate severity of the illness, but this is far ahead of our current knowledge about schizophrenia.

The symptoms during this phase of illness are not particularly specific to schizophrenia. They often resemble, in many respects, depression or even one of the Cluster A personality disorders. The decision to initiate antipsychotic medication at this stage depends on the degree of certainty of the diagnosis, the severity of the symptoms, and the risk and benefits of the medication.

In cases where there is a strong family history of schizophrenia and the symptoms are particularly ominous, many clinicians will recommend antipsychotic treatment during the prodromal phase. Low doses of an atypical antipsychotic (other than clozapine) probably offer the best promise of a treatment response with a minimal risk of problematic side effects.

4.6.2 Acute Phase

The goals of treatment during the acute phase of illness are to reduce the positive symptoms of schizophrenia and to plan for extended treatment during the maintenance phase. Reducing the positive symptoms quickly is important for at least two reasons. First, the erratic behavior of an acutely psychotic patient can take a tremendous toll, risking arrest, loss of job, suicide, and the alienation of friends and family. Second, there is some evidence that psychosis itself is harmful to the brain. In other words, it may be that the longer the patient is actively psychotic, the worse the prognosis becomes.

First Break. The first acute episode of schizophrenia is commonly called the "first break." Hospitalization is almost always needed during this period. There are several reasons for this. First, the patient needs a thorough yet expeditious medical evaluation to rule out serious medical causes of psychosis. Second, antipsychotic medication can be dosed more aggressively in the hospital with the goal of rapid symptom relief. During an inpatient hospitalization, the potential side effects of a newly started antipsychotic are more easily monitored. Third, the patient may briefly need the safety and structure of an inpatient stay if his/her judgment is compromised by the illness, as it often is. Finally, hospitalization provides an opportunity for the patient to begin building a trusting therapeutic alliance with caregivers. This alliance will be crucial to continued treatment success once the patient is discharged from the hospital.

We recommend initiating treatment with one of the atypical antipsychotics (other than clozapine) for the first episode. If the patient is extremely paranoid or disorganized and prone to agitation or combativeness, injectable formulations may be required. Injectable formulations are currently available for olanzapine and ziprasidone and are under development for the other agents. When an atypical antipsychotic that is not available in an injectable form is being used in the inpatient setting, it is common practice to coadminister injectable doses of a typical antipsychotic, usually 5 mg haloperidol, to manage aggressive or agitated behavior.

It usually takes several days to a few weeks before the symptoms of psychosis noticeably improve. During that period, benzodiazepines (usually lorazepam or clonazepam) can also be used to calm the agitated patient.

An adequate trial of an antipsychotic is defined as treatment with a demonstrable therapeutic dose for at least 6 weeks. We generally recommend a full 6 week trial of an antipsychotic before switching to another antipsychotic when the response is unsatisfactory. One exception may be the rare circumstances when there is absolutely no improvement after 2–3 weeks of treatment. In this case, we believe that it often makes sense to go ahead and switch to another antipsychotic rather than wait the full 6 weeks.

One area of debate is whether an acetylcholine-blocking (anticholinergic) medication should be routinely started for EPS prophylaxis whenever a typical antipsychotic is used. Anticholinergics are no doubt overprescribed for schizophrenia patients, and they can worsen the cognitive impairment of the illness. Nevertheless, some practitioners believe that there is some justification for routinely coprescribing anticholinergics when treating a first episode patient with a typical antipsychotic. The emotional impact of severe EPS at this critical point of treatment when one is trying to gain a paranoid patient's trust can seriously undermine any commitment to treatment.

Subsequent Acute Exacerbations. When a patient with schizophrenia experiences another acute phase of illness, two questions must be answered. First, is hospitalization needed? Second, why has this happened?

The decision regarding hospitalization depends on the severity of the episode. If the illness is seriously threatening the patient's well-being, then the patient should be hospitalized.

The second question has the greater impact on treatment choice. There are four major possibilities to consider when trying to determine why the patient has relapsed. First, it may have been treatment failure due to inadequate dosing of the antipsychotic. Second, a psychosocial stressor may have triggered the exacerbation despite otherwise adequate antipsychotic treatment. Third, the patient may not be adherent with the antipsychotic. Finally, this may represent the natural course of this patient's illness.

If the patient is not adherent, one needs to investigate further to determine why (s)he is not taking the medication. It could be due to poor insight; that is, the patient may not believe the diagnosis of schizophrenia and therefore may question the need for an antipsychotic. Early in the course of illness, it is also not terribly unusual for friends or family who do not understand schizophrenia to discourage the patient from taking antipsychotic medication. The patient may refuse medication because of some delusional thoughts about it. For example, the patient might think the antipsychotic drug is a poison. Finally, the antipsychotic may have caused bothersome side effects. It is obviously very important to determine why the exacerbation has occurred before choosing a new treatment regimen.

If the patient has done well on a previous antipsychotic for an extended period of time, and is willing to continue taking it, then it usually makes the most sense to restart or continue the same medication. This keeps the patient from unnecessarily starting on a merry-go-round of constant medication changes. An increase in dose or the addition of new psychosocial therapies may, however, be required.

If the relapse is due to nonadherence that resulted from poor insight (either on the part of the patient or his/her friends and family), then an aggressive psychosocial intervention is warranted. Again, it often makes sense to continue the same medication in this scenario. If poor insight remains a problem, then serious consideration should be given to a depot form of antipsychotic.

In other cases, it makes sense to switch medications. If the previous medication was a typical antipsychotic, then we recommend switching to an atypical antipsychotic to take advantage of a different mechanism of action and a different side effect profile. If the previous medication was an atypical, then switching to another atypical is reasonable.

Only after a patient has failed two adequate antipsychotic trials should clozapine or augmentation with a second medication be considered. Refer to Section 4.7 for more information on handling treatment resistance.

4.6.3 Maintenance Phase

The goals of maintenance treatment are to prevent new exacerbations of the illness while minimizing the burden of side effects. One additional goal is to reduce the impairment in all four of the symptom clusters and thus improve the patient's social functioning. After a single acute episode of illness, maintenance treatment should continue for least 1 year. If there is no recurrence of acute illness and there are no persistent negative symptoms after 1 year, then one might consider tapering and eventually discontinuing the antipsychotic. In such cases, the original diagnosis of schizophrenia should be revisited.

However, when there is clear evidence of persistent illness or when the patient endures several acute episodes of illness, treatment should be indefinite and probably lifelong. Except in the residual phases of illness, discontinuing antipsychotic medication exposes the schizophrenia patient to a serious risk of relapse. However, there is evidence that gradually decreasing the dose of antipsychotic in 4 week intervals can still provide good protection from relapse while lowering the risk of side effects.

Some researchers have investigated the notion of intermittent treatment. Patients are intensively monitored off medication, and a medication is started once prodromal signs of an impending acute exacerbation are detected. One thought is that this minimizes the risk of side effects such as tardive dyskinesia. Although in theory this may sound attractive, unfortunately, it rarely is successful in practice. Patients receiving intermittent treatment are at exceptionally high risk for relapse.

During the maintenance phase, treatment can be fine-tuned. If persistent side effects (especially EPS) are a problem, then the antipsychotic can be gradually switched or countermeasures such as anticholinergic therapy can be taken. In addition, maintenance therapy is also an appropriate time to address the less dramatic but nonetheless troublesome symptoms such as a mood disturbance. Antidepressants are often used to treat depressed mood in patients with schizophrenia. Likewise, benzodiazepines are commonly used with an antipsychotic to treat persistent yet subsyndromal anxiety in schizophrenia patients.

For patients in whom treatment noncompliance is a recurring problem, the success of maintenance therapy can greatly be enhanced by administering a depot formulation of the antipsychotic. Depot formulations are currently available for haloperidol (which must be administered once every 4 weeks) and risperidone or fluphenazine (each of which must be administered once every 2 weeks).

4.6.4 Residual Phase

Decades after the onset of illness, some patients experience a distinct improvement and enter a residual phase of the disorder. In this phase, positive symptoms wane or disappear altogether. Negative symptoms, mood disturbance, and cognitive impairment may, however, persist.

In the residual phase, the patient is unlikely to have an acute exacerbation even if (s)he stops taking an antipsychotic. Nevertheless, (s)he may still require treatment for residual symptoms. If medications are continued during a residual phase of schizophrenia, an atypical antipsychotic is preferred. Because positive symptoms are no longer a prominent aspect of the illness, there is usually little justification for using a typical antipsychotic and thereby exposing a patient to the risk of tardive dyskinesia. Moreover, atypical antipsychotics likely better treat the remaining negative symptoms of residual schizophrenia.

4.7 TREATMENT RESISTANT SCHIZOPHRENIA

We define treatment resistance as the failure to respond fully to an adequate trial (6 weeks of recognized therapeutic doses) of at least two different antipsychotics. With the recent introduction of several atypical antipsychotics, we furthermore suggest that there should be failed treatment with at least one typical *and* one atypical antipsychotic before being considered treatment resistant.

What are the best treatments for resistant schizophrenia? If the disease has shown little or no improvement with the previous antipsychotics, then a trial of clozapine is warranted. This is a difficult and expensive medication that requires a motivated patient who is willing to report for weekly blood draws. Taken altogether, clozapine is a difficult drug. Nevertheless, it is the one antipsychotic that has clearly been shown to help schizophrenia that is resistant to other antipsychotics.

When there is a partial response to an antipsychotic but more improvement is needed, then the decision becomes more complicated. Even in this setting, clozapine is an option.

One question that we commonly hear is: "Can you give two antipsychotics together for synergistic effects?" This is a reasonable question with little to no data to guide choices. Situations such as this emphasize more the "art" of medicine and less of the "science." It is harder to justify the combination of two "typical" antipsychotics except perhaps if a depot and an oral preparation are being coadministered. What about combining two atypical antipsychotic agents? The jury is still out. Combinations can be helpful in some patients. The rapid progression to medication combinations may be a warning sign that a consultation with an experienced psychopharmacologist is advised. When we say that a patient has had a partial response, we mean that they have either prominent residual positive or negative symptoms, but nevertheless that clear improvement has occurred. Once appropriate switching from one antipsychotic to another has been tried, then augmentation may make sense. For persistent positive symptoms, we recommend adding a mood stabilizer to the antipsychotic. Lithium augmentation studies in patients treated with antipsychotics have largely been disappointing. However, valproate (Depakote) is safer (except in women of childbearing age in whom valproate should be avoided due to its significant risks during pregnancy) and easier to tolerate and, in at least one clinical trial, successfully augmented the antipsychotic drug response.

When negative symptoms are persistent despite using an atypical antipsychotic, we recommend adding an antidepressant. Although there are no clear studies to support this practice, our experience has found that this strategy can be helpful.

ADDITIONAL READING

Bergman RN, Ader M. Atypical antipsychotics and glucose homeostasis. *J Clin Psychiatry* 2005; 66: 504–514.

Correll CU, Leucht S, Kane JM. Lower risk for tardive dyskinesia associated with second-generation antipsychotics: a systematic review of 1-year studies. *Am J Psychiatry* 2004; 161: 414–425.

Geddes J, Freemantle N, Harrison P, et al. Atypical antipsychotics in the treatment of schizophrenia: systematic overview and meta-regression analysis. *BMJ* 2000; 321(7273): 1371–1376.

Kablinger AS, Freeman AM. Prodromal schizophrenia and atypical antipsychotic treatment. *J Nerv Ment Dis* 2000; 188(10): 642–652.

Kapur S. Psychosis as a state of aberrant salience: a framework linking biology, phenomenology, and pharmacology in schizophrenia. *Am J Psychiatry* 2003; 160(1): 13–23.

Kapur S, Remington G. Serotonin–dopamine interaction and its relevance to schizophrenia. *Am J Psychiatry* 1996; 153(4): 466–476.

Kelleher JP, Centorrino F, Albert MJ, et al. Advances in atypical antipsychotics for the treatment of schizophrenia: new formulations and new agents. *CNS Drugs* 2002; 16(4): 249–261.

McElroy SL, Keck PE, Strakowski SM. An overview of the treatment of schizoaffective disorder. *J Clin Psychiatry* 1999; 60(Supplement 5): 16–21.

Miyamoto S, Duncan GE, Marx CE, et al. Treatments of schizophrenia: a critical review of pharmacology and mechanisms of action of antipsychotic drugs. *Mol Psychiatry* 2005; 10: 79–104.

Rascol O, Fabre N. Dyskinesia: L-dopa-induced and tardive dyskinesia. *Clin Neuropharmacol* 2001; 24(6): 313–323.

Scatton B, Sanger DJ. Pharmacological and molecular targets in the search for novel antipsychotics. *Behav Pharmacol* 2000; 11(3–4): 243–256.

Van Harten PN, Hoek HW, Kahn RS. Acute dystonia induced by drug treatment. *BMJ* 1999; 319(7210): 623–626.

5

ANXIETY DISORDERS

5.1 INTRODUCTION

5.1.1 History of Anxiety Disorders

Freud coined the term "anxiety neurosis" approximately 100 years ago, and all forms of anxiety would be subsumed under that collective diagnostic entity for decades to come. In 1980, based on an emerging literature DSM-III classified anxiety disorders into several discrete syndromes including panic disorder, obsessive–compulsive disorder (OCD), and generalized anxiety disorder (GAD).

Subsequent delineation of specific syndromal anxiety disorders coincided with a surge of research regarding the diagnostic classification, biology, and treatment of anxiety. The heightened interest undoubtedly stems from the results of large-scale epidemiological studies revealing the surprisingly high prevalence rates of these disorders and the considerable disability of these disorders. In fact, anxiety disorders rival substance use disorders as the most common of the psychiatric syndromes in the United States.

The irony is that anxiety disorders, which were for so long consolidated into a single diagnostic entity and as recently as two decades ago were treated primarily

Principles of Psychopharmacology for Mental Health Professionals
By Jeffrey E. Kelsey, D. Jeffrey Newport, and Charles B. Nemeroff

with a single class of psychiatric medications, the benzodiazepines, now arguably represent the category of psychiatric disorders with the most diversified pharmacological treatment options. In fact, accurately diagnosing the specific anxiety syndrome that is being treated can be crucial to the ultimate success of treatment.

5.1.2 Anxiety Symptoms

Under certain circumstances, anxiety is an appropriate emotional response. We expect a person to feel sad after a significant loss such as the death of a loved one, and it is equally reasonable for a person to feel fearful and anxious when faced with a frightening situation such as a painful or risky medical procedure. Indeed, in the context of the "fight or flight" reaction readily witnessed in nature when a predator is lurking near its intended prey, the physical and mental symptoms of anxiety can indeed be adaptive. This anxiety clearly serves as an appropriate alarm that potential danger is nearby and readies the individual for a self-protective response.

However, there are situations in which anxiety is maladaptive and thereby represents a symptom of a psychiatric disorder. There are three major signs that anxiety has become pathological. First, anxiety is disabling when it lasts too long. Chronic and unremitting anxiety ultimately leads to severe untoward mental and physical consequences. Second, anxiety is a problem when it occurs at inappropriate times. For example, a person who is extremely anxious in public places such as restaurants or shopping malls may become homebound for fear of encountering any situation that potentially triggers anxiety. Finally, anxiety is maladaptive when its magnitude is disproportionate to the triggering event. For example, the city dweller who experiences panic attacks when driving in freeway traffic can be limited in vocational and social opportunities. In all of these cases, anxiety interferes with social and/or occupational functioning.

The symptoms of anxiety are both mental and physical. Mentally, anxious people often describe themselves as worried, keyed up, restless, or on edge. They experience difficulty concentrating and often describe their minds as going blank. Anxious people also describe a variety of physical symptoms that impact on nearly every organ system (see Table 5.1).

TABLE 5.1. Physical Manifestations of Anxiety

Organ System	Symptoms
Cardiovascular	Rapid pulse, bounding heartbeat, palpitations, profuse sweating, clammy hands
Gastrointestinal	Nausea, vomiting, diarrhea, dry mouth, lump in throat, "butterflies"
Musculoskeletal	Restlessness, muscle tension, pacing, muscle pain
Neurological	Dizziness, lightheadedness, fainting, headache, tremulousness, tingling in extremities
Respiratory	Shortness of breath, smothering sensation
Urinary	Frequent urination, difficulty initiating urination

5.1.3 Brief Overview of the Anxiety Disorders

Anxiety disorders are generally classified according to both the predominant symptoms manifested and the precipitating situations or objects (see Table 5.2). One class of anxiety disorders, the phobias, is characterized by the presence of irrational fear. The most common of the phobias, specific phobias, consist of the irrational fear of certain objects such as spiders (i.e., arachnophobia) or blood, certain activities such as flying in airplanes, or certain places such as tall buildings or mountaintops (i.e., acrophobia). Also common is social phobia, also known as social anxiety disorder, which is the fear of judgment or scrutiny by others. It typically occurs in situations such as public speaking, parties, or restaurants leading the sufferer to avoid such settings. Finally, agoraphobia is the fear of being in situations from which escape may be embarrassing or difficult. Agoraphobia is frequently a complicating factor in panic disorder and like social phobia leads to avoidant behavior.

Panic disorder is characterized by the occurrence of panic attacks that occur spontaneously and lead to persistent worry about subsequent attacks and/or behavioral changes intended to minimize the likelihood of further attacks. Sporadic panic attacks are not limited, however, to those with syndromal panic disorder as they do occur occasionally in normal individuals and in those with other syndromal psychiatric disorders. The hallmark of panic disorder is that the panic attacks occur without warning in an unpredictable variety of settings, whereas panic attacks associated with other disorders typically occur in response to a predictable stimulus. For example, a person with acrophobia might experience a panic attack when on a glass elevator. A patient with obsessive–compulsive disorder (OCD) with contamination fears may have a panic attack when confronted with the sight of refuse, and a combat veteran with post-traumatic stress disorder (PTSD) may experience a panic attack when a helicopter flies overhead or an automobile backfires.

The stress disorders, PTSD and acute stress disorder (ASD), occur in the aftermath of exposure to traumatic events such as combat, violent crimes, natural

TABLE 5.2. Anxiety Disorders

A. Phobias
  1. Specific Phobia
  2. Social Phobia (Social Anxiety Disorder)
  3. Agoraphobia
B. Panic Disorder
C. Obsessive–Compulsive Disorder
D. Generalized Anxiety Disorder
E. Trauma Associated Anxiety Disorders
  1. Post-traumatic Stress Disorder
  2. Acute Stress Disorder
F. Other Anxiety Disorders
  1. Anxiety Disorder Due to Medical Condition
  2. Substance-Induced Anxiety Disorder
  3. Adjustment Disorder with Anxiety
  4. Anxiety Disorder not Otherwise Specified

disasters, or terrible accidents. These disorders are comprised of a wide assortment of symptoms including fear and anxiety, panic, depression, dissociation, and impulsivity.

OCD is manifested by persistent unwanted thoughts (obsessions) that intrude on the mind and thus engender anxiety. To cope with this anxiety, the individual attempts to ignore or suppress the obsessive thoughts. Alternatively, the person might try to neutralize the thoughts through ritualistic, repetitive behaviors known as compulsions. The compulsive behaviors can become excessive and time-consuming and interfere with the day-to-day activities of life.

Finally, generalized anxiety disorder (GAD) is characterized by a chronic, unremitting yet uncontrollable worry that disturbs emotional well-being and interferes with social and occupational functioning.

5.1.4 History of Pharmacological Treatment for Anxiety

As noted earlier, prior to the advent of DSM-III in 1980, the anxiety disorders were collectively subsumed under some variation of the single diagnostic entity, anxiety neurosis. Consequently, the "history" of pharmacological treatment for the discrete anxiety syndromes is relatively brief, only approximately 20 years. Prior to 1980, we can only speak in a general manner as to how well medicines relieved "anxiety" in the broad sense of the term. Consequently, we'll present the more extensive history of pharmacological treatment for anxiety in this broader sense before launching into a more detailed discussion of the treatment of the individual anxiety disorders.

Alcohol. Along with several bromide preparations and paraldehyde, alcohol has often been used to relieve anxiety. Due to the marked untoward social and medical consequences of frequent use, alcohol has no place in the treatment of anxiety. Unfortunately, the inappropriate use of alcohol to self-medicate anxiety, depression, insomnia, or other symptoms often leads to alcoholism and therefore contributes to a significant public health problem.

Barbiturates. The first barbiturate, barbital, was introduced in 1903 and was followed a few years later by phenobarbital. The barbiturates effectively relieve anxiety, but they are never used as anxiolytics today due to toxicity and abuse concerns. However, several barbiturates, including phenobarbital (Luminal), secobarbital (Seconal), and pentobarbital (Nembutal), remain available and are occasionally used to treat epilepsy and rarely to manage acute alcohol withdrawal.

The side effects of barbiturates include sedation, poor physical coordination, and impaired mental performance. They also potentiate the intoxicating effects of alcohol. Barbiturates can be extremely dangerous in overdose, causing anesthesia, coma, and even death. In addition, barbiturates can cause dangerous suppression of breathing in patients with sleep apnea or other respiratory disorders. With repeated use over just a few weeks, physical dependence and tolerance to their effects can develop, leading to increasing doses to maintain the desired therapeutic effect. If a patient abruptly stops taking a barbiturate, withdrawal symptoms, ranging from mild anxiety to severe seizures and death, can occur.

Nonbarbiturates. After the introduction of the barbiturates, there was little progress in the medical treatment of anxiety until meprobamate (Equanil, Miltown) was introduced in 1950. Soon after its introduction, a series of similar medicines entered the market, including carisoprodol (Soma), glutethimide (Doriden), methaqualone (Qaalude, Sopor), methyprylon (Noludar), and ethchlorvynol (Placidyl). These medications have all been used to treat anxiety, insomnia, and muscle spasms.

Although they were initially thought to represent a major breakthrough in the treatment of anxiety, it was soon learned that these medicines, like their predecessors, the barbiturates, were highly addictive and dangerous in overdose. Methaqualone and methyprylon have consequently been removed from the market, and meprobamate and glutethimide are seldom prescribed today. Although these medications have largely disappeared from use, carisoprodol, which is metabolized to meprobamate, continues to be prescribed as a muscle relaxer, though it is not used in the treatment of anxiety.

Benzodiazepines. A major advance in the treatment of anxiety was the introduction of the next class of anxiolytics, the benzodiazepines, introduced in the late 1950s and early 1960s. The first benzodiazepine, chlordiazepoxide (Librium), was followed a few years later by diazepam (Valium). Benzodiazepines act at the GABA receptor complex in much the same manner as the barbiturates. As modulators of the GABA receptor, benzodiazepines do not directly stimulate the receptor. Instead, they bind a site adjacent to the GABA receptor, producing three-dimensional changes in the conformation of the receptor that in turn increases its affinity for GABA. As a result, GABA neurotransmission is enhanced.

Despite their pharmacological similarities to barbiturates, benzodiazepines are considerably safer in intentional or accidental overdose. This enhanced safety profile undoubtedly contributed to the widespread use of the benzodiazepines in the decade following their introduction. In fact, the ubiquitous prescribing of benzodiazepines in the 1960s led the Rolling Stones to immortalize the little yellow pill, presumably diazepam (Valium), in their song, "Mother's Little Helper." The subsequent recognition that benzodiazepines, while safer than their predecessors, possessed dependence and addiction liability led to more restrained prescribing practices in subsequent decades.

Benzodiazepines have a wide array of clinical uses. In addition to relieving anxiety, they can be used to treat epilepsy, alcohol withdrawal, insomnia, agitation, and perhaps impulsivity. They can also be used as muscle relaxants or to produce "conscious sedation" during certain medical procedures such as cardiac catheterization and colonoscopy.

Benzodiazepines are virtually identical from a pharmacodynamic standpoint (refer to Chapter 2 for a comprehensive discussion of pharmacodynamics and pharmacokinetics). Specifically, they all act by activating the GABA-A receptor complex. Despite their similarity, the benzodiazepines are not wholly interchangeable as a result of their pharmacokinetic differences. The speed with which they begin to act, the duration of their action, and the ease with which they can be metabolized and eliminated vary considerably from medicine to medicine. As a result, each benzodiazepine has evolved a particular set of one or more preferred uses in routine clinical practice. Refer to Table 5.3 for a summary of the characteristics of the currently available benzodiazepines.

It does bear special mention that many mental health practitioners consider lorazepam (Ativan) to be the most versatile of the benzodiazepines. Lorazepam has an intermediate onset and duration of action. Because it is easily metabolized, lorazepam is preferred when a benzodiazepine must be used to treat medically compromised or elderly patients. Most importantly, lorazepam is the only benzodiazepine that can be administered via oral, intramuscular, and intravenous routes. As a result, the transition between inpatient and outpatient care is rendered much easier with lorazepam than other benzodiazepines.

Side effects of benzodiazepines include sedation, dizziness, poor coordination, and, at higher doses, amnesia. Benzodiazepines also increase the effects of alcohol; therefore, alcohol use should be avoided or markedly curtailed. Benzodiazepines can also exacerbate the breathing problems of patients with sleep apnea and other respiratory disorders such as emphysema. Like the barbiturates, long-term use of benzodiazepines can lead to physical dependence, and abrupt discontinuation can produce an unpleasant, or even dangerous, withdrawal syndrome.

Monoamine Oxidase Inhibitors (MAOIs). Developed in the 1950s, the MAOIs were the first class of antidepressants. Subsequently, in the 1960s, the MAOIs were also found to be effective anxiolytics. Unlike benzodiazepines and barbiturates, the MAOIs are not addictive; however, their onset of action is delayed not by minutes or hours but by 3 weeks or more.

There are currently three approved MAOIs in the United States: phenelzine (Nardil), tranylcypromine (Parnate), and isocarboxizide (Marplan). These medications are all nonselective, irreversible inhibitors of the MAO enzymes. Being irreversible, the MAOIs permanently deactivate the MAO enzyme molecule when they bind it, and being nonselective, they block the actions of both the MAO-A and MAO-B enzyme subtypes. By deactivating the MAO-A enzyme, MAOIs increase the activity of both norepinephrine and serotonin. Blocking the MAO-B enzyme adds little to their effectiveness but causes many problematic side effects.

Besides the delayed onset, MAOIs are plagued by numerous side effects including dizziness from orthostatic hypotension, drowsiness, insomnia, palpitations, rapid pulse, sexual dysfunction, and weight gain. Of greater concern are the potentially dangerous interactions of the MAOIs with certain foods and medications that can lead to dangerously high blood pressure that can in turn cause severe headaches, strokes, or heart attacks. Despite their effectiveness, MAOIs are seldom used because of these food and drug interactions. For these reasons, newer more selective and/or reversible MAOIs remain an active avenue of investigation. For additional information regarding the MAOIs, refer to Chapter 3.

TABLE 5.3. Benzodiazepines

Generic	Trade	Route(s)	Duration of Action	Daily Dose (mg/day)	Common Use(s)
Alprazolam	Xanax Xanax XR	Oral	Short	0.75–10	Anxiety disorders
Chlordiazepoxide	Librium	Oral	Long	15–100	Anxiety disorders, alcohol withdrawal
Clonazepam	Klonopin	Oral	Long	0.5–4	Anxiety disorders, epilepsy, mania
Clorazepate	Tranxene	Oral	Long	15–60	Anxiety disorders, alcohol withdrawal
Diazepam	Valium	Oral, IV	Long	4–40	Anxiety disorders, alcohol withdrawal
Estazolam	ProSom	Oral		1–2	Insomnia
Flurazepam	Dalmane	Oral	Long	15–30	Insomnia
Halazepam	Paxipam	Oral	Long	60–160	Anxiety disorders, alcohol withdrawal
Lorazepam	Ativan	Oral, IV, IM	Intermediate	1–10	Anxiety disorders, alcohol withdrawal, insomnia
Midazolam	Versed	IV	Short	N/A	Conscious sedation
Oxazepam	Serax	Oral	Intermediate	30–120	Anxiety disorders, alcohol withdrawal
Prazepam	Centrax	Oral	Long	20–60	Anxiety disorders
Quazepam	Doral	Oral	Intermediate	7.5–15	Insomnia
Temazepam	Restoril	Oral	Intermediate	15–30	Insomnia
Triazolam	Halcion	Oral	Short	0.125–0.5	Insomnia

Tricyclic Antidepressants (TCAs). The TCAs were also introduced in the 1950s, and some were discovered to be effective anxiolytics in the 1960s. For example, early studies pioneered by Donald Klein and his colleagues indicated that imipramine (Tofranil) effectively relieved panic attacks. Like the MAOIs, the TCAs are not addictive but also require over 3 weeks to begin to achieve significant therapeutic benefit for anxiety.

TCAs primarily act by blocking the reuptake of norepinephrine and/or serotonin. TCAs are unfortunately plagued by numerous side effects including sedation, weight gain, constipation, dry mouth, urinary hesitancy, and blurred vision. Furthermore, safety is of great concern with TCAs. Toxic TCA levels can produce lethal cardiac arrhythmias, seizures, and suppression of breathing. An overdose of as little as a 1–2 week supply of most TCAs is often fatal. Furthermore, drug interactions, through the cytochrome P_{450} 2D6 enzyme, can unexpectedly produce toxic TCA levels. Please refer to Chapter 3 for more information regarding TCAs.

Other Antidepressants. Antidepressant refinements for the next 30 years primarily consisted of the development of new TCAs. However, in 1988, a novel antidepressant class, the selective serotonin reuptake inhibitors (SSRIs), was introduced in the United States. The chief innovation of the SSRIs was that they afforded the comparable effectiveness of the TCAs with fewer side effects and minimal toxicity. The debut of the SSRIs coincided with the reworking of the nosology of the anxiety disorders in DSM-III and DSM-IV. As a result, the SSRIs have been studied extensively in each of the respective anxiety disorders and in many cases have obtained FDA approval for the treatment of one or more of these anxiety syndromes. The SSRIs currently available in the United States include citalopram (Celexa), escitalopram (Lexapro), fluoxetine (Prozac), fluvoxamine (Luvox), paroxetine (Paxil), and sertraline (Zoloft).

Being serotonin selective does not mean that the SSRIs are totally devoid of side effects. Common side effects of SSRIs include nausea, diarrhea, headache, diminished libido, and delayed orgasm. When starting treatment, the SSRIs can also produce a transient increase in nervousness that is especially difficult for anxious patients to tolerate. SSRI-induced anxiety can be minimized by starting the medication at about one-half the dose normally used when treating depression and then gradually adjusting the dose higher. At the opposite end of the treatment spectrum, abruptly stopping a SSRI (or SNRI), particularly those with a short half-life such as paroxetine or venlafaxine, can produce an unpleasant discontinuation syndrome. This syndrome is not life threatening or otherwise dangerous but can produce symptoms of malaise, nausea, abdominal pain, irritability, anxiety, and shock-like sensations in the arms and/or legs. The symptoms of SSRI/SNRI discontinuation syndrome can be minimized by gradually tapering the dose over weeks to months when a decision has been made to discontinue treatment.

In the past decade, other antidepressants have been introduced. Many of these act, at least in part, via serotonin-mediated mechanisms and, as such, have been tested in the treatment of one or more anxiety disorders. These additional antidepressants include two dual serotonin–norepinephrine reuptake inhibitors (SNRIs), duloxetine (Cymbalta) and venlafaxine (Effexor, Effexor XR), mirtazapine (Remeron), and nefazodone (Serzone). Please refer to Chapter 3 for additional information regarding the SSRIs, SNRIs, and other antidepressants.

Azapirones. Though several azapirones have been developed and tested in the laboratory setting, only one, buspirone (Buspar), is currently on the market. Buspirone is the first nonsedating, nonbenzodiazepine anxiolytic, other than the antidepressants described earlier. It has no dependence or addictive liability and is not lethal in overdose. Buspirone is also devoid of many of the problems of the benzodiazepines such as sedation, motor impairment, addiction, physical dependence, or withdrawal. Yet, doubts remain in the minds of many practitioners regarding the effectiveness of buspirone. This will be discussed in more detail later in this chapter.

Antihistamines. Some clinicians have prescribed the antihistamine, hydroxyzine (Vistaril, Atarax) to treat anxiety. A typical regimen is 25 mg administered one to three times per day as needed for anxiety. The use of hydroxyzine to treat anxiety is largely driven by concern regarding the addictive potential of benzodiazepines. In reality, hydroxyzine does little to relieve anxiety other than produce drowsiness. Because other nonaddictive anxiolytics are available, we do not recommend routine use of this largely ineffective treatment.

Newer GABA-Related Medications. Despite the unqualified anxiolytic efficacy of benzodiazepines, they are not without drawbacks including cognitive and sedative side effects and dependence liability. This has served as a major impetus for the ongoing search for alternative anxiolytic agents that, like benzodiazepines, act to increase GABA activity but do so via novel mechanisms that might avoid the problems associated with benzodiazepines. For example, β-carboline (abecarnil), a partial agonist at the GABA receptor, was shown more effective than placebo in controlled trials for GAD. However, abecarnil was outperformed in head-to-head comparisons with both benzodiazepines and buspirone, dimming initial enthusiasm that it might prove to be an effective anxiolytic.

Another approach to increasing GABA activity is to slow its degradation and elimination. Vigabatrin (Sabril), approved outside the United States for the management of epilepsy, acts in just this manner. It blocks the activity of GABA transaminase (GABA-T), the enzyme that metabolizes GABA. Although initial studies suggest that vigabatrin might be effective for panic disorder, reports that it has been associated with visual field constriction will likely preclude its approval in the United States.

Yet another approach to heightening GABA activity is to block the reuptake of the neurotransmitter in a fashion analogous to the blockade of serotonin reuptake by SSRIs. Tiagabine (Gabitril), approved in the United States for the management of seizures, acts via this mechanism. Initial results from controlled studies for GAD and PTSD have been encouraging. Furthermore, tiagabine has been well tolerated with complaints chiefly comprised of mild-to-moderate headaches, nausea, dizziness, and anorexia. Larger scale studies of tiagabine for anxiety disorders are being implemented.

Finally, two anticonvulsants that are structurally similar to GABA, gabapentin (Neurontin) and pregabalin (Lyrica), were initially utilized with the mistaken notion that they worked, as their names would imply, via direct GABA-mediated mechanisms. However, despite their similarity to GABA, neither of these agents interacts with GABA receptors. Instead, they act by modulating the neuronal influx of calcium, which, in turn, may influence GABA neurotransmission in the brain. Gabapentin, introduced a decade ago as an adjunctive treatment for epilepsy, has been shown in controlled studies to be effective for both panic disorder and social anxiety disorder. The most common side effects are dizziness, drowsiness, headache, nausea, and dry mouth. Although gabapentin reportedly has limited addictive potential, physical dependence can develop, leading to rebound anxiety and insomnia if gabapentin therapy is abruptly discontinued. In 2004, the FDA approved pregabalin for the treatment of neuropathic pain. It is approved in Europe for the management of epilepsy. Randomized controlled trials indicate that pregabalin is effective in the treatment of GAD and social anxiety disorder.

Miscellaneous. In recent years, other medication classes have been tested in the treatment of specific anxiety syndromes. For example, atypical antipsychotics have been used as adjunctive treatments for OCD and GAD, and mood stabilizers have been used to treat PTSD. These syndrome-specific regimens will be discussed in the following sections.

5.2 PANIC DISORDER

5.2.1 Brief Description and Diagnostic Criteria

The most dramatic presentation of anxiety is the panic attack. In contrast to other forms of anxiety, panic is characterized by an abrupt onset and rapid escalation. Many people mistakenly refer to any significant level of apprehension as an anxiety attack or panic attack. For purposes of accurate diagnosis and treatment selection, a panic attack is a very specific entity with well-delineated characteristics. A true panic attack has an abrupt, unmistakable onset and reaches peak severity within 10 minutes. It is usually accompanied by a sense of impending doom. Panic attacks then typically resolve spontaneously within 30 minutes to one hour. Thus, "anxiety attacks" described as gradual in onset or lasting several hours likely do not represent genuine panic attacks. Instead, a true panic attack requires the presence of four or more specific symptoms occurring during a brief yet extremely intense period of fear (see Table 5.4).

As you might expect, the diagnostic criteria for panic disorder requires the presence of recurrent panic attacks, but panic attacks alone are not sufficient for the diagnosis of panic disorder. Those with other anxiety disorders, for example, can experience panic attacks when confronted by the situation or object that they fear.

TABLE 5.4. Panic Attack Criteria

1. Palpitations, pounding heart, or rapid heart rate
2. Sweating
3. Trembling or shaking
4. Shortness of breath or smothering sensation
5. Choking sensation
6. Chest discomfort
7. Nausea or abdominal distress
8. Dizziness, lightheadedness, faintness
9. Feeling that things are unreal or that one is detached from oneself
10. Fear of going crazy or losing control
11. Fear of dying
12. Numbness or tingling
13. Chills or hot flushes

Four or more of above symptoms develop abruptly and reach peak in 10 minutes or less.

Source: Adapted from DSM-IV.

TABLE 5.5. Diagnostic Criteria for Panic Disorder

A. Repeated and unexpected panic attacks followed by at least one of the following for 1 month:
   1. Worrying about having more attacks
   2. Worrying about losing control or becoming seriously ill or dying in a future attack
   3. Avoiding situations that might trigger attacks
B. May occur with or without agoraphobia.
C. Not due to a medicine, an illicit drug, or a medical illness.
D. Not due to another mental illness.

Source: Adapted from DSM-IV.

Furthermore, DSM-IV does not specify a minimum number of panic attacks or a minimum frequency of panic attacks. The hallmark of panic disorder is that the panic attacks are unpredictable. They must occur without warning in a variety of settings, and they inexorably lead to a persistent anticipatory worry about the meaning of the attacks or the possibility of having more attacks. See Table 5.5 for the diagnostic criteria for panic disorder.

Although the delineation of panic disorder as a unique diagnostic entity is a relatively recent development, references to what would today be known as panic attacks commonly appeared in the annals of medical and psychiatric literature. For example, cardiologists, who frequently encounter patients with panic disorder due to the dramatic presentation of cardiac symptoms in association with panic, have numerous terms for panic including cardiac neurosis, DaCosta's syndrome, soldier's heart, and neurocirculatory asthenia.

The functional impairment associated with panic disorder is often underestimated. This may in part be due to the fact that the panic attacks themselves are brief and occupy only a small fraction of the patient's waking hours. However, the intensely noxious symptoms of a panic attack often lead to extensive efforts to avoid situations that might precipitate future attacks. In this manner, panic disorder commonly lays the foundation for the development of agoraphobia. As the panic attacks recur in a variety of contexts, the scope of the avoidance becomes ever widening. Consequently, many persons with panic disorder and incrementally more severe agoraphobia become increasingly isolated from the world.

The result is that panic disorder, particularly when associated with agoraphobia, confers considerable social impairment. Patients with panic disorder are less productive at work, are prone to absenteeism, are less satisfied in family roles, and have higher mortality and suicide rates. In addition, the physical symptoms of panic disorder are frequently misattributed to medical conditions such as emphysema or heart disease and lead to the costly and inappropriate use of emergency room and other medical services. Panic disorder is costly both from an economic and a social perspective.

5.2.2 Prevalence and Risk Factors

Panic disorder is a common clinical problem. Over the course of their lives, about 1 of every 5 people experience at least one panic attack. Less than half of these have a spontaneous or "unexpected" panic attack in a situation in which they would not have expected to be anxious, but even those do not necessarily fulfill the diagnostic criteria for panic disorder, which requires a persistent worry about the consequences of attacks or the possibility of having future attacks. The lifetime incidence of panic disorder is 2–4%. It is evenly distributed among all races and ethnic groups, but women are twice as likely to be affected as men. Early childhood trauma, such as sexual abuse, markedly increases the risk for the development of panic disorder in adulthood.

Panic disorder usually begins during adolescence or early adulthood with the mean age of onset in the early twenties. New onset panic disorder in the elderly is relatively uncommon, though panic attacks may be seen in those with medical illnesses such as emphysema or heart disease.

As noted above, panic disorder is commonly accompanied by agoraphobia as avoidant behaviors develop in what are usually partially successful attempts to reduce the frequency and intensity of panic attacks. Estimates for the co-occurrence of agoraphobia in patients with panic disorder range from 30% to 50%.

5.2.3 Presentation and Clinical Course

The symptoms of a panic attack are so frightening that an unusually large number of those with panic disorder (in comparison to other psychiatric illnesses) seek treatment on their own accord. However, easily half of those who seek treatment do so in general medical settings such as hospital emergency rooms and the offices of primary care physicians. Easily mistaken for severe and even life-threatening medical conditions such as asthma attacks and heart attacks, panic disorder results in disproportionately higher health care utilization than other anxiety disorders.

The referral for mental health care is often not made until an extensive medical evaluation has been completed. This medical assessment is often warranted, but a delay in recognizing the presence of panic disorder can result in an unending battery of expensive, unnecessary, and sometimes unpleasant medical tests.

Panic disorder is typically a chronic condition, but its severity often waxes and wanes over time. Some experience continuous symptoms whereas others have long periods of remission interspersed with periodic outbreaks of panic attacks. When agoraphobia accompanies panic disorder, it usually begins within the first year or so of panic attacks. The course of agoraphobia varies. The severity of the agoraphobic avoidance can either fluctuate with the frequency of panic attacks or remain constant despite changing severity in the panic attacks themselves.

5.2.4 Initial Evaluation and Differential Diagnosis

The differential diagnosis of panic disorder includes other psychiatric illnesses, medical illnesses, and substances that can cause panic attacks. Also included are medical illnesses that cause symptoms resembling panic attacks. It should be mentioned that these other conditions, which are described below, and panic disorder are not necessarily mutually exclusive. In fact, there is a high rate of comorbidity between panic disorder, other anxiety disorders, and mood disorders. Because panic disorder is frequently accompanied by agoraphobia, the differential diagnosis also includes illnesses that are associated with symptoms resembling the avoidance of the agoraphobic patient.

Generalized Anxiety Disorder (GAD). Theoretically, panic disorder and GAD should be fairly easy to distinguish. The symptoms of a panic attack are known for their intensity and their brevity, whereas the symptoms of GAD tend to be somewhat milder and considerably more persistent. Nevertheless, patients commonly confuse the two when describing their symptoms. It is not at all unusual for a patient to describe an "anxiety attack" or "panic attack" that comes on gradually and lasts several hours (or even days). This does not represent a true panic attack but a periodic fluctuation in the severity of their anxiety.

Social Anxiety Disorder (Social Phobia). The patient with social phobia can experience panic attacks though the condition is relatively easy to distinguish from panic disorder. You'll recall that patients with social phobia experience anxiety only when anticipating or confronting the feared social situation(s), but those with panic disorder experience spontaneous panic attacks, at least some of the time, in situations in which they did not expect to be nervous or anxious. Discriminating social phobia from agoraphobia, however, is somewhat more challenging. In both conditions, the patient typically avoids large gatherings. The distinction lies in the underlying reason. Patients with social phobia specifically wish to avoid being watched by others. They either literally (in the case of performance anxiety) or figuratively fear being "put on a stage" where they will be subject to the scrutiny of others. Patients with agoraphobia do not so much fear being watched by others, as they fear being trapped in a situation from which it will be difficult or embarrassing to escape.

In particular, they often fear having a panic attack or panic-like symptoms before being able to remove themselves from the crowd.

Obsessive–Compulsive Disorder (OCD). Like those with social phobia, patients with OCD can also experience a panic attack when confronted by the object of their fear. Again, the distinction from panic disorder lies in discriminating such stimulus-induced panic attacks from spontaneous panic attacks.

Post-traumatic Stress Disorder (PTSD). The same distinction holds true for PTSD. Reminders of the trauma (e.g., sexual intimacy for a rape survivor; loud noises for a combat veteran) can trigger panic attacks. Furthermore, PTSD is associated with a variety of avoidant behaviors that can resemble agoraphobia. In the case of PTSD, the avoidance is specifically targeted at reminders of the trauma. For example, places or people who in some way cue memories of the traumatic event are avoided. As for agoraphobia, the avoidance tends to be less specific. It is any situation from which it would be difficult to escape should a panic attack occur that is avoided.

Major Depressive Disorder (MDD). Depressed patients, like those with agoraphobia, often shun social interaction. The high rate of comorbidity of panic disorder with both depression and agoraphobia can complicate efforts to distinguish the two. The distinction, of course, lies in the reason that social gatherings are being avoided. The depressed patient is typically either uninterested in social interaction (anhedonic) or cannot muster the energy to engage in it. Those with agoraphobia typically would like to be able to enjoy interacting with others but are unable to do so because they fear being trapped in a situation in which they'll experience a panic attack.

Substance-Induced Anxiety Disorder. Numerous medicines and drugs of abuse can produce panic attacks. Panic attacks can be triggered by central nervous system stimulants such as cocaine, methamphetamine, caffeine, over-the-counter herbal stimulants such as ephedra, or any of the medications commonly used to treat narcolepsy and ADHD, including psychostimulants and modafinil. Thyroid supplementation with thyroxine (Synthroid) or triiodothyronine (Cytomel) can rarely produce panic attacks. Abrupt withdrawal from central nervous system depressants such as alcohol, barbiturates, and benzodiazepines can cause panic attacks as well. This can be especially problematic with short-acting benzodiazepines such as alprazolam (Xanax), which is an effective treatment for panic disorder but which has been associated with "between dose" withdrawal symptoms.

Anxiety Disorder Due to a General Medical Condition with Panic Attacks. Many medical illnesses are associated with anxiety and even recurrent panic attacks. These include endocrine disorders, such as hyperthyroidism, hyperparathyroidism, hypoglycemia, and pheochromocytomas, inner ear (vestibular) dysfunction, seizure disorders, and cardiac (heart) disorders such as supraventricular tachycardia, mitral valve prolapse, and various arrhythmias, and carcinoid. A general physical examination, routine laboratory studies including electrolytes and thyroid profile, and a careful medical history can generally identify these medically caused panic attacks.

General Medical Conditions that Resemble Panic Attacks. Panic attacks are characterized by the abrupt onset of characteristic physical symptoms such as chest pain, shortness of breath, profuse sweating, dizziness, and nausea. Such symptoms may also be caused by severe and even life-threatening medical conditions such as asthma, emphysema, strokes, aneurysms, and heart attacks. It is, in fact, the fear that they're having a heart attack or some other severe medical problem that leads many patients to seek treatment after a panic attack.

What's often overlooked is that such medical conditions and panic disorder are not mutually exclusive. For example, those with asthma or heart disease become conditioned to monitoring bodily signals very closely. At times, they may misinterpret a physical symptom as an impending attack of asthma or angina. This may result in an escalating spiral of anxiety that leads to a panic attack. Thus, those with true medically verified asthma or heart disease can also suffer from panic disorder as an indirect consequence of their medical condition.

5.2.5 History of Pharmacological Treatment

Monoamine Oxidase Inhibitors (MAOIs). Shortly after their introduction, MAOIs, such as phenelzine (Nardil), were found to reduce the frequency of panic attacks. It became a standard treatment for what is now known as panic disorder until supplanted by the benzodiazepines and SSRIs. Although all MAOIs are presumably effective for panic disorder, phenelzine is the best studied and has been shown to be effective at daily doses ranging from 45 to 90 mg. When used to treat panic disorder, phenelzine should be initiated at a dose of 15 mg/day and gradually increased in 15 mg increments until reaching a therapeutic dose.

One drawback to MAOI therapy is that the therapeutic benefit typically does not begin until after the third week of treatment at the earliest. This is, of course, generally true of all antidepressants that are used to treat panic disorder and other anxiety syndromes. Of greater concern are the potentially dangerous food and drug interactions of the MAOIs (cf. Chapter 3), which have relegated the use of MAOIs for those panic disorder patients who do not respond to other treatments.

Tricyclic Antidepressants (TCAs). The TCAs, particularly imipramine (Tofranil), were also discovered soon after their introduction to be effective in the treatment of panic attacks. Imipramine, the best-studied TCA in the treatment of panic disorder, is most often helpful at daily doses of 150–250 mg, though it must be started at 10–25 mg, usually at bedtime, and gradually increased over 2–4 weeks. Although they are not as well studied, many clinicians prefer to use the secondary amine TCAs, desipramine (Norpramin) and nortriptyline (Pamelor), because they have milder side effects than imipramine. Clomipramine (Anafranil), though probably the TCA with the greatest side effect burden, is often said to be most effective in patients with refractory disease.

Like the MAOIs, TCAs are hindered by a delayed onset of action that can be especially intolerable for those with frequent and severe panic attacks. When starting treatment, TCAs, like SSRIs, may also produce a transient nervousness that is especially uncomfortable for those with panic disorder. When this occurs, the starting dose should be reduced by half, and the pace of subsequent dose increases should be even slower than usual. Because they produce prominent side effects and can be dangerous in overdose, TCAs are also now reserved for patients unresponsive to other treatments. Refer to Chapter 3 for a more extensive discussion of the TCAs.

Benzodiazepines. The introduction of the benzodiazepines represented a significant advance in the treatment of panic disorder. In contrast to MAOIs and TCAs, the benzodiazepines begin to provide relief the very first day of treatment, and many patients experience a complete response by the end of the second week of therapy. All benzodiazepines should theoretically alleviate the symptoms of a panic attack at comparable doses, but the benzodiazepines of choice are alprazolam (Xanax, Xanax XR) and clonazepam (Klonopin). It likely is not coincidental that these two are among the highest potency benzodiazepines. However, they differ considerably from a pharmacokinetic standpoint. If clonazepam is the tortoise of benzodiazepines, then alprazolam is the hare.

Alprazolam has an especially rapid onset of action and can therefore provide rapid relief when a panic attack is impending. In addition to its rapid onset, alprazolam also has a brief duration of action. Thus, it's often necessary to administer alprazolam several times per day, and patients are more likely to complain of breakthrough anxiety in between doses. Without careful discussion prior to initiating alprazolam, this breakthrough anxiety can lead to a rapid escalation in dose. This problem, however, can be minimized by a newly available sustained-release preparation of alprazolam. Alprazolam should be started at 0.25–0.50 mg given three times daily. The dose can be increased every 5–7 days as necessary. The typical daily dose is 2–4 mg per day given in three to five divided doses. A long-acting preparation (Xanax XR) is now available that can be administered one to three times daily. Xanax XR is typically started at a dose of 0.5–1 mg/day and gradually increased to a therapeutic dose of 3–6 mg/day.

In contrast to alprazolam, clonazepam has a gradual onset of action and a relatively longer duration of action. Whereas clonazepam is less effective than alprazolam at providing rapid relief when a panic attack is underway, it provides more consistent symptom relief during the course of the day with less potential for interdose breakthrough anxiety. Clonazepam should be started at 0.5–1.0 mg/day and increased every 3–5 days as needed to a maximum dose of 4 mg/day. Due to its long duration of action, clonazepam can be administered two to three times per day and provide adequate symptom control throughout the day for patients with panic disorder. A clonazepam wafer that is rapidly dissolving is believed to provide a more rapid onset of action than the usual oral preparation.

As noted earlier, the principal advantage of the benzodiazepines is that they provide faster relief than the MAOIs, TCAs, and SSRIs (which were introduced later). They are also considerably safer than the MAOIs, TCAs, and barbiturates.

However, there are disadvantages to benzodiazepines. They produce sedation and can impair short-term memory and coordination (psychomotor function such as driving). They can magnify the effects of alcohol and are subject to abuse and withdrawal syndromes. Refer to Section 5.1 for a more extended discussion of benzodiazepines.

Beta Blockers. Beta blockers such as propranolol (Inderal) and atenolol (Tenormin) act by blocking the activity of the neurotransmitter norepinephrine. They have been used in the treatment of patients with panic disorder in an effort to alleviate the physical (autonomic) symptoms of the panic attack, but they proved no better than placebo and have no place in the treatment of panic disorder.

Clonidine (Catapres). Like the beta blockers, clonidine acts by reducing norepinephrine activity, though by a different mechanism. Studies show that clonidine can provide early relief from the symptoms of a panic attack, but patients unfortunately relapse with continued treatment. Therefore, clonidine is not used in the treatment of panic disorder.

Newer Generation Antidepressants. All SSRIs have been shown effective in the treatment of panic disorder. Of these, fluoxetine (Prozac), paroxetine (Paxil), and sertraline (Zoloft), as well as the SNRI venlafaxine ER (Effexor XR), have received FDA approval for the treatment of panic disorder. Because they are safer and easier to tolerate, SSRIs/SNRIs have largely supplanted the MAOIs and TCAs as standard treatments (along with benzodiazepines) for panic disorder.

As noted earlier, SSRIs/SNRIs can produce transient nervousness during the start-up phase of treatment. A "start low and go slow" approach is therefore advisable when treating patients with panic disorder. Nevertheless, panic disorder is often best controlled only after attaining daily doses at the upper end of the dose range. Please refer to Chapter 3 for additional discussion of the SSRIs/SNRIs.

Buspirone (Buspar). The azapirone, buspirone, has been tested in the treatment of panic disorder and found to be ineffective.

Anticonvulsants. Scattered case reports suggest that carbamazepine (Tegretol) and valproic acid (Depakote, Depakene) may be helpful in the treatment of panic disorder. This has yet to be verified in systematic studies. Furthermore, because these anticonvulsants are hindered by toxicity and side effect concerns (cf. Chapter 3), they should only be considered if other better studied and more tolerable treatment options have failed.

5.2.6 Current Approach to Treatment

Acute Phase Treatment. The short-term objective when treating panic disorder is to optimize symptom relief. This primarily consists of reducing the severity and frequency of panic attacks but also includes the anticipatory anxiety and secondary agoraphobic avoidance associated with the disorder. The long-term objectives are to safeguard against future panic attacks while continuing to address the phobic avoidance, which often takes considerably longer to resolve.

The first-line treatments for panic disorder are (1) cognitive-behavioral therapy (CBT), (2) benzodiazepines, and (3) SSRIs/SNRIs. Each of these three treatment modalities can be used independently or in combination. The selection of the primary treatment depends on several factors including severity and frequency of the panic attacks, comorbid illnesses, and patient preference.

When treating mild-to-moderate panic disorder, we recommend avoiding benzodiazepines in favor of CBT or antidepressants. Because CBT and antidepressants are both effective for panic disorder and major depression (commonly comorbid with panic disorder), the choice between the two largely rests on patient preference. Antidepressants are preferred for those who are pessimistic regarding the potential benefit of CBT, cannot afford CBT, or are unable (or unwilling) to invest the time necessary to complete a course of CBT. In our experience, some patients may accrue significant benefit from the combined treatment, particularly those with more moderate symptoms who struggle with the exposure aspects of therapy.

For those with more severe panic disorder, pharmacotherapy is preferred, though CBT can be introduced once the medication has afforded some degree of symptomatic relief. In choosing between antidepressants and benzodiazepines, antidepressants are preferred when treating elderly patients who may have difficulty tolerating benzodiazepines and are essential when treating those with comorbid depression. Benzodiazepines are now largely reserved for those patients with panic disorder whose symptoms are so severe that they are unable to tolerate waiting several weeks for an antidepressant to take effect.

One increasingly popular approach when treating those with severe panic disorder is to begin treatment with both a benzodiazepine and an antidepressant. In this combined approach, the benzodiazepine provides the initial symptom relief during the first 2 weeks of therapy. Meanwhile, the antidepressant is gradually titrated to an effective antipanic dose. After about 8 weeks of treatment, when the antidepressant has had sufficient time to produce its therapeutic benefit, the benzodiazepine can be tapered and discontinued, leaving only the antidepressant for long-term maintenance treatment. Because it is easier to taper long-acting benzodiazepines without producing unpleasant withdrawal symptoms, we prefer using clonazepam as opposed to alprazolam when implementing the combined strategy. Extended-release alprazolam is a suitable alternative.

Maintenance Phase Treatment. Because panic disorder tends to be a chronic condition, the appropriate duration of therapy is a critically important question. Conventional practice is to continue treatment for 6–9 months after remission has been achieved and then to taper medicines gradually over several weeks to months. The relapse rate is extremely high with over one-half of those treated with medications alone experiencing a relapse within a few months of discontinuing treatment. There is some evidence that CBT may reduce this relapse rate. When relapse occurs, it is usually advisable to restart the medication that was previously used.

Unfortunately, some patients respond poorly to these first-line interventions. In particular, patients with a long duration of illness, extreme agoraphobic avoidance, and comorbid personality disorders are more likely to exhibit a poor treatment response. For such patients, TCAs such as imipramine or clomipramine and MAOIs such as phenelzine remain viable strategies.

5.3 GENERALIZED ANXIETY DISORDER

5.3.1 Brief Description and Diagnostic Criteria

Generalized anxiety disorder (GAD) lies at the opposite end of the anxiety spectrum from panic disorder. Whereas panic attacks are noteworthy for their abrupt onset and dramatic presentation, the symptoms of GAD are characterized by their chronicity and pathognomonic sign of pathological worry. If a panic attack is a raging wildfire, then GAD is a smoldering ember that refuses to dissipate. The principal symptom of GAD is pervasive worry about a variety of issues that persists for at least 6 months. This worry is focused on everyday concerns such as health, finances, job performance, or family safety. Those with GAD feel unable to control their worrying and are plagued by any of a number of accompanying symptoms such as tension, fatigue, irritability, and insomnia. See Table 5.6 for the diagnostic criteria for GAD. Although not included in the diagnostic criteria, patients with GAD may also complain of frequent tremulousness, dry mouth, sweating, clamminess, nausea, diarrhea, a lump in the throat, and a variety of other annoying physical symptoms.

5.3.2 Prevalence and Risk Factors

Often unrecognized by primary care physicians and mental health professionals alike, GAD is surprisingly common. Estimates of the lifetime prevalence of GAD

TABLE 5.6. Diagnostic Criteria for Generalized Anxiety Disorder

A. Exaggerated worry about several real-life concerns on most days for at least 6 months.
B. Finds it hard to stop worrying.
C. Accompanied by at least three of the following symptoms:
   1. Feels keyed up
   2. Tires easily
   3. Finds it hard to concentrate
   4. Feels irritable
   5. Muscles are tense
   6. Insomnia
D. Worries are not solely related to another mental illness.
E. Worrying causes significant distress.
F. Not due to a medicine, an illicit drug, or a medical illness.

Source: Adapted from DSM-IV.

range from 4% to 9%. The disorder is twice as common among women. The onset of GAD is typically during adolescence or early adulthood; however, a pediatric equivalent of GAD, known as overanxious disorder of childhood (ODC), is also common with 3–7% fulfilling criteria in any given year.

5.3.3 Presentation and Clinical Course

In contrast to panic disorder, the somewhat more subtle and persistent symptoms of GAD do not always command immediate attention. Although patients with GAD may present with a primary complaint of anxiety, they are more likely to complain of a physical ailment or another psychiatric condition or symptoms, for example, depression or insomnia. As such, many patients with GAD will seek treatment from a primary care physician long before recognizing the need for mental health care despite readily acknowledging that they have been anxious virtually all of their lives.

GAD tends to be a persistent illness, though its severity can fluctuate over time. Without treatment, few patients with GAD experience complete remission of symptoms. When GAD does remit, it is highly prone to recurrence. A declining course has been described among some patients who gradually experienced more and more functional disability as the illness endures. GAD has a high rate of comorbidity with some studies estimating that over 90% of those with GAD also fulfill diagnostic criteria for another DSM-IV Axis I disorder. Depression is by far the most common comorbidity confronting patients with GAD, and those with comorbid depression typically have a poorer prognosis. Many consider GAD to be a significant risk factor for the development of major depression.

5.3.4 Initial Evaluation and Differential Diagnosis

Primary care physicians are critical to the successful identification of GAD. Characterized by often-vague physical complaints, GAD must be distinguished from medical illnesses and other psychiatric disorders, though the high rate of comorbidity requires that a thorough evaluation for GAD be completed even when another disorder has been identified. GAD warrants particular consideration for those patients with nonspecific physical complaints who nevertheless have an urgent need for relief that has resulted in repeated office visits. The differential diagnosis for GAD includes other anxiety disorders, depression, and a variety of medical conditions and substance-induced syndromes.

Panic Disorder. As previously noted, panic disorder and GAD should in theory at least be fairly easy to distinguish. Yet, patients commonly confuse the two when describing their symptoms. It is common that a patient with GAD will describe an "anxiety attack" or "panic attack" that comes on gradually and lasts several hours (or even days). This does not represent a true panic attack but a periodic fluctuation in the severity of their generalized anxiety. It should be noted, however, that patients with a principal diagnosis of GAD might occasionally experience panic attacks. In addition, those with panic disorder may experience "persistent worry" that they will have another panic attack. If the persistent worry is exclusively anticipatory anxiety concerning the possibility of another panic attack, then the diagnosis of GAD is not warranted.

Social Anxiety Disorder (Social Phobia). Patients with social anxiety disorder can similarly experience "persistent worry" regarding a potentially embarrassing social interaction. In contrast, the patient with GAD worries about a variety of activities or events.

Obsessive–Compulsive Disorder (OCD). The excessive worry of GAD can be confused with the intrusive thoughts of OCD. Whereas GAD entails an exaggerated concern regarding real-life concerns, the obsessional focus of OCD is on senseless yet intrusive, ego-dystonic thoughts and images. Moreover, the obsessions of OCD are typically accompanied by ritualistic, compulsive behaviors that aim to alleviate the anxiety triggered by the obsession. Those with GAD are fretful and tense, but they do not typically engage in compulsive behaviors to relieve their anxiety.

Post-traumatic Stress Disorder (PTSD). Persistent anxiety is an invariable feature of both GAD and PTSD. In the case of GAD, the worry relates to a wide array of situations. As for PTSD, the worry relates to a perceived threat that is often directly, or at least indirectly, reminiscent of the previous trauma.

Major Depressive Disorder (MDD). Although there is some degree of symptomatic overlap (e.g., sleep disturbance and poor concentration), distinguishing GAD from MDD and other depressive disorders is usually not especially problematic. The dilemma is that many clinicians, both those in primary care and those working in mental health care, having determined that a depressive disorder is present, terminate the diagnostic evaluation and fail to determine whether comorbid GAD is present. Recognizing the considerable comorbidity between GAD and MDD, and the poorer prognosis when both disorders are present, this failure can carry grave clinical consequences.

Substance-Induced Anxiety Disorder. Many of the same medicines and drugs of abuse known to trigger panic attacks can also produce symptoms of anxiety resembling GAD. This keyed up state can be caused by central nervous system stimulants such as cocaine, methamphetamine, caffeine, over-the-counter herbal stimulants such as ephedra, and prescription psychostimulants such as methylphenidate (Ritalin) or dextroamphetamine (Dexedrine) as well as modafinil (Provigil). Thyroid hormone supplementation can also rarely cause generalized anxiety. Acute withdrawal from central nervous system depressants such as alcohol, barbiturates, and benzodiazepines can also cause generalized anxiety, though, left untreated, this can rapidly escalate to panic attacks, seizures, and delirium. Mild opioid withdrawal can also produce symptoms resembling GAD.

Anxiety Disorder Due to a General Medical Condition with Generalized Anxiety. Generalized anxiety can be produced by numerous medical conditions, including endocrine disorders such as hyperthyroidism, hyperparathyroidism, hypoglycemia, and pheochromocytomas, complex partial seizures, central nervous system tumors, multiple sclerosis, strokes and transient ischemic attacks, and menopause. Gastrointestinal disorders, such as peptic ulcer disease and carcinoid, can produce generalized anxiety, as can cardiovascular and pulmonary disorders, though the latter two are more often associated with panic attacks.

5.3.5 History of Pharmacological Treatment

Benzodiazepines. Shortly after their introduction in the 1960s, benzodiazepines emerged as the treatment of choice for those experiencing generalized anxiety, though syndromal GAD would not be identified in the psychiatric nosology for nearly 20 years. Compared to other alternatives, they offer the prominent advantage of rapid symptom relief. They do not appear, however, to provide effective relief from the core symptoms of worry experienced by those with GAD, and some patients, particularly the elderly, have difficulty tolerating certain of their side effects such as sedation, impaired physical coordination increasing the risk for falls, poor concentration, and potentiation of the effects of alcohol. We consequently avoid using benzodiazepines in such patients; however, when benzodiazepines must be used in susceptible patients, agents that can be more readily cleared, that is, those without active metabolites and without very long half-lives, including lorazepam (Ativan) and oxazepam (Serax), are preferred. Finally, the dependence and addictive liability of benzodiazepines must be factored into any treatment decision regarding these agents.

Unlike the intermittent nature of panic attacks, the symptoms of GAD persist throughout the day. Consequently, longer-acting benzodiazepines, for example, chlordiazepoxide (Librium), clonazepam, clorazepate (Tranxene), and diazepam (Valium), have been most widely used. Longer-acting agents minimize both the need for multiple doses during the course of the day and the potential for interdose symptom reemergence. Surprisingly, the short-acting agent alprazolam (Xanax) has also found widespread use for GAD, typically administered in three to four divided doses per day. The recent introduction of extended-release alprazolam (Xanax ER) is likely suitable for GAD.

When initiating benzodiazepine treatment for GAD, tolerability can be improved by starting at a low dose and gradually titrating to the effective dose range over the course of several days. Most patients with GAD respond well to 1–3 mg/day of extended-release alprazolam, 1–2 mg/day of clonazepam, or 10–20 mg/day of diazepam. Elderly patients often do best at approximately half these daily doses.

Because GAD is a chronic illness, benzodiazepines are often used in long-term maintenance therapy, leading to physical dependence over the course of several weeks. Consequently, abrupt discontinuation of a benzodiazepine can result not only in rebound anxiety and a rapid relapse but an acute benzodiazepine withdrawal syndrome as well. Refer to Chapter 6 for a more extensive discussion of benzodiazepine withdrawal. A very slow tapering over several weeks, if not months, is often required in order to discontinue a benzodiazepine so that the patient does not experience prominent withdrawal symptoms. An inpatient admission for benzodiazepine detoxification is sometimes necessary.

TCAs. Although the TCAs were introduced in the 1950s and 1960s, they were not formally tested in the treatment of GAD until the late 1980s. Controlled studies demonstrated that imipramine and clomipramine are effective in the treatment of GAD. They were outperformed by benzodiazepines at the end of the initial 2 weeks of therapy but actually provided greater benefit than benzodiazepines after 6 or more weeks of treatment. Due to the prominent side effects and danger in toxicity associated with TCAs, they have been supplanted by the newer generation of antidepressants, such as the SSRIs and SNRIs, as preferred agents in the treatment of generalized anxiety disorder. Refer to Chapter 3 for more information regarding TCAs.

SSRIs and SNRIs. The SSRI antidepressants, together with venlafaxine, have replaced the benzodiazepines as treatments of choice for GAD. Paroxetine and escitalopram are FDA approved for GAD, though it is generally believed that all SSRIs and SNRIs are effective for GAD. Similar to the TCAs, SSRIs/SNRIs appear to be most effective for the intrapsychic symptoms of GAD but less effective than benzodiazepines for the somatic manifestations of the disorder.

SSRI and SNRI onset of action is delayed by several weeks, and transient anxiety or agitation can be experienced during the first week of treatment. This problem can be avoided when treating GAD, as in other anxiety disorders, by initiating these agents at a daily dose that is approximately half that used when treating depression. This transient agitation aside, SSRIs and SNRIs are generally well tolerated by patients with GAD, and initial reports indicate that they are safe and effective as a long-term maintenance treatment for the disorder. Refer to Chapter 3 for a more extensive discussion of these agents.

Extended-release venlafaxine (Effexor XR), an antidepressant that blocks the reuptake of both serotonin and norepinephrine, has also obtained FDA approval for the treatment of GAD. Controlled studies indicate that venlafaxine is effective both in the acute treatment of GAD and as a longer-term maintenance therapy. Indeed, as noted earlier, like the SSRIs, venlafaxine has a delayed onset of action and can cause transient anxiety and agitation during the first week of therapy, particularly if the dose is too aggressively increased. When treating GAD, extended-release venlafaxine should be started at 37.5 mg taken as a single daily dose in the morning. It can gradually be titrated, as tolerated, to the effective dose range of 75–300 mg/day. Venlafaxine side effects are similar to those witnessed with SSRIs. Clinically significant blood pressure elevation can arise when the daily dose of venlafaxine exceeds 300 mg/day. Refer to Chapter 3 for more information regarding venlafaxine.

A controlled trial of duloxetine (Cymbalta)—like venlafaxine a dual serotonin–norepinephrine reuptake inhibitor—in the treatment of GAD is currently underway. Anecdotal data suggests that nefazodone (Serzone) and mirtazapine (Remeron) may be effective in the treatment of GAD, though no controlled data is available. In addition, recent concerns regarding nefazodone and liver toxicity have limited this medication's utility. Please refer to Chapter 3 for more information regarding these antidepressants.

Buspirone (Buspar). The first nonsedating, nonbenzodiazepine specifically introduced as an anxiolytic, buspirone is FDA approved for the treatment of GAD. This medication acts as a partial agonist at the postsynaptic serotonin (5HT)-1A receptor. Like the antidepressants, buspirone has a delayed onset of action and effectively relieves the intrapsychic symptoms of GAD. Devoid of the muscle-relaxing properties of benzodiazepines, buspirone does not as effectively relieve the physical symptoms of GAD. Buspirone is not effective in the treatment of depression. Furthermore, its utility for the treatment of anxiety disorders other than GAD appears to be limited.

Buspirone does not share any of the problematic benzodiazepine properties such as sedation, motor impairment, addiction, physical dependence, or withdrawal. The most common side effects of buspirone include dizziness, nausea, headache, fatigue, and dry mouth. Despite its activity in the serotonin system, buspirone is not associated with the sexual side effects that plague the SSRIs, SNRIs, MAOIs, and TCAs.

There are two principal disadvantages of buspirone therapy. First, it must be administered two or three times daily. Long-term patient compliance is notoriously poor for medications that cannot be administered in a single daily dose. Second, buspirone is not an effective treatment for depression or any of the other comorbidities that frequently accompany GAD. As a result, buspirone monotherapy is only an alternative for GAD patients who have no comorbid illness.

The typical starting dose for buspirone is 15–20 mg/day, administered either as a regimen of 5 mg taken three times each day or 10 mg taken twice daily. The efficacy of buspirone is typically maximized at a daily dose of 30–60 mg. The maximal daily dose of 60 mg can be administered either as 20 mg taken three times daily or 30 mg taken twice daily.

Other Medications. A recent controlled GAD study revealed that pregabalin at a daily dose of 600 mg/day outperformed placebo and compared favorably to lorazepam, 6 mg/day. After 4 weeks of treatment, the participants assigned to pregabalin reportedly tolerated a 1 week taper better than those taking lorazepam. The most common pregabalin side effects reported in this study were sedation, weight gain, and dizziness. Although it is too early to recommend pregabalin for routine use for GAD, it may emerge as a favorable alternative to the benzodiazepines. It already warrants consideration for GAD patients who have not responded to other treatments.

Controlled studies of tiagabine in the treatment of GAD are currently underway.

Antihistamines. The antihistamine hydroxyzine (Vistaril, Atarax) has been used to manage anxiety. A typical regimen is 25 mg hydroxyzine administered one to three times per day as needed for anxiety. There is no evidence that hydroxyzine acts in any way to relieve anxiety other than by producing drowsiness. We do not recommend routine use of this treatment.

5.3.6 Current Approach to Treatment

The short-term goal when initiating treatment for GAD is to optimize symptom relief. The duration of the acute phase of GAD treatment can be quite variable. Achieving an optimal response may require 3–6 months. The rapidity of the treatment response can be influenced by the choice of pharmacotherapy, the severity and chronicity of the disorder, and the ongoing presence of psychosocial stressors. Due to the paucity of formal longitudinal studies of GAD therapy, guidelines for long-term GAD treatment are largely dictated by anecdotal evidence and conventional practice. Once a satisfactory treatment response has been achieved, maintenance therapy is typically continued for an additional 6–9 months.

First-line GAD treatments include (1) cognitive-behavioral therapy (CBT), (2) antidepressants, (3) buspirone, and (4) benzodiazepines. Treatment selection is determined by the severity of the illness, the presence of any comorbid illnesses, previous patient treatment responses, and patient preference. When treating mild GAD, we recommend eschewing psychotropic medication altogether in favor of CBT. Moderate-to-severe GAD usually requires pharmacotherapy, though combined CBT–pharmacotherapy is highly encouraged.

Due to the extensive comorbidity of GAD with depression, when pharmacotherapy is indicated, antidepressant therapy is preferred. At present, only escitalopram, paroxetine, and venlafaxine are approved by the FDA for the treatment of GAD. It is generally accepted that all SSRIs represent effective treatments for GAD. Due to the transient exacerbation of anxiety that can be experienced when initiating treatment with a SSRI or SNRI, initial doses should be low, and dose titration should be gradual. For GAD patients, escitalopram should be started at 5 mg/day, fluoxetine at 10 mg/day, paroxetine at 10 mg/day (12.5 mg/day for the controlled-release preparation of paroxetine), sertraline at 12.5–25 mg/day, and venlafaxine XR at 37.5 mg/day. Some patients with GAD may respond at these low doses that are seldom effective for treating depression. For those requiring higher doses, dose increments can usually be scheduled every 7 days, though some sensitive patients will require even less frequent dose increases. If there is no benefit experienced with these first-line antidepressants, then other antidepressants including tricyclic antidepressants, nefazodone, or mirtazapine are reasonable alternatives.

The subset of patients with GAD who do not have a comorbid depressive illness can be treated with buspirone in lieu of an antidepressant. Like the antidepressants, the buspirone treatment response is delayed by several weeks; however, opting for buspirone is less likely to cause the transient exacerbation of anxiety or the sexual side effects commonly witnessed with antidepressants. Unfortunately, the usefulness of buspirone is severely limited by its requirement that it be administered two to three times each day. When buspirone is used, it can be started at 10 mg/day and gradually titrated to an effective dose of 20–60 mg/day.

We do not use benzodiazepines as readily when treating GAD as we do when treating panic disorder. In comparison to those with panic disorder, most patients with GAD can more easily tolerate the delay in treatment response and even any transient exacerbation of anxiety associated with antidepressant therapy. Benzodiazepines are reserved for those who present with especially severe anxiety that necessitates more rapid relief than an antidepressant can afford and for those who do not achieve a satisfactory response to antidepressant or buspirone therapy. Due to the persistent nature of the anxiety experienced by patients with GAD, short-acting benzodiazepines such as alprazolam are not especially helpful unless dosed 3–4 times per day. Instead, we prefer long-acting agents such as clonazepam. When used to treat GAD, clonazepam should be started at a low dose (0.25–0.5 mg/day) and titrated to higher doses (1–4 mg/day) if clinically necessary.

In the event that these conventional GAD therapies prove ineffective, other alternatives merit attention. In particular, the GABA-related agents, pregabalin, tiagabine, or vigabatrin, can be used though data regarding their effectiveness for generalized anxiety remains preliminary.

5.4 OBSESSIVE–COMPULSIVE DISORDER

5.4.1 Brief Description and Diagnostic Criteria

Obsessive–compulsive disorder (OCD) is a disturbing and at times debilitating illness characterized by persistent obsessions and compulsions. By obsession, we mean unwanted ideas or urges that are difficult to dismiss. Compulsions are highly repetitious behaviors aimed at alleviating the anxiety produced by the obsessions. These compulsions sometimes evolve into highly complicated and time-consuming rituals. Although DSM-IV requires only the presence of obsessions or compulsions, patients with OCD nearly always demonstrate both. In fact, because a compulsion is typically intended to relieve the anxiety produced by an obsession, the two are commonly paired in a fairly predictable pattern. Refer to Table 5.7 for the DSM-IV diagnostic criteria for OCD.

The most common obsessions faced by patients with OCD involve fears of contamination. This fear may focus on germs and infectious diseases, household chemicals, environmental pollutants, or bodily wastes. These contamination obsessions most often result in washing compulsions but may also produce compulsive visits to health care providers. Obsessional doubts (e.g., "Did I remember to . . . ?") are typically associated with checking compulsions. Another common obsession, need for symmetry and exactness, leads to compulsive arranging, ordering, or counting. Obsessions may also be aggressive, somatic, or sexual in content.

The distinction between an obsession and delusion is an important one. Both represent over-valued ideas. The conceptual difference lies in the patient's insight into the senselessness of those ideas. By definition, patients with delusions are

TABLE 5.7. Diagnostic Criteria for Obsessive–Compulsive Disorder

A. Has either obsessions *OR* compulsions:
   1. Obsessions (must include all four of the following):
      i. Repeated and unwanted thoughts
      ii. Not just exaggerated worry about real-life problems
      iii. Tries to ignore or stop having the thoughts
      iv. Realizes thoughts are a product of his/her own mind
   2. Compulsions (must include both of the following):
      i. Repeated acts performed in response to an obsession or in accordance with some strict ritual
      ii. Acts represent unsuccessful attempts to reduce anxiety and/or to prevent some imagined tragedy
B. Realizes (at least at some point in the illness) that the obsessions and/or compulsions are unreasonable.
C. Causes considerable distress, consumes more than an hour per day, and/or interferes with normal daily routine.
D. Obsessions and/or compulsions are not solely related to another mental illness.
E. Not due to a medicine, an illicit drug, or a medical illness.

Source: Adapted from DSM-IV.

unaware that their false beliefs are unreasonable. Patients with obsessions, by contrast, have historically been said to recognize the unreasonableness of their recurrent thoughts. We now know that this distinction is not wholly reliable. Although the DSM-IV criteria specify that the OCD patient realized "at some point" that the thoughts and rituals of the disorder were unreasonable, this insight may be lost. Hence, the diagnostic specifier for OCD "with poor insight."

When a patient with OCD has impaired insight, the distinction between obsession and delusion becomes blurred. We would argue that such a patient is in fact delusional. The "with poor insight" specifier is therefore the OCD equivalent to the "with psychotic features" specifier applied to the mood disorders. There may in fact be a continuum of insight in patients with OCD that fluctuates over time. For example, patients with OCD may recognize that their preoccupation with an obsessional idea or compulsive ritual is excessive, yet they may remain insistent that the premise underlying their anxiety is entirely reasonable.

5.4.2 Prevalence and Risk Factors

Believed historically to be a relatively rare disorder, large-scale epidemiological research undertaken during the last 20 years indicates that OCD is in fact quite common. The lifetime prevalence of OCD is 2–3%, making it more common, in fact, than bipolar disorder, schizophrenia, and most psychiatric illnesses other than depression and the substance use disorders.

OCD affects both genders in nearly equal rates, with most studies showing the disorder to be only slightly more common among women than men. Child psychiatrists interestingly report that the rate among boys doubles that of girls. It remains unclear whether childhood onset OCD is a different illness or simply a precocious onset of the same illness seen during adulthood. Some cases of childhood onset OCD and comorbid tic disorders are related to a prior strep infection through mechanisms that are not completely understood.

5.4.3 Presentation and Clinical Course

Patients with panic disorder or GAD commonly seek treatment on their own initiative, though they may not recognize that the underlying problem for which they're seeking relief is an anxiety disorder. This is in stark contrast to OCD, an illness that often persists for years before coming to clinical attention. Patients with OCD, often ashamed by their frustrating inability to control the unwanted intrusive thoughts and compulsive behaviors of the disorder, exert considerable effort to hide their symptoms. Suffering in secrecy, patients with OCD are often able to conceal their illness from friends and co-workers.

Eventually, those with OCD, fed up with the constant pressure of their ego-dystonic thoughts and behaviors, might seek treatment on their own accord. Alternatively, they might seek treatment with encouragement, or coercion, from concerned family members who are frustrated with the impact of the patient's illness on family life. Children with OCD, for whom the obsessions are more likely to be ego-syntonic, seldom seek treatment but are virtually always forced into treatment by understandably worried parents.

The precise nature of the clinical presentation is determined by the content of the obsessions and compulsions. Refer to Table 5.8 for a list of the recognized OCD subtypes.

The symptoms of OCD generally arise in an insidious manner, though acute onset of OCD has been reported. Considerable evidence indicates that OCD, once it arises, is a chronic lifetime disorder. Even with treatment, only a small fraction of OCD sufferers experience complete remission of their symptoms. Although patients with OCD are seldom, if ever, completely symptom free, the severity of the illness fluctuates over time. During periods of heightened stress, patients with OCD are especially prone to symptomatic exacerbation. For example, the postpartum period,

TABLE 5.8. Obsessive-Compulsive Disorder Subtypes

Obsessions	Compulsions
Aggression	Cleaning/washing
Contamination	Counting
Sexual	Repetition
Hoarding	Ordering/arranging
Religious	Somatic
Symmetry	Miscellaneous
Somatic	
Miscellaneous	

an extraordinarily stressful event in a woman's life, is increasingly recognized as a time when women are vulnerable to not only depression but also obsessive–compulsive symptoms.

5.4.4 Initial Evaluation and Differential Diagnosis

Panic Disorder. Over half of OCD patients will at some time during the course of their illness experience a panic attack. This does not necessarily mean that they have comorbid panic disorder. The distinction is that those with panic disorder sometimes experience spontaneous attacks whereas patients with OCD experience panic attacks only when confronted by a specific feared trigger that is associated with the content of the obsessions.

Generalized Anxiety Disorder. The obsessions of OCD in some respects resemble the persistent and excessive worry of GAD. However, GAD entails an exaggerated preoccupation regarding real-life concerns, whereas the obsessions of OCD are senseless ego-dystonic thoughts and images. In addition, the obsessions of OCD are typically accompanied by compulsive behaviors that aim to alleviate the anxiety triggered by the obsession. Patients with GAD do not usually engage in compulsive behaviors to relieve tension.

Schizophrenia. The obsessions and compulsive rituals of OCD must be distinguished from the delusions and behavioral peculiarities of schizophrenia. Usually, the OCD patient recognizes the excessive nature of the obsessions and wishes to be rid of them. This is in contrast to the delusional patient with schizophrenia who clings tenaciously to his/her false beliefs, unaware that they are not based in reality. Distinguishing OCD patients with insight from those with schizophrenia is typically straightforward; however, some OCD patients lose the insight that their obsessions are excessive, blurring the distinction between an obsession and a delusion.

Several clues can clarify the diagnosis. First, hallucinations commonly occur in schizophrenia; they are not associated with OCD, though very strong obsessions are sometimes described as voices or a tape playing in the person's head. Second, even severe cases of OCD do not exhibit the disorganized thinking (e.g., loose associations) of schizophrenia. Finally, the odd rituals of OCD are purposeful; they are intended to alleviate the anxiety created by the obsession. The odd posturing of schizophrenia is generally purposeless.

Impulse Control Disorders. It can be challenging to distinguish the repetitious behaviors of certain impulse control disorders (e.g., kleptomania) from the compulsions of OCD. However, whereas the compulsive behaviors of OCD are ego-dystonic and driven by an obsessional fear, the behaviors associated with the impulse control disorders provide a transient ego-syntonic sense of gratification and are not motivated by an underlying fear.

Tourette's Disorder. The compulsions of OCD in many respects resemble the complex motor tics exhibited by patients with Tourette's disorder. However, although the tics of Tourette's disorder are preceded by an urgency to perform the motor tic, this irresistible urge is distinct from the obsessional fear that drives the compulsive behaviors of OCD.

Somatoform Disorders. Similarities also exist between OCD and certain somatoform disorders. For example, somatic obsessions occurring in OCD resemble hypochondriasis. These can usually be distinguished in that those with OCD have typically experienced other nonsomatic obsessions during the course of their illness and typically engage in classic compulsive behaviors to alleviate, albeit temporarily, their somatic concerns.

In addition, patients with body dysmorphic disorder experience a preoccupation with an imagined defect in appearance that leads to repetitive checking behaviors to assess their appearance. The symptoms of body dysmorphic disorder, essentially equivalent to the obsessions and compulsions of OCD, have led some to propose that the former syndrome is not a distinct disorder but a subtype of the latter. Again, a key distinguishing factor is that OCD will typically have been associated with some other nonsomatic obsession during the course of the illness.

Cluster A Personality Disorders. The obsessions and compulsive rituals of OCD can sometimes resemble the odd behavior of a Cluster A personality disorder. The most helpful difference may be that the rituals of OCD are ego-dystonic while the eccentricity of Cluster A personality disorder tends to be ego-syntonic. Usually, the patient with OCD is aware of the excessive nature of the obsessions and wishes to be rid of them. The Cluster A patient tends to embrace the odd behavior and draw comfort from it.

Obsessive–Compulsive Personality Disorder (OCPD). OCD and OCPD are often confused, though their similarities are not as extensive as their names might suggest. OCD is defined by the distressing presence of ego-dystonic obsessions and compulsions. Conversely, the "obsessionality" of OCPD is not comprised of discrete obsessions and repetitive compulsions but a rigid, perfectionistic character structure that is overattentive to detail to the extent that it becomes difficult to complete tasks. Furthermore, the characteristics of OCPD are ego-syntonic. Nevertheless, features of OCPD are sometimes observed in patients with OCD, with as many as 20% of those with OCD also fulfilling diagnostic criteria for OCPD.

5.4.5 History of Pharmacological Treatment

Clomipramine (Anafranil). Initially described as an effective treatment for OCD in the 1960s, clomipramine would later become the first FDA approved treatment for the disorder. To this day, it remains the best studied, and thereby the gold standard, treatment for OCD. Other TCAs have not proved effective for OCD. Because clomipramine is unique among the TCAs for particularly potent blockade of the serotonin transporter, subsequent theories regarding the neurobiology of OCD have largely emphasized this neurotransmitter system.

The effective dose range for treating OCD is 150–300 mg/day. Side effects associated with clomipramine are similar to or slightly more severe than those observed with other TCAs and are described in more detail in Chapter 3.

Despite its considerable efficacy, clomipramine has given way to the SSRIs as a result of their more favorable side effect and safety profiles. Clomipramine, however, is often used as an augmentation strategy for OCD patients who are partial responders to SSRI therapy. The effectiveness of this approach has not been verified in controlled trials. Furthermore, coadministration of clomipramine with some of the SSRIs can result in potentially dangerous drug interactions.

SSRIs. SSRI antidepressants have also received considerable scrutiny in the treatment of OCD. Fluoxetine, fluvoxamine, paroxetine, and sertraline are all approved by the FDA for the treatment of OCD. Current studies suggest that each of these medications is more effective for OCD when administered at the higher end of the therapeutic dose range, that is, fluoxetine 60–80 mg/day, fluvoxamine 200–300 mg/day, paroxetine 40–60 mg/day, and sertraline 150–200 mg/day. No controlled studies are yet available regarding the use of citalopram or escitalopram for OCD. Refer to Chapter 3 for more information regarding SSRI antidepressants.

Monoamine Oxidase Inhibitors (MAOIs). Controlled trials comparing the MAOI phenelzine to clomipramine or fluoxetine have produced mixed results. Given the limited data regarding any efficacy of MAOIs in the treatment of OCD coupled with their potentially dangerous interactions, we cannot recommend MAOIs in the treatment of OCD until other approaches have been tried.

Atypical Antidepressants. Preliminary open label studies suggested that venlafaxine and trazodone might be effective for OCD. However, controlled studies have not yet been completed for venlafaxine, and a controlled study of trazodone (100–200 mg/day) did not find it an effective treatment for OCD.

Pindolol (Visken). A beta blocker known to potentiate serotonin activity via a distinct action on serotonin autoreceptors, pindolol has been reported in a controlled study to augment SSRI treatment in OCD patients who are partial responders. Pindolol is administered at a dose of 2.5 mg three times daily. It is generally well tolerated but low blood pressure, dizziness, and sedation can occur.

Lithium. Known to increase serotonergic neurotransmission during antidepressant treatment, lithium has also been tested as an augmentation strategy for OCD. Although preliminary open label trials were promising, a subsequent controlled study demonstrated no benefit of lithium augmentation in SSRI-treated OCD patients. Refer to Chapter 3 for more information regarding lithium.

Buspirone (Buspar). Studies of buspirone augmentation for OCD have produced conflicting results. It remains a common augmentation strategy for the disorder.

Started at 15–20 mg/day, the ultimate therapeutic range is 30–60 mg/day administered in two to three divided daily doses. Refer to Section 5.1.4 for more information regarding buspirone.

L-Tryptophan. Open label studies suggest that tryptophan, the amino acid precursor to serotonin, administered at 500–2000 mg/day, may be effective for OCD. This has not been tested in controlled studies. Furthermore, the clinical utility of tryptophan supplementation has been limited by the association of one batch of tryptophan with the eosinophilia myalgia syndrome. Therefore, we cannot recommend the routine use of tryptophan supplementation for OCD.

Benzodiazepines. Although a cornerstone of anxiety disorder pharmacotherapy, in general, there is surprising little data regarding benzodiazepine therapy for OCD. Controlled studies of clonazepam have produced mixed results. Consequently, benzodiazepines are seldom used in the treatment of OCD.

Triiodothyronine (Cytomel). A reportedly effective augmentation strategy for major depression, though two recent studies are negative, a controlled study for OCD, utilizing a daily dose of 25–50 μg, did not find triiodothyronine to be effective.

Antipsychotics. It was recognized some years ago that high potency typical antipsychotics, that is, haloperidol (Haldol) and pimozide (Orap), were effective in treating OCD patients who had a comorbid tic disorder. The efficacy of these agents, however, is primarily in reducing the tics rather than the core symptoms of OCD.

More recently, trials of atypical antipsychotics for OCD have largely been instigated by the realization that they, at least in part, act by modulating serotonergic activity. In addition, some have argued that the quasipsychotic state of OCD patients with poor insight might warrant antipsychotic therapy in any event. The earliest such studies, including one controlled trial, revealed that risperidone (Risperdal), administered at 2–4 mg/day in two daily doses, is an effective augmentation therapy for those with OCD who are partial responders to SSRI therapy. Similarly, a controlled augmentation study of olanzapine (Zyprexa), 5–20 mg/day, found it to be effective. Controlled augmentation trials of quetiapine (Seroquel) and ziprasidone (Geodon) are currently underway.

Psychosurgery. Numerous brain procedures, which can now be performed in a much less invasive manner via techniques such as the gamma knife, can be beneficial for patients who are resistant to all other forms of treatment.

5.4.6 Current Approach to Treatment

Acute Phase Treatment. There is considerable-evidence that cognitive-behavioral therapy (CBT) is effective in the treatment of OCD. Some studies have even suggested that CBT may provide enduring prophylactic benefit against OCD recurrence. Consequently, we strongly encourage inclusion of CBT in any treatment program for OCD.

Psychotherapy often produces symptomatic improvement but incomplete resolution of OCD, necessitating pharmacotherapy. The first-line agent for OCD is a SSRI. When treating OCD, SSRIs are initiated at a low dose that is approximately one-half the starting dose for depression; however, successful treatment for OCD usually requires that the dose be gradually titrated to or even above the higher reaches of the particular SSRI's therapeutic dose range. A full treatment response might not be expected until 8–12 weeks or often longer after treatment initiation.

In the event that the initial SSRI provides an unsatisfactory treatment response, preferred alternatives include (1) switching to another SSRI, (2) switching to venlafaxine or duloxetine, or (3) switching to clomipramine. Despite limited data to date regarding their efficacy, SNRIs are included as alternatives prior to considering clomipramine due to their more favorable safety and side effect profiles.

When a satisfactory therapeutic response cannot be achieved with any single agent in conjunction with concomitant psychotherapy, augmentation strategies warrant consideration. Preferred augmentation strategies include (1) an atypical antipsychotic (risperidone, olanzapine), (2) clomipramine, (3) buspirone, and (4) pindolol.

When other alternatives have failed, psychosurgical procedures, conducted at a few specialty centers in the United States, may warrant consideration for severe, intractable OCD.

Maintenance Phase Treatment. OCD is typically a lifelong disorder that rapidly recurs when treatment is discontinued. Consequently, maintenance therapy lasting at least 1–2 years is recommended for all patients with OCD. During medication discontinuation, periodic CBT sessions are commonly used to increase the likelihood of sustained remission. Long-term pharmacotherapy is recommended after only two moderately severe episodes of OCD.

5.5 SOCIAL ANXIETY DISORDER (SOCIAL PHOBIA)

5.5.1 Brief Description and Diagnostic Criteria

There is something distinctly human about social anxiety. Mark Twain once remarked, "Man is the only animal that blushes—or needs to." Although there are other mammalian species with complex social pecking orders, we, as humans, are particularly sensitive to how we are perceived by others. This sensitivity, when marked by a fear of evaluation by others, can become maladaptive. If that fear is transient and leads to little or no avoidance of social interactions, then it is considered normal shyness. However, when the social consequences of that fear become more pronounced, then the diagnosis of social phobia, now more commonly referred to as social anxiety disorder, is warranted.

DSM-IV defines social anxiety disorder as an excessive fear of scrutiny by others in social situations. Refer to Table 5.9 for the diagnostic criteria for social anxiety

TABLE 5.9. Diagnostic Criteria for Social Anxiety Disorder

A. Fear of being embarrassed while being watched by others.
B. Almost always becomes anxious in the feared social situation.
C. Realizes that this fear is unreasonable.
D. Avoids social situations that cause anxiety or at least endures them with considerable distress.
E. The fear interferes with normal daily function.
F. If under 18 years old, the symptoms must have lasted at least 6 months.
G. Not due to a medicine, an illicit drug, or a medical illness.
H. Not due to embarrassment about the symptoms of another medical or mental illness.

Source: Adapted from DSM-IV.

disorder. Commonly feared situations include public speaking, meeting strangers, attending large social gatherings, eating in public, or even writing in public.

There are two generally accepted diagnostic subtypes: specific and generalized. The specific subtype applies when the anxiety is only engendered by one or two social situations, most commonly, public speaking. When the anxiety is present in most social situations, then the generalized type specifier applies. Only the generalized diagnostic specifier is included in DSM-IV.

5.5.2 Prevalence and Risk Factors

Recent evidence now indicates that social anxiety disorder, long overlooked in both routine clinical practice and the scientific literature, might be the third most common psychiatric syndrome, after major depression and alcohol dependence, with a lifetime prevalence of over 13%. Social anxiety disorder is only slightly more common among women than men.

The etiology of social anxiety remains unclear; however, evidence suggests that developmental and genetic factors may predispose some individuals to social anxiety disorder. Adults with social anxiety disorder are more likely to report a history of childhood shyness and separation anxiety, limited social interaction during adolescence, and having had parents who placed great emphasis on the importance of the opinion of others.

5.5.3 Presentation and Clinical Course

Historically, few people with social anxiety disorder have sought treatment. Because the symptoms of the disorder can be confused with normal shyness, many could simply be unaware of the presence of the disorder. Others might recognize that they have the disorder but remain reluctant to seek treatment because that would require them to endure an anxiety-provoking social encounter with a health care professional.

Patients with social anxiety disorder often come to clinical attention as a result of other frequent comorbid illnesses. In particular, those with social anxiety disorder commonly present for treatment of depression or an alcohol use disorder. The onset of the social anxiety disorder usually predates that of the comorbid condition and might contribute to the development of the second disorder. Screening for social anxiety disorder should always be conducted for patients with (1) depression, (2) alcohol or other substance abuse, (3) a history of childhood anxiety, or (4) complaints of anxiety-related physical symptoms such as tremor, blushing, or sweating, difficulty eating in public, or using public restrooms.

Social anxiety disorder usually begins during adolescence, though it is commonly preceded by a history of childhood anxiety. It may begin insidiously or abruptly in the immediate aftermath of a particularly humiliating experience. Social anxiety disorder is typically a persistent, lifelong illness, though symptom severity may vary over time. The illness can appear to lie dormant for a period of time only to reemerge when social demands change, for example, promotion to a new job that requires public speaking.

The often overlooked functional disability associated with social anxiety disorder underscores the importance of identifying and treating it. Adults with social anxiety disorder are more likely to have never married and to be living with their parents. They are generally less educated and have lower incomes. As previously mentioned, they are more likely to suffer from depression or abuse alcohol, and they are also at increased risk for suicidal behavior.

5.5.4 Initial Evaluation and Differential Diagnosis

Because few patients with social anxiety present seeking treatment for that disorder, the first task in the evaluation is to include social anxiety disorder in the differential diagnosis when interviewing the patient. We recommend that a screening for social anxiety should be performed for all patients presenting with depression, alcohol abuse, or anxiety-related physical symptoms. This screening can be very brief. It is important to ask, "Do you get more anxious than most people during public speaking? What about when you're meeting strangers?" Those who respond negatively to these two questions are very unlikely to fulfill criteria for social anxiety disorder. Having completed this screening, differential diagnoses can now be ruled out.

Normal Introversion. As previously noted, normal shyness exists on a severity continuum with social anxiety disorder. The social anxiety experienced by normal introverts is transient and does not lead to avoidance of important social interactions or having to endure such encounters with tremendous discomfort though some degree of discomfort is often present. Among those with social anxiety disorder, these symptoms are more severe and/or persistent, and they by definition interfere with social or occupation functioning.

Agoraphobia. Patients with agoraphobia, like those with social anxiety disorder, typically avoid large social gatherings. The distinction lies in the underlying reason. Those with social anxiety disorder specifically wish to avoid being watched and scrutinized by others. Agoraphobic patients do not so much fear being watched by others, as they fear being trapped in a situation from which escape will be difficult or embarrassing.

Major Depressive Disorder (MDD) with Atypical Features. The anhedonia of MDD is often manifested by social withdrawal. In contrast to social anxiety disorder, the social withdrawal of MDD is desired by the patient, at least during the major depressive episode, and does not persist when the episode remits. Atypical depression is characterized by another symptom reminiscent of social anxiety disorder—a longstanding pattern of sensitivity to interpersonal rejection. The interpersonal sensitivity associated with atypical depression is often characterized by stormy relationships and overly emotional responses to perceived slights. Such social lability is seldom observed in patients with social anxiety disorder.

Cluster A Personality Disorders. These personality disorders, especially schizoid personality disorder, share the tendency toward social withdrawal and isolation observed among those with social anxiety disorder. However, whereas patients with social anxiety disorder are greatly troubled by the fact that they feel very uncomfortable around others, those with schizoid personality disorder are indifferent to their social isolation. They prefer it that way. Those with schizotypal personality disorder are in a more intermediate position, feeling anxious around others and perhaps wanting more friends, but finding it easy to withdraw into a life of isolated fantasy.

Avoidant Personality Disorder (APD). APD is virtually indistinguishable from the generalized subtype of social anxiety disorder. APD is typically diagnosed when the social inhibition pervades almost all social interaction and has been present since childhood. Some have suggested that it is, in fact, the most severe manifestation of generalized social anxiety disorder and does not warrant inclusion as a separate diagnostic entity.

5.5.5 History of Pharmacological Treatment

Although social anxiety disorder garnered little attention in the psychiatric literature until the past decade, remarkable strides have been made in its treatment. Cognitive-behavioral therapies, both individual therapy (CBT) and group therapy (CBGT), are important tools in the treatment of social anxiety disorder. These treatments incorporate relaxation training, cognitive restructuring of negative thoughts, and graduated exposure including both in-session role playing exercises and intersession homework exercises confronting the fear inducing situations in real life.

Poorer responses to psychotherapy can be expected for those with more severe symptoms or the generalized subtype of social anxiety disorder, those who are poorly compliant with homework assignments, and those who enter therapy with little expectation of benefit. Furthermore, psychotherapy may not be readily available for all patients. Consequently, treatment with medications is commonly recommended.

Beta Blockers. Most often used to treat hypertension, beta blockers also alleviate many of the readily visible physical (i.e., autonomic) symptoms of anxiety. Namely, these medications decrease the sweating, palpitations, racing pulse, dry mouth, and tremulousness that can accompany anxiety. Although beta blockers do not remedy the emotional aspects of anxiety, they can circumvent the spiraling anxiety of patients with social phobia who during performance situations become self-conscious of their readily evident physical symptoms.

Both atenolol and propranolol have been used in the treatment of social anxiety disorder. Early reports suggested that atenolol was helpful for both the generalized and specific subtypes, but subsequent studies indicate that regular doses of antidepressants or benzodiazepines are much more effective in the generalized subtype. Beta blockers remain helpful, however, for patients with specific social anxiety whose symptoms are infrequent and predictable, for example, performance anxiety. Doses of 10–40 mg of propranolol or 50–150 mg of atenolol can be administered about 1–2 hours before a scheduled anxiety-provoking event such as a public speaking engagement.

The side effects of beta blockers include decreased blood pressure, dizziness, and sedation. They are also believed by some to worsen symptoms of depression in vulnerable individuals, though how beta blockers such as atenolol that do not enter the brain might do so is not readily understandable. In addition, beta blockers should be avoided in diabetic patients because they may dangerously mask the symptoms of hypoglycemia. Finally, beta blockers should not be taken by patients with emphysema (COPD) or asthma.

It's generally wise to instruct patients to take a test dose of the beta blocker in the safety of their homes before the performance situation, to be certain that they can tolerate any side effects, especially potential dizziness.

The utility of another beta blocker, pindolol, as an augmentation strategy for generalized social anxiety disorder has been assessed in a controlled study. Pindolol was not found to be effective and is not used to treat social anxiety disorder. It bears noting that the theoretical basis for utilizing pindolol in this manner was not due to its beta receptor blocking activity but because it potentiates serotonergic activity through an action on serotonin autoreceptors.

Benzodiazepines. The best studied of the benzodiazepines for social anxiety disorder, clonazepam has been demonstrated in controlled trials to be effective during both acute treatment (at an average dose of 2.4 mg/day) and long-term maintenance therapy lasting up to 2 years. A controlled study of another high potency benzodiazepine, alprazolam, also proved effective, though it was outperformed by the MAOI antidepressant phenelzine and exhibited response rates lower than those reported with clonazepam.

Benzodiazepines offer several advantages over alternative treatments. They act quickly, can be dose-adjusted in an expeditious manner, and can be administered both in scheduled doses and on an as-needed basis. Despite their rapid action, however, one controlled study of clonazepam showed that some patients did not experience a satisfactory treatment response for 6–8 weeks. One important limitation is that benzodiazepines are not effective in the treatment of depression, a frequent comorbidity for those with social anxiety disorder. They are also associated with concerns regarding dependence liability and potential addiction in addition to troublesome side effects such as sedation and poor motor coordination. Refer to Section 5.1.4 for more information.

Clonazepam should initially be administered at 0.25–1 mg/day and titrated every 3–7 days to an effective dose of 0.5–4 mg/day in one to two daily doses. Shorter-acting alprazolam is initiated at 0.5–1 mg/day in two to four divided daily doses and titrated to 1–8 mg/day in two to four divided daily doses. The extended release formulation of alprazolam permits less frequent dose administration. Initiating the benzodiazepines at a low dose and titrating in a stepwise fashion minimizes the potential for excessive sedation during treatment initiation.

Monoamine Oxidase Inhibitors (MAOIs). Many, though not all, antidepressants are effective treatments for social anxiety disorder. Although they do not provide rapid symptom relief and may even transiently worsen anxiety symptoms during the first 1–2 weeks of treatment, antidepressants have the advantage of treating comorbid depression.

Early controlled studies demonstrated the effectiveness of irreversible MAOIs, particularly phenelzine and tranylcypromine, for generalized social anxiety disorder. Prior to the advent of the SSRIs, MAOIs were considered the gold standard treatment for social anxiety disorder. The best studied of the MAOIs, phenelzine, has proved superior to both beta blockers and the benzodiazepine alprazolam in treating generalized social anxiety disorder.

Phenelzine therapy is initiated at a dose of 15 mg/day. The daily dose can be increased in 15 mg increments on a weekly basis until a therapeutic dose of 45–90 mg/day is attained. Tranylcypromine doses are titrated in a similar fashion. Started at 10 mg/day, the daily dose of tranylcypromine can be increased each week by 10 mg/day until a therapeutic dose of 30–40 mg/day is achieved.

Although the MAOIs are highly effective, their usefulness is limited by their potential for dangerous interactions with certain medications and foods. Please refer to Chapter 3 for a more complete discussion of MAOIs.

The so-called reversible MAOIs, moclobemide and brofaromine, appear to obviate these problematic interactions, though the latter was never approved and the former is not available in the United States. Controlled studies of these agents in the treatment of social anxiety disorder have produced mixed results.

Tricyclic Antidepressants (TCAs). There has been surprisingly little study of TCAs in the treatment of social anxiety disorder. Early trials with imipramine and clomipramine suggested they might be beneficial; however, subsequent controlled studies indicate that TCAs are no more effective than placebo. Consequently, they are not used to treat social anxiety disorder.

SSRIs and SNRIs. The introduction of the SSRIs and SNRIs has provided treatments for social anxiety disorder that are not only equally effective but safer and more tolerable than their counterparts. At present, paroxetine, sertraline and venlafaxine ER have been approved by the FDA in the treatment of social anxiety disorder. Other SSRIs are also effective treatments as shown by a combination of controlled and open label studies. Open label studies indicate that fluoxetine and citalopram are also likely to be effective for social anxiety disorder.

Current studies indicate that considerable dosing flexibility is required when using a SSRI/SNRI to treat social anxiety disorder. Many patients respond at the lower end of the therapeutic range at doses that are comparable to those used for MDD; however, a substantial number of patients will only experience a satisfactory response at the higher end of the published therapeutic range. Nevertheless, a low initial dose and a slow titration schedule is recommended when treating social anxiety disorder, as with other anxiety disorders, due to the possibility that aggressive SSRI/SNRI dosing can transiently worsen anxiety during the initial phase of treatment. Please refer to Chapter 3 for a more extensive discussion of the SSRI/SNRI antidepressants.

Atypical Antidepressants. Initial open label studies of nefazodone and mirtazapine have been conducted and offer promise, though one negative controlled study with the former has been reported. Further studies are needed.

Buspirone. Although initial open label results were promising, a controlled study of buspirone, approved by the FDA for treatment of GAD, failed to demonstrate any effectiveness in the treatment of social anxiety disorder. However, a subsequent controlled study indicated that buspirone administered at 30–60 mg/day is an effective augmentation strategy for patients with social anxiety disorder who have only experienced a partial response to SSRI therapy.

Buspirone therapy is typically initiated at 15–20 mg/day, administered either as a regimen of 5 mg taken three times each day or 10 mg taken twice daily. The target dose range is 30–60 mg/day. The maximal daily dose of 60 mg can be administered either as 20 mg taken three times daily or 30 mg taken twice daily.

Other Medications. There has been limited study of other nonbenzodiazepine agents that act by increasing GABA activity by any of several mechanisms. Please refer to Section 5.1.4 for more information regarding these agents.

A single controlled study of gabapentin demonstrated modest effectiveness. A high gabapentin dose, 3600 mg/day, was required to achieve this modest degree of success. Similarly, high dose pregabalin (600 mg/day) was effective in a recent controlled study for social anxiety disorder.

A recent open label retrospective report indicates that tiagabine, which acts by blocking GABA reuptake, might be an effective augmentation strategy for patients who are only partially responsive to antidepressant therapy.

Psychosurgery. Case series have been reported of patients with severe treatment resistant social anxiety disorder undergoing surgical procedures including capsulotomy and endoscopic transthoracic sympathectomy. Given the limited evidence for the effectiveness of these interventions in conjunction with the significant associated surgical risk, we cannot recommend such procedures, though they would understandably warrant consideration by those patients who are especially disabled by the disorder and who have not responded to either psychotherapy or pharmacotherapy.

5.5.6 Current Approach to Treatment

Specific Social Anxiety Disorder, Acute Phase Treatment. Different strategies have evolved for treating specific social anxiety disorder versus generalized social anxiety disorder. Less complicated is the management of the specific subtype. Exposure-based psychotherapy is a mainstay of treatment, and as-needed medication doses prior to scheduled performances are also widely used. Preferred agents for performance anxiety are alprazolam or propranolol.

Generalized Social Anxiety Disorder, Acute Phase Treatment. CBT is also important in the treatment of generalized social anxiety disorder. Far more complex is the management of pharmacotherapy for generalized social anxiety disorder. Initial treatment should be guided by the severity of the social anxiety and the presence of any comorbid illnesses, particularly major depression. For the majority of patients, SSRIs particularly paroxetine or sertraline, or the SNRI venlafaxine ER, all FDA approved for social anxiety disorder, are the treatment of choice. As previously noted, when treating an anxiety disorder, the starting dose should be approximately one-half that used when starting treatment for depression. The dose is then titrated as tolerated every 5–7 days. Considerable attention must be paid to dose titration as many, though not all, patients with social anxiety disorder will not respond until receiving higher doses.

The long-acting benzodiazepine clonazepam can be used as a first-line agent for those patients with particularly severe symptoms who are unable or unwilling to wait for the delayed therapeutic benefit of an antidepressant. Clonazepam can be initiated as a monotherapy for those without comorbid depression or in conjunction with an antidepressant for those who are also depressed. In the latter case, clonazepam can be used transiently with a plan to taper and discontinue it once sufficient time has elapsed to experience benefit from antidepressant therapy.

Generalized Social Anxiety Disorder, Treatment Resistance. A significant minority of patients will not experience a satisfactory treatment response to antidepressant therapy, even after a trial of adequate duration at full strength doses. For those with comorbid depression who are experiencing no benefit from SSRI treatment for either the anxiety or depression, then switching treatment is advisable. The options include switching to another SSRI, a SNRI (venlafaxine or perhaps duloxetine), or, when other alternatives fail, phenelzine.

Other alternatives are available for those with comorbid depression who are experiencing a satisfactory antidepressant response but whose anxiety is not satisfactorily improving. Switching to another SSRI or venlafaxine, which preserves the monotherapy, can still be considered, but we recommend an augmentation strategy before resorting to phenelzine therapy. The principal augmentation strategy in this context is to add the long-acting benzodiazepine clonazepam. In the event that clonazepam is unhelpful, poorly tolerated, or to be avoided due to a history of substance abuse, alternative augmentation strategies with controlled evidence supporting their efficacy include buspirone, gabapentin, or pregabalin. If the residual anxiety to be addressed by the augmentation treatment is mild-to-moderate in severity, then we recommend buspirone. For more severe residual anxiety, we prefer pregabalin.

Generalized Social Anxiety Disorder, Maintenance Phase Treatment. There has been little formal study of maintenance therapy for social anxiety disorder. Limited data indicates that continued pharmacotherapy provides significant prophylactic protection against relapse. Furthermore, growing evidence indicates that patients with social anxiety disorder experience a high rate of relapse after treatment discontinuation. CBT, however, may afford continued prophylactic benefit long after conclusion of the therapy, though the data to support this contention is limited.

The conventional recommendation is to continue pharmacotherapy for at least 9–12 months after achieving remission. Medication might then be tapered slowly over several weeks, if not months. In the event of relapse after discontinuation of maintenance therapy, long-term therapy is advised.

5.6 POST-TRAUMATIC STRESS DISORDER

5.6.1 Brief Description and Diagnostic Criteria

Previously known by a variety of combat-related colloquialisms such as shell shock, war neurosis, and battle fatigue, post-traumatic stress disorder's (PTSD) inclusion in DSM-III produced considerable controversy. Some contended that PTSD so overlaps other anxiety and mood disorders that it is superfluous to psychiatric nosology. There were even implications that political pressures in the aftermath of the Vietnam War unduly contributed to its inclusion in DSM-III. Others debated whether PTSD belongs among the anxiety disorders, the mood disorders, or a unique class of stress response disorders. Ironically, emerging data regarding the neurobiology of PTSD not only supports its validity as a psychiatric disorder but might ultimately clarify its place within the larger diagnostic classification scheme.

The DSM-IV diagnostic criteria for PTSD (cf. Table 5.10) requires that the patient has been exposed to a traumatic stressor. In this context, the concept of traumatic stress is specifically defined as an event involving actual or threatened death or serious injury, or a threat to physical integrity. Such traumatic events include sexual abuse (e.g., rape, molestation), life-threatening accidents, interpersonal violence, natural disasters, and combat.

The symptoms of PTSD are grouped into three symptom clusters: (1) reexperiencing symptoms, (2) avoidance/numbing symptoms, and (3) hyperarousal symptoms. To fulfill the diagnostic criteria for PTSD, these symptoms must have persisted

TABLE 5.10. Diagnostic Criteria for Post-traumatic Stress Disorder

A. Has been exposed to a traumatic event in which both of the following occurred:
   1. Experienced a death, serious injury, or a threat to the physical integrity of self or someone else
   2. Felt helpless, horrified, and/or intensely afraid at the time of the trauma
B. Keeps reexperiencing the trauma in at least one of the following ways:
   1. Intrusive and unwanted thoughts about the trauma
   2. Nightmares about the trauma
   3. Flashbacks in which it seems as if the trauma is happening again
   4. Becoming very upset when reminded about the trauma
   5. Developing physical symptoms of anxiety when reminded about the trauma
C. Avoids reminders of the trauma in at least three of the following ways:
   1. Tries not to think or talk about the trauma
   2. Avoids people or places that trigger memories of the trauma
   3. Cannot remember parts of what happened when the trauma occurred
   4. Not interested in taking part in major activities
   5. Avoids becoming emotionally close to others
   6. Cannot have loving feelings
   7. Doesn't expect much of a future (no career, no marriage, no children, short life span)
D. Has at least two of the following persistent symptoms of heightened arousal:
   1. Insomnia
   2. Irritability or angry outbursts
   3. Poor concentration
   4. On guard all the time
   5. Startles easily
E. Symptoms last more than 1 month.
F. Causes significant distress or loss of function.

Source: Adapted from DSM-IV.

for at least 1 month and caused considerable functional impairment. The disorder is termed "acute" if the symptoms have lasted 1–3 months. It is considered "chronic" when the symptoms have persisted for more than 3 months.

5.6.2 Prevalence and Risk Factors

Trauma is unfortunately and remarkably common in the modern world. At least 40% of adults in the United States have been exposed to a traumatic life event. The prevalence of PTSD is also considerably higher than typically assumed with an overall lifetime rate in the United States of approximately 8%.

Certain individuals are especially likely to experience, or to have already experienced, a traumatic event. Trauma exposure is more likely among military personnel or those working in emergency services, for example, police officers, firefighters, or emergency medical technicians. In addition, those who have recently emigrated from war zones or regions of civil unrest are likely to have been exposed to a traumatic event.

Identifying who will or will not develop PTSD in the aftermath of a traumatic event is a complex and inexact science requiring consideration of multiple interactive risk factors. Beyond the required exposure to a trauma, the risk factors for PTSD include the characteristics of both the trauma and the individual experiencing the trauma. The probability that PTSD will develop is decided in part by the severity of the trauma as determined by (1) the perceived likelihood that death, serious injury, or some other loss will occur, (2) a greater sense of loss of control during the event, and/or (3) the occurrence of an actual as opposed to only a threatened loss. The risk for developing PTSD is also shaped by qualitative aspects of the trauma. In particular, sexual traumas such as rape or childhood sexual abuse are more likely to lead to the development of PTSD than other traumas such as natural disasters. It has been suggested that vulnerability to PTSD is greater after traumas such as rape because they are more likely to precipitate feelings of humiliation and guilt.

Individual characteristics can determine how a person reacts to a trauma and thereby contribute to the risk for developing PTSD. These include neurosis, limited social support, a family history of an anxiety disorder, and a personal history of previous significant stressors, particularly childhood sexual or physical abuse.

Gender is another important risk factor for PTSD. Although men are more likely to experience a traumatic event, PTSD is at least twice as common among women. This apparent gender discrepancy, however, provides an opportunity to examine the manner in which varied risk factors might interact. The gender difference might be explained, at least in part, by the nature of the traumatic stressors that are more likely to be experienced by women. In particular, women are disproportionately victimized by sexual traumas, such as rape or childhood sexual abuse. Sexual traumas, in both men and women, are more likely to lead to the development of PTSD than other traumas such as natural disasters.

5.6.3 Presentation and Clinical Course

Patients can present for clinical care either in the immediate aftermath of a trauma or months to years later. Immediately after a trauma, the patient may be seeking medical care for injuries suffered during the traumatic event or psychiatric care for the disturbing emotional symptoms. In addition to physical injury, trauma can produce a variety of emotional sequelae including dissociative symptoms and disorganized behavior. This has led to the inclusion of acute stress disorder in DSM-IV. Such symptoms typically resolve over a few days to weeks; however, some patients will go on to develop PTSD. Less often, the onset of PTSD can be delayed by months or even years from the original traumatic experience. This delayed onset is most likely to arise when a more recent life event, not necessarily a trauma, triggers recall of the prior trauma. For example, a young mother who is a survivor of childhood abuse can suddenly develop symptoms of PTSD when her own children approach the age at which she was victimized.

The course of PTSD is variable. Typical estimates are that 50% of those who develop acute PTSD will ultimately suffer a persistent form of the illness that warrants lifelong treatment. Among those who recover and do not develop chronic PTSD, many remain susceptible to periodic symptomatic exacerbations that can arise in the context of novel stressors.

5.6.4 Initial Evaluation and Differential Diagnosis

With the notable exception of the Veteran's Administration (VA) hospital system, health care providers, both in primary care and mental health care, do a relatively poor job of identifying PTSD. There are two basic steps to diagnosing PTSD: (1) determining that the patient has been exposed to a traumatic event, and (2) determining that the trauma-exposed patient is experiencing symptoms that fulfill diagnostic criteria for the disorder.

In view of the fact that at least 40% of American adults have experienced a traumatic life event, screening for trauma should yield a large number of patients with PTSD. Screening for trauma is typically a straightforward exercise, though it should obviously be conducted with sensitivity.

Once it has been determined that a patient has been exposed to a trauma, the next step is to disentangle the anxiety and mood symptoms of PTSD from those of other syndromes.

Adjustment Disorder. Like PTSD, an adjustment disorder is a maladaptive response to a stressful life event that is characterized by anxiety and mood symptoms. The distinction is that the stressor need not fulfill the DSM-IV criterion for a traumatic event. The adjustment disorder diagnosis is appropriate when (1) symptoms consistent with PTSD occur in the aftermath of a stressful event that does not fulfill the DSM-IV trauma criterion, or (2) the symptomatic criteria for PTSD are not fulfilled after an event that does fulfill the DSM-IV trauma criterion.

Malingering. When eligibility for disability benefits or other financial remuneration is at stake, the possibility that the patient is malingering must be considered.

Panic Disorder. Panic attacks are commonly experienced by patients with PTSD. In addition, the avoidant symptoms of PTSD resemble agoraphobia, and the hyperarousal symptoms of PTSD bear some semblance to certain panic symptoms. The key discriminating factor is that patients with panic disorder will, at some point in the course of the illness, experience spontaneous panic attacks arising in the absence of any traumatic reminder or other precipitating stressor.

Generalized Anxiety Disorder. The symptoms of GAD overlap with certain hyperarousal symptoms of PTSD, such as insomnia and poor concentration. The distinction between GAD and PTSD lies in the object of the worry. Patients with GAD worry about an array of everyday concerns, whereas those with PTSD specifically ruminate about the trauma and events related to the trauma.

Obsessive–Compulsive Disorder. The obsessions of OCD resemble the intrusive thoughts of PTSD. For those with OCD, however, these intrusive thoughts are not limited to recollections of a traumatic event.

Specific Phobia. This diagnosis is appropriate when exposure to a traumatic event leads to a phobic avoidance of some specific reminder of the trauma in the absence of other PTSD symptoms. For example, a survivor of a terrible automobile accident might avoid driving on freeways or traveling in cars altogether. If such avoidance occurs in the absence of other PTSD symptoms, then a specific phobia, rather than PTSD, could indeed be diagnosed.

Major Depressive Disorder. The symptoms of depression can overlap with many of the avoidant/numbing or hyperarousal symptoms of PTSD. For example, those with either disorder can experience insomnia, poor concentration, irritability, diminished interest in activities, or a restricted range of affect. Furthermore, comorbid depression is very common among those with PTSD.

Psychotic Disorders. Patient descriptions of flashback experiences occasionally resemble those of auditory or visual hallucinations. In addition, the numbing and affective restriction of PTSD can resemble the affective flattening of schizophrenia. Finally, some evidence indicates that those with chronic psychotic disorders such as schizophrenia are more vulnerable to trauma, creating the possibility of comorbid PTSD and psychosis. Flashbacks can be distinguished from hallucinations in that the sounds and visions described by a patient with PTSD during a flashback represent a reexperiencing of an earlier traumatic event. The content of the flashback, therefore, is either directly or indirectly tied to the trauma.

Dissociative Disorders. Many of the reexperiencing symptoms of PTSD are, in fact, dissociative phenomena. The numbing symptoms of PTSD also resemble the depersonalization and derealization experienced by those with dissociative disorders. Furthermore, dissociative symptoms are the principal manifestation of acute stress disorder, the predecessor to PTSD that arises in the first month after a trauma. The diagnosis of a dissociative disorder is warranted when dissociative symptoms exceeding the PTSD criteria, (e.g., amnesia or profound identity disturbance) are present.

5.6.5 History of Pharmacological Treatment

PTSD pharmacotherapy has been an area of intense research interest over the past decade. This has been complemented by a plethora of studies regarding the neurobiology of the disorder that may ultimately serve to inform the development and refinement of novel therapies. Pharmacotherapy is used to target one or more of the main PTSD symptom clusters, that is, reexperiencing symptoms, avoidance/numbing symptoms, and hyperarousal symptoms.

Tricyclic Antidepressants (TCAs). Because of their effectiveness not only for depression but for anxiety disorders such as panic disorder as well, TCAs were the first medications formally tested in the treatment of PTSD. Three TCAs, amitriptyline, imipramine, and desipramine, have been studied in small trials, producing modest benefit for reexperiencing and hyperarousal symptoms, without any relief of avoidance/numbing symptoms. Given this limited benefit in conjunction with the side effect burden and potential for toxicity in a suicide prone population, TCAs are infrequently used in the treatment of PTSD. Please refer to Chapter 3 for more information regarding TCAs.

Monoamine Oxidase Inhibitors (MAOIs). Early studies also evaluated the effectiveness of the MAOI phenelzine. Phenelzine, relative to TCAs, provided greater benefit for PTSD; however, its usefulness is limited by its potential for drug and food interactions. A recent open label study suggests that the reversible MAOI moclobemide might be helpful for PTSD. It is not available in the United States.

SSRIs and SNRIs. SSRIs and SNRIs have rapidly emerged as first-line treatments for PTSD. The two best-studied, sertraline and paroxetine, have shown effectiveness in large multisite studies for all three PTSD symptom clusters, obtaining FDA approval for PTSD. Dose ranges for sertraline and paroxetine parallel those used in the treatment of depression. These studies indicate that the PTSD treatment response for SSRIs may lag behind that of depression with benefit becoming evident after 4 weeks and the maximal response requiring 8–12 weeks. Preliminary studies suggest that fluoxetine, citalopram, escitalopram, *and* fluvoxamine might also be effective as treatment for PTSD. Refer to Chapter 3 for more information regarding SSRIs.

An initial controlled study of venlafaxine, a SNRI, indicated that it is as effective as sertraline for overall PTSD symptoms at a mean dose of approximately 225 mg/day.

Atypical Antidepressants. Among the so-called atypical antidepressants, the earliest PTSD studies evaluated nefazodone and trazodone. Open label studies suggest that nefazodone might be helpful for PTSD reexperiencing and hyperarousal symptoms, with particular effectiveness for PTSD-related sleep disturbance. However, recent findings regarding potential toxic effects of nefazodone on liver function have diminished enthusiasm for these agents, and it is unlikely that additional controlled studies of nefazodone will be conducted. Trazodone has not proved particularly helpful for PTSD symptoms, though it is commonly used in conjunction with a SSRI to manage PTSD-related insomnia.

A single controlled PTSD study has also been conducted using mirtazapine, an antidepressant that increases serotonergic and noradrenergic activity by a variety of mechanisms. Mirtazapine outperformed placebo in this study, producing a moderate level of benefit for overall PTSD symptoms.

Finally, a single open label trial of bupropion, a novel antidepressant with an obscure mechanism, found it helpful for depressive symptoms in PTSD patients but largely ineffective for the core symptoms of PTSD itself.

In summary, early evidence indicates that mirtazapine holds promise in the treatment of PTSD, but nefazodone, trazodone, and bupropion offer little benefit.

Benzodiazepines. These agents, particularly alprazolam and clonazepam, have been widely used in the treatment of PTSD, despite little evidence to demonstrate their effectiveness. The few studies exploring the effectiveness of benzodiazepines for PTSD suggest that they provide modest relief for anxiety in general but offer no benefit for the core symptoms of PTSD, namely, intrusive recollections and emotional numbing. Furthermore, a small controlled study investigating prophylactic treatment with a benzodiazepine in the immediate aftermath of trauma exposure failed to protect patients from the subsequent development of PTSD symptoms. Consequently, we do not recommend benzodiazepines for the routine management of PTSD.

Buspirone. A nonbenzodiazepine anxiolytic, buspirone is an effective treatment for generalized anxiety disorder but not other anxiety disorders. There are as yet no published controlled studies of buspirone for PTSD, though a small open label series suggested it might be effective for the core symptoms of PTSD. In the absence of more definitive evidence regarding its effectiveness, we do not routinely use buspirone when treating PTSD.

Blocking Norepinephrine Activity. Studies regarding the biology of PTSD have consistently documented excessive noradrenergic activity. Consequently, it seems reasonable to conclude that medications that interfere with norepinephrine signaling in the central nervous system might be effective in the treatment of PTSD. One such agent, propranolol, which blocks postsynaptic beta adrenergic receptors, has produced mixed results when used in the treatment of chronic PTSD. Some studies, though not all, have reported that propranolol therapy provides modest benefit for the hypervigilance and reexperiencing symptoms of PTSD. More intriguing are reports regarding the administration of propranolol immediately after exposure to a traumatic stressor. Trauma survivors who completed a 10 day course of propranolol (10 mg three times daily) therapy that began within hours after the traumatic event experience less physiological arousal when reminded of the trauma 3 months later.

Other agents, clonidine and guanfacine, reduce norepinephrine activity by reducing its release. Open label studies suggest these agents might be helpful for the impulsivity that often accompanies PTSD, but the lone controlled study did not find guanfacine to be effective.

Antipsychotics. Similar to benzodiazepines, the so-called typical antipsychotics have been widely used in the management of PTSD in the absence of data supporting their utility for the core symptoms of PTSD. Low doses of a high potency antipsychotic such as haloperidol, however, have been reported to alleviate the disorganization that can arise in PTSD patients during periods of acute decompensation. Thus, although haloperidol is not recommended for the long-term management of PTSD, it can be helpful when used as a short-term strategy in low doses of 0.5–2.0 mg/day during acute crises.

In contrast to the typical antipsychotics, early evidence suggests that the newer atypical antipsychotics might be helpful for the core symptoms of PTSD. Although there have been some negative studies, several small controlled studies of olanzapine (5–20 mg/day), quetiapine (25–300 mg/day), and risperidone (0.5–3 mg/day) have demonstrated improvement in PTSD reexperiencing symptoms.

Anticonvulsants. Several antiseizure medicines have been studied in the treatment of PTSD, and some results have been encouraging. Open label studies, first with carbamazepine (800–1200 mg/day) and later with valproate (500–2000 mg/day), demonstrated overall improvement in PTSD patients, though not for intrusive recollections per se. Recent open label studies of gabapentin, lamotrigine, tiagabine, and topiramate have suggested these anticonvulsants might also be helpful for some PTSD symptoms.

Small controlled PTSD studies have now been conducted for valproate, lamotrigine, and tiagabine. The valproate study suggests that it relieves PTSD avoidant symptoms though it did not outperform placebo for PTSD reexperiencing symptoms. The small lamotrigine (50–500 mg/day) and tiagabine (4–16 mg/day) studies indicate that they might be helpful for both reexperiencing and avoidant symptoms.

5.6.6 Current Approach to Treatment

Immediate Aftermath of Trauma. We recommend instituting, whenever possible, a 10 day course of propranolol (10 mg three times daily) within hours of exposure to a severe traumatic stressor. Although the data supporting it remains limited, the brief duration of therapy coupled with the relative tolerability of propranolol supports use of this intervention. This medication therapy should, of course, be implemented in conjunction with appropriate crisis intervention services. Benzodiazepines should be avoided if possible during this critical window of vulnerability.

Acute Phase Treatment. Clinical improvement can be maximized when medication is combined with cognitive-behavioral therapy. SSRIs are the pharmacological mainstay of the initial phase of treatment. Controlled studies support their effectiveness for the core symptoms of PTSD, they are effective for the comorbid depression frequently experienced by those with PTSD, and they are well tolerated and safe. Because SSRIs can transiently exacerbate preexisting anxiety during treatment initiation, the starting dose should be no more than one-half that used when initiating SSRI therapy for depression. The SSRI dose is then titrated upward as tolerated every 5–7 days. Patience is required when treating PTSD because the full response to therapy may require 12 weeks or longer.

Treatment Resistance. Many patients with PTSD remain symptomatic despite antidepressant treatment and psychotherapy. Thus, augmentation strategies are commonly employed when treating PTSD. Although promising data are beginning to emerge with respect to numerous agents from various classes, these data as yet are not sufficient to permit definitive guidelines. At present, the most commonly used augmentation strategies include atypical antipsychotics, buspirone, and certain anticonvulsants.

The nature of the residual symptoms should guide the selection of an augmentation strategy. For example, when the patient continues to experience prominent impulsivity or lability, an atypical antipsychotic or an anticonvulsant/mood stabilizer would be preferred. If depressive symptoms remain evident, then adding a second antidepressant or switching to a different antidepressant is a reasonable option. For residual anxiety of mild-to-moderate severity, buspirone augmentation is a preferred strategy. For severe anxiety, a benzodiazepine can be used, though we prefer to avoid using benzodiazepines when treating PTSD, especially in the acute phase treatment. In the event that a benzodiazepine is chosen, we recommend using a long-acting agent such as clonazepam or extended-release alprazolam. The benzodiazepine should be administered one to two times daily. As-needed benzodiazepine dosing is not recommended as this will tend to undermine the exposure therapy techniques commonly used in PTSD psychotherapy.

ADDITIONAL READING

Blanco C, Antia SX, Liebowitz MR. Pharmacotherapy of social anxiety disorder. *Biol Psychiatry* 2002; 51: 109–120.

Davidson JRT. Long-term treatment and prevention of posttraumatic stress disorder. *J Clin Psychiatry* 2004; 65(Supplement 1): 44–48.

Dougherty DD, Rauch SL, Jenike MA. Pharmacotherapy for obsessive-compulsive disorder. *J Clin Psychol* 2004; 60: 1195–1202.

Dunner DL. Management of anxiety disorders: the added challenge of comorbidity. *Depress Anx* 2001; 13: 57–71.

Eddy KT, Dutra L, Bradley R, et al. A multidimensional meta-analysis of psychotherapy and pharmacotherapy for obsessive–compulsive disorder. *Clin Psychol Rev* 2004; 24: 1011–1030.

Goodman WK. Selecting pharmacotherapy for generalized anxiety disorder. *J Clin Psychiatry* 2004; 65(Supplement 13): 8–13.

Gorman JM. Treating generalized anxiety disorder. *J Clin Psychiatry* 2003; 64 (Supplement 2): 24–29.

Greist JH, Bandelow B, Hollander E, et al. Long-term treatment of obsessive–compulsive disorder in adults. *CNS Spectr* 2003; 8(Supplement 1): 7–16.

Hidalgo RB, Davidson JRT. Diagnostic and psychopharmacologic aspects of posttraumatic stress disorder. *Psychiatr Ann* 2004; 34: 834–844.

Hollander E, Bienstock CA, Koran LM, et al. Refractory obsessive–compulsive disorder: state-of-the-art treatment. *J Clin Psychiatry* 2002; 63(Supplement 6): 20–29.

Husted DS, Shapira NA. A review of the treatment for refractory obsessive–compulsive disorder: from medicine to deep brain stimulation. *CNS Spectr* 2004; 9: 833–847.

Nemeroff CB. Anxiolytics: past, present, and future agents. *J Clin Psychiatry* 2003; 64 (Supplement 3): 3–6.

Nemeroff CB. The role of GABA in the pathophysiology and treatment of anxiety disorders. *Psychopharmacol Bull* 2003; 37: 133–146.

Pollack MH, Allgulander C, Bandelow B, et al. WCA recommendations for the long-term treatment of panic disorder. *CNS Spectr* 2003; 8(Supplement 1): 17–30.

Rickels K, Rynn M. Pharmacotherapy of generalized anxiety disorder. *J Clin Psychiatry* 2002; 63(Supplement 14): 9–16.

Rynn MA, Brawman-Mintzer O. Generalized anxiety disorder: acute and chronic treatment. *CNS Spectr* 2004; 9: 716–723.

Schoenfeld FB, Marmar CR, Neylan TC. Current concepts in pharmacotherapy for post-traumatic stress disorder. *Psychiatr Serv* 2004; 55: 519–531.

Sheehan DV. The management of panic disorder. *J Clin Psychiatry* 2002; 63(Supplement 14): 17–21.

Slaap BR, den Boer JA. The prediction of nonresponse to pharmacotherapy in panic disorder: a review. *Depress Anx* 2001; 14: 112–122.

Stevens JC, Pollack MH. Benzodiazepines in clinical practice: consideration of their long-term use and alternative agents. *J Clin Psychiatry* 2005; 66(Supplement 2): 21–27.

Van Ameringen M, Mancini C, Pipe B, et al. Optimizing treatment in social phobia: a review of treatment resistance. *CNS Spectr* 2004; 9: 753–762.

6

SUBSTANCE USE DISORDERS

6.1 INTRODUCTION

6.1.1 The Illness Model of Substance Abuse

Substance abuse as an illness remains a controversial topic in society. Some perceive substance abuse or dependence as a criminal activity or a character deficit and, moreover, believe that its treatment legitimizes or absolves abusers of responsibility for their actions. We strongly disagree with such views.

A number of chronic conditions such as high blood pressure or diabetes bear certain similarities to substance use disorders. These illnesses produce a variety of physical symptoms that, if left untreated, can result in significant medical complications and even death. Complications of uncontrolled diabetes include blindness, kidney failure, neuropathies, and limb amputation. Similarly, inadequately controlled hypertension is a risk factor for stroke, heart attack, and other serious complications. Recognizing that these are diseases does not relieve the patient of responsibility; indeed, the knowledge that one has such an illness imposes significant responsibility. For example, knowing the likely outcome of uncontrolled diabetes is hopefully an impetus for the diabetic to exercise, take medication, and

Principles of Psychopharmacology for Mental Health Professionals
By Jeffrey E. Kelsey, D. Jeffrey Newport, and Charles B. Nemeroff

regularly monitor blood sugars. Patients who take responsibility in this way live longer and relatively healthier lives and decrease the chances of experiencing the worst consequences of the illness. Unfortunately, patients who do not take responsibility for managing their illness are likely to encounter the serious adverse outcomes of poorly controlled diabetes or high blood pressure.

The illness model of substance abuse imposes a similar responsibility. Patients with substance use disorders learn of their genetic predisposition and lifelong vulnerability to relapse. Furthermore, they must learn the measures and strategies to employ in order to maximize continued sobriety and to resist using when craving arises. Like the nonadherent patient with diabetes or hypertension, the substance abuser who does not take responsibility for managing his/her illness is unfortunately likely to succumb to it. Poor insight precipitates relapse, and the serious consequences of untreated addiction include loss of employment, disruption of family life, legal problems, and a host of medical complications.

Does applying the illness model to addiction provide a crutch for the addict? In a word, no. When properly implemented, this model, in fact, readily explains the addict's vulnerability to abusing substances, predicts the course of illness should treatment either be sought out or not, and helps to guide rational therapy decisions that will increase the probability of keeping the illness in remission.

6.1.2 Glossary of Terms

One of the difficulties in discussing substance use disorders is that people from different disciplines use the terminology in a variety of ways, with the end result being considerable confusion. For this reason, we think it is important to review some of the more commonly used terms.

Abuse. We have all heard the terms substance abuse, drug abuse, alcohol abuse, cocaine abuse, and so on. In one sense, any illicit use of a substance is abuse. For example, from the legal point of view, whenever someone smokes crack (even if it is the only time), (s)he has broken the law and abused cocaine. Likewise, if you borrow a prescription sedative or pain reliever from a friend, then you have similarly abused that medication. That is an appropriate use of the term in many cases, but this is not customarily the way that mental health specialists use the term. From our perspective, substance abuse involves a pattern of repeated use over time that results in problems in one or more areas. These include compromised physical health and well-being, legal proceedings, job status, and relationships as well as overall day-to-day functioning.

Dependence. The term dependence has at least two meanings in the context of substance use. First, it can refer to physical (i.e., physiological) dependence. This is a pharmacological property of the drug and is typically a predictable consequence of repeated substance use. Physiological dependence implies either tolerance (more of the drug is required for the previously obtained effect) or the propensity for withdrawal upon discontinuation of the substance. The phenomenon of physical withdrawal contributes to the difficulty many have in halting their substance of abuse. In comparison, when psychiatrists and other mental health professionals refer to dependence, they are instead referring to psychological dependence, a pattern of substance misuse that is even more pervasive than substance abuse. In this context, dependence is often synonymous with the term addiction. This behavior is defined as a continuing use of a substance in the presence of serious adverse consequences (legal, medical, social, occupational) that are becoming obvious to everyone including the addict.

It is important to recognize that someone can be physically dependent on a substance but not addicted; that is, (s)he would not meet the psychiatric definition of substance dependence. On the other hand, someone can be psychologically dependent but yet not physically dependent.

Let's use the cancer patient as an example. Cancer patients often have intractable pain and need strong pain-relieving medication. They may require high doses of narcotic analgesics such as morphine to control their severe pain. The overwhelming majority of cancer patients use their pain medication appropriately. They take it as prescribed and only to relieve their severe pain. They do not go to extreme measures (such as doctor-shopping or prescription-forging) to obtain medication. Such a patient in no way meets criteria for a substance use disorder. Nevertheless, they can become physically dependent on the pain medication. Tolerance not uncommonly develops such that it requires higher doses to achieve the same degree of pain relief. Were the narcotic analgesic to be discontinued abruptly, there would almost certainly be an unpleasant withdrawal syndrome. But being physically dependent does not mean that the cancer patient is addicted. When the cancer is brought into remission and the need for pain medication ceases, the medication can safely be tapered and in all likelihood the patient will not experience cravings for the analgesic. Clearly, this is a case where a patient is physically dependent on a medication but is not psychologically dependent on it. Addiction therefore implies that there is an element of abuse present. Another example are benzodiazepines such as alprazolam (Xanax) and clonazepam (Klonopin). They are quite effective in the treatment of certain anxiety disorders such as panic disorder, social anxiety disorder, and generalized anxiety disorder. One of the early, but usually transient, side effects of therapy with benzodiazepines is sedation. Tolerance to sedation quickly develops, but tolerance to the anxiety-reducing properties of the benzodiazepines usually does not develop. Thus, the benzodiazepines can be prescribed to treat anxiety disorders successfully without the patient becoming too sleepy. In contrast, the person who is seeking out benzodiazepines for the sedating effect as a "high" finds that the rapid development of tolerance requires ever escalating doses in order to achieve the desired degree of sedation. These are patients who "lose" their prescriptions, have multiple physicians prescribing for them, or who invariably finish a prescription earlier than it should have been completed. The abuse potential of benzodiazepines unfortunately has led some physicians to be reluctant to prescribe this class of medications even when it is medically appropriate to do so. The predictable development of physiological dependence to benzodiazepines also correctly predicts that when these compounds are discontinued, it should be done in a very gradual fashion.

In contrast, some drugs of abuse produce intense craving and are highly addictive but do not produce physical dependence. The absence of physical dependence indicates the relative lack of physiological withdrawal. This is not synonymous with meaning that discontinuation of these compounds may not be psychologically uncomfortable. Two examples are marijuana and cocaine. One need only look to the recent crack epidemic to see evidence of the way these substances can destroy lives, but they do not produce tolerance or risk of withdrawal to the same extent as alcohol or heroin. As a result, we would say that the daily crack or marijuana user meets the definition of substance dependence but does not exhibit true physical (or physiological) dependence.

6.2 BRIEF DESCRIPTION AND DIAGNOSTIC CRITERIA

In DSM-IV parlance, psychiatric illnesses that result from substance use are called substance-related disorders. Within this broad spectrum are two distinct categories: substance use disorders and substance-induced disorders. The substance use disorders consist of abusive patterns of use that produce a myriad of problems in relationships, employment, medical or physical well-being, and legal matters. There is no predefined amount or frequency of substance use that defines these disorders; instead, they are diagnosed when the consequences of substance use include an adverse impact on other areas of life. As noted earlier, in some instances, substance use disorders lead to physical dependence that is manifested by tolerance and the potential for withdrawal symptoms. When anyone talks about addiction, it is typically substance use disorders to which they refer.

The other category is known as the substance-induced disorders. These illnesses are also caused by a substance but not necessarily from a long-term pattern of abusing it. Nonetheless, patients who do abuse a substance will by definition be at greater risk for experiencing a concomitant substance-induced disorder. The substance-induced disorders include intoxication, withdrawal, substance-induced delirium, substance-induced dementia, substance-induced amnesia, substance-induced psychosis, substance-induced mood disorder, substance-induced anxiety disorder, substance-induced sexual dysfunction, and substance-induced sleep disorder. As we mentioned earlier, substance-induced disorders can sometimes occur after only a single use of the offending substance. This is obviously true of intoxication and can be true of substance-induced psychotic disorder, substance-induced mood disorder, and substance-induced anxiety disorder as well. Other substance-induced disorders such as substance withdrawal and substance-induced dementia tend to occur only after prolonged use and usually only in those who are abusing the substance. In many cases, when a patient with a substance-induced disorder stops using the substance, the substance-induced disorder gradually resolves. This can often occur quickly but may take several days or even weeks for full resolution. In the case of substance-induced dementia, the damage that has been done is often irreversible. Nevertheless, stopping further use of the substance should halt further progression. Sometimes the substance-induced disorder is a consequence of appropriate and required medical treatment. Examples of this include mania or psychosis from steroid administration for the treatment of emphysema or multiple sclerosis and therapy with interferon for hepatitis C or malignant melanoma. The onset of depression associated with interferon therapy is now well recognized and some practitioners recommend prophylactic treatment with antidepressants prior to the initiation of interferon therapy, especially in individuals prone to depression.

In this chapter, we will focus primarily on treatments for the substance use disorders. However, because detoxification during a substance-induced withdrawal is often the first step in treating a substance use disorder, we will discuss withdrawal states to some extent. The substance use disorders include both substance abuse and the more serious substance dependence. Substance abuse consists of a pattern of misuse that causes recurring problems in at least one aspect of life. This can be a failure to fulfill responsibilities at home or work, reckless use of the substance such as drunken driving, repeated substance-related arrests, and ongoing substance use despite resulting problems in family relationships. See Table 6.1 for the diagnostic criteria for substance abuse.

A more pervasive pattern of misuse occurs in substance dependence. This often includes symptoms of physical dependence such as tolerance or withdrawal (although these are not necessary). Other symptoms of substance dependence include spending so much time using or acquiring the substance that other responsibilities and activities are neglected, persistent unsuccessful attempts to cut down or stop using the substance, and progressively increasing use of the substance over time. Table 6.2 lists the diagnostic criteria for substance dependence.

TABLE 6.1. Diagnostic Criteria for Substance Abuse

Misuse of a substance over a 12 month period that causes one of the following problems:

1. Neglecting responsibilities at work, school, or home
2. Using substances in dangerous situations (such as drunken driving)
3. Repeated legal problems due to substance use
4. Repeated substance use in spite of it causing problems in relationships

Source: Adapted from DSM-IV.

TABLE 6.2. Diagnostic Criteria for Substance Dependence

Misuse of a substance over a 12 month period that causes at least three of the following problems:

1. Tolerance requiring more of the substance to produce the same pleasurable effects
2. Withdrawal symptoms when the patient stops taking the substance
3. Using progressively larger amounts of the substance
4. Repeated yet unsuccessful efforts to stop or cut down substance use
5. Spending a lot of time using, obtaining, or recovering from the substance
6. Neglecting work or leisure activities in order to use
7. Continuing to use despite its causing physical or psychological problems

Source: Adapted from DSM-IV.

One important point is that substance dependence is a lifetime diagnosis. Once someone has substance dependence, they will always have it. It may be in a state of remission, but the risk of relapse remains indefinitely. Proper treatment, however, will enable many patients to recover from the devastating consequences of dependence. For this reason, DSM-IV includes diagnostic specifiers for remission. These specifiers describe both how long and to what extent the substance misuse has been in remission. Early remission is arbitrarily attained when substance use has been stopped or curtailed for 1–12 months. Remission is considered sustained when the patient has been abstinent for over 12 months. In addition, remission can be specified as full or partial. Partial remission occurs when some substance dependence symptoms are still present but the full criteria for the illness are no longer met. As a result, the remission specifiers for substance dependence include early full remission, early partial remission, sustained full remission, and sustained partial remission.

When diagnosing a substance use disorder, it is named in accordance with the substance that is being misused. Patients can be said to have alcohol abuse or dependence, cocaine abuse or dependence, opiate abuse or dependence, and so forth. In severe cases when the patient is misusing several substances, (s)he is diagnosed with polysubstance dependence. The complete list of DSM-IV substance use disorders is shown in Table 6.3. Although the diagnostic criteria for the specific substance use disorders are uniform from substance to substance, certain features of the addiction are specific to the substance being misused. The typical age of onset, the course of the disorder, and the treatment of the disorder vary by substance. Nevertheless, many features of substance abuse and substance dependence are similar across substances.

This chapter is organized somewhat differently than previous chapters. Because there are so many aspects of the clinical course and treatment that are common to all substances of abuse, we will first review the features of substance abuse and dependence that are common to all substances. This will include a general description of risk factors, clinical course, evaluation, and treatment recommendations. What follows is a review of treatment recommendations specific to each substance of abuse.

TABLE 6.3. List of Substance Use Disorders Included in DSM-IV

Alcohol Abuse, Alcohol Dependence
Amphetamine Abuse, Amphetamine Dependence
Cannabis Abuse, Cannabis Dependence
Cocaine Abuse, Cocaine Dependence
Hallucinogen Abuse, Hallucinogen Dependence
Inhalant Abuse, Inhalant Dependence
Nicotine Dependence
Opiate Abuse, Opiate Dependence
Phencyclidine Abuse, Phencyclidine Dependence
Sedative/Hypnotic/Anxiolytic Abuse, Sedative/Hypnotic/Anxiolytic Dependence
Polysubstance Dependence

6.3 PREVALENCE AND RISK FACTORS

The prevalence of substance use disorders varies widely from culture to culture. In addition, the rates of abuse within a given culture also tend to change over time. In the United States heroin abuse was epidemic in the 1960s but subsided in the late 1970s and 1980s only to resurface in more recent years. Other drugs such as marijuana and cocaine have seen similar fluctuations over the years. The epidemic of "crack" cocaine in recent years was primarily a result of this new and "more efficient" delivery system for the drug. In general, the faster a substance enters the brain, the higher the abuse potential is. Crack cocaine is smoked and this method of use allows for a more rapid delivery system to the central nervous system than does inhalation of powdered cocaine. The other factors contributing to the abuse of crack cocaine included good affordability per dose and that smoking is easier than injecting as a method of administration. Were one to attempt to develop a compound with the potential to be highly addictive, crack cocaine is about as good a model as one might come up with. These trends of drug use/abuse in large part also depend on fads among drug users. Methamphetamine is the most recent example of emerging drugs of abuse.

Overall, the highest rates of substance use occur during late adolescence and early adulthood. In those who will eventually have a substance use disorder, the pattern of use moves from "experimentation" to overt substance abuse fairly quickly. The more serious problems resulting from substance dependence typically lag behind by 5–10 years, though such behavior can start significantly sooner.

On the whole, substance use disorders are at least twice as common in men, but this discrepancy does vary somewhat from substance to substance. Furthermore, this difference has been disappearing in recent years.

A variety of genetic, psychological, and social factors contribute to the risk for developing a substance use disorder. There is an inherited basis for susceptibility that has been demonstrated repeatedly across a variety of studies. Most of this research has focused on the genetic risk for alcoholism, but inheritance also appears to be a factor in other substance use disorders as well.

Psychological factors also contribute to the risk of developing substance abuse. Patients with depression and/or anxiety disorders are at a higher risk for abusing one or more substances. There are, however, large numbers of patients with these disorders who have minimal risk for substance abuse. Individuals who tend to be thrill seekers or who are prone to agitation and aggression are also at greater risk for abusing substances. While the substance use problems arguably contribute to the propensity for aggression and recklessness, there is evidence that aggressive and reckless traits in substance abusers often date back to childhood and therefore predate the onset of substance use. In fact, the substance use itself may be an attempt to self-medicate these behavioral traits or other psychiatric disorders, and this is a good reason to ask patients with any of the above-mentioned disorders whether or not they have found anything that seems to help. The abuse of substances as an attempt at self-medication must be recognized and addressed if treatment is to be at all successful.

Social factors such as peer pressure at school or work as well as family patterns of substance use can also contribute to the risk. Teenagers who respond to pressure to use "gateway" drugs such as alcohol, tobacco, and marijuana in their early teens are more likely to develop substance dependence disorders than those who refrain from doing so until their late teens.

6.4 PRESENTATION AND CLINICAL COURSE

The first experiences with substance use usually occur in early adolescence about the time of puberty. At this point, it is extremely difficult to determine who will go on to develop a substance use disorder and who will not. With the passage of time, however, teenagers who are headed for trouble involving substances typically become preoccupied with substance use and associate almost exclusively with others who abuse drugs. Family conflicts often arise, school performance suffers, and the teen who is beginning to abuse may become disruptive. In most cases, a full-blown substance use disorder will have developed by the late teens or early twenties.

A crisis often will precipitate presentation for treatment. Relationship issues, job or school difficulties, court mandated treatment, or medical complications are commonly cited reasons to the question: "Why treatment now?" Acute intoxication either currently or at least recently is not uncommon. There may in fact already be evidence of withdrawal by the time the patient is evaluated. This initial visit usually occurs in one of three contexts. First, the patient may realize that (s)he has reached rock bottom. When a crisis leads someone to seek treatment on his/her own, (s)he should be well-motivated, but practitioners must realize that this motivation may be fragile and may not withstand the challenges that lie ahead, and there might be a very narrow window of opportunity to initiate treatment. At other times, a concerned friend, family member, or the police will bring a patient to treatment. Sometimes, this is the result of a so-called intervention in which several loved ones have confronted the substance abuser with the consequences of that substance use. Typical scenarios might involve potential loss of employment or ending of relationships including marriage, child custody, or visitation rights. In these cases, the patient is seeking treatment, but only after considerable coaxing and pressure from others. The patient may be following advice only begrudgingly. Finally, some patients may come seeking help for another problem, but a careful evaluation reveals the presence of substance abuse. Often, these patients have little insight and refuse substance abuse treatment altogether. No matter how the patient presents, his/her dedication to, and motivation for, treatment can be highly variable both between seemingly similar patients and within the same patient simply with the passage of time or changing circumstances. Once treatment begins, craving often sets in and can readily undermine motivation to see the treatment through.

In early adulthood, the first crisis might be sufficient to shake some patients out of a pattern of substance abuse. Maybe they have been fired or failed classes at school due to repeated hangovers. For some, these first problems are sufficient to bring them out of the downward spiral of abusing drugs or alcohol. Others, unfortunately, do not sustain sobriety and go on to develop substance dependence entering the cycle of repeated relapses and remissions.

The dynamics of friendships and family relationships play a key role in the clinical course of substance dependence. When substance use is so prevalent, it may become the foundation on which friendships are built. If drinking or using cocaine is the most rewarding part of one's life, then that person will naturally be surrounded by friends or associates who do likewise. Breaking the cycle of relapse therefore often requires changing the patient's circle of friends and acquaintances, as well as the environments in which (s)he spends time, which are conducive to substance use. As a result, departing a life of substance abuse often leaves a tremendous void in the addict's life. This vacancy has to be filled by other interests, activities, or relationships; otherwise, the substance abuser will soon return to a group of friends who share an interest in getting high together. By contrast, a shared dedication to sobriety is a key component to the success of 12 step groups such as Alcoholics Anonymous and Narcotics Anonymous.

Families may also play an unwitting role in fostering ongoing substance use. This is known as the "enabling phenomenon." As the toll of substance use becomes more apparent, the substance abuser begins to neglect responsibilities both inside the home and outside it. Desperate to preserve their family, spouses, parents, and even children begin to take on responsibilities being neglected by the substance abuser. This is understandable, but it is also ultimately counterproductive. By assuming the substance abuser's obligations, family members allow the drug abuser to avoid facing the consequences of the illness. As a result, the addict is helped or "enabled" to continue using, remaining oblivious to the impact the abuse is having on their loved ones. The patient's substance use then becomes a precious family secret. The secret is closely guarded not just to protect the reputation of the substance abuser but to protect the reputation of the family as well. Again, this may be understandable, but it is ultimately fruitless. Eventually, most families reach a crisis when they recognize that they cannot keep the secret any longer. They are forced to confront the effects that the substance abuse has had on their family. This is an important juncture, because at this point, some substance abusers will recognize that their problem is out of control. This can serve as a final impetus to break the cycle of substance dependence. Many families and relationships that are caught up in the cycle of enabling the substance user will acknowledge significant problems, but quickly rationalize their ongoing actions with an endorsement of the substance users' good qualities when they are not using, or the qualities that were genuinely attractive early on in the relationship prior to the onset of the difficulties substance abuse presented.

The good news is that treatment can have a profound impact on the clinical course of substance dependence. Most patients who have been treated are eventually able to stop their pattern of compulsive misuse. Some abstain altogether while others are able to manage long periods of sobriety with only brief episodes of substance use. Those who are able to maintain periods of sustained abstinence from substance abuse and dependence also find improvement in job performance and social functioning. Those who do the best had little comorbid psychiatric illness, were able to develop new relationships that were not founded on shared drug use, and made consistent use of 12 step groups such as Alcoholics Anonymous. A not insignificant number of patients with substance use disorders may require multiple attempts at treatment before it is successful, so initial failures or relapses should not be seen as an indication to abandon treatment. Rather, repeated failures suggest the need for a rethinking of the overall approach that is being utilized and perhaps a reformulation of the treatment plan.

6.5 INITIAL EVALUATION AND DIFFERENTIAL DIAGNOSIS

The initial evaluation should consist of a comprehensive medical, social, and psychiatric assessment. First and foremost, it is important to have a clear idea of the circumstances that have precipitated the patient's decision to seek treatment. This includes having a good sense as to whether or not treatment was sought on one's own or whether pressure has been applied by others. Having a firm sense of this crisis will be invaluable as treatment proceeds. The initial commitment to treatment can be very tenuous, but having a clear history enables us to remind the patient of the misery that brought him/her into treatment in the first place, and might provide leverage when the commitment to treatment begins to waver.

Both past and present patterns of substance use need to be assessed along with an estimation of how often and how much of the substance is being used. Substance abusers are notorious for underreporting consumption. One favored approach is to inquire about substance use and then ask for an endorsement of substance use starting at a very high level and proceeding downward. In the case of alcohol abuse or dependence, for example, if the patient is drinking beer, one might ask if they can drink two cases of beer a day, then one and a half cases per day, a case a day, and so on. By the time the patient admits to one case of beer per day, they seem relieved to admit to drinking less then the high level of abuse initially suggested. Another item to watch is the unit of use. Should a patient be having only "two" drinks per day, it is important to note the size of each drink, for example, 4 ounces versus 24 ounces! In addition, one needs to know if the patient is mixing the drug of choice with other substances. Consumption is important, but we also need to ask about the social and physical impact of the substance use. This includes asking about legal and employment history, as well as relationships. Using the example of alcohol use, these questions include: Have there been any DUIs (DWIs)? Has the patient ever been fired because of drinking? What about going to work with a hangover? How does the family feel about the substance use?

It is also important to know about comorbid psychiatric disorders. If these are overlooked, treating the substance use disorder becomes significantly more difficult. Recognizing this, most treatment centers have developed dual diagnosis programs to treat those patients who have another major psychiatric illness in addition to a substance use disorder. It may be virtually impossible to discern at first, but the other psychiatric illnesses might either contribute to or be a result of substance use. The social toll of alcoholism alone can trigger a severe clinical depression. However, a severe depression can precipitate alcohol abuse in a misguided attempt to alleviate suffering. It becomes a chicken and egg problem: Which came first, the depression or the drinking? In the short term, answering that question is less important than ensuring that the patient's treatment is comprehensive and addresses all aspects of his/her illness. To focus your treatment on one (i.e., drinking vs. depression) while ignoring the other is almost certainly doomed to failure. Alcohol abuse/dependence is seen at a higher than expected rate in a number of anxiety disorders. It is easy to understand how this might occur. In social anxiety disorder there is a fear of being judged, scrutinized, or embarrassing oneself. In young adults who want to socialize, but find it a painful experience, they might discover that alcohol makes it easier. Without recognizing this attempt at self-treatment, trying to achieve abstinence and prolonged sobriety, in the absence of treatment for the anxiety disorder, becomes an often insurmountable challenge for both the patient and the clinician.

A family and social history is also important. In particular, it is important to assess the family patterns of substance use to know whether or not there is a sustained family history of substance abuse. This will aid not only in identifying genetic risk factors but also in understanding the family setting in which your patient's drug abuse problems arose. Family patterns of relatedness can often unwittingly foster ongoing substance abuse (e.g., "enabling").

Other important components of the initial evaluation include a medical evaluation including both a medical history and physical examination. This can identify medical consequences of substance abuse, such as liver impairment from chronic alcohol abuse or sinus complications from cocaine use, as well as reveal needle tracks from a variety of self-injection sites that might not be readily apparent to casual observation.

Laboratory testing should be used to complete the assessment and includes urine drug screens, as well as general medical screening tests to rule out underlying substance-induced medical illness. The specific tests vary somewhat depending on the substance that is being abused.

Diagnosing substance use disorders is often relatively straightforward. One can typically gather enough information to determine the severity of substance abuse. When conducting this assessment, there are other important differential diagnoses to keep in mind.

Socially Appropriate Use. Who decides how much use is socially appropriate? In some cultural settings, any substance use is inappropriate; conversely in others there may be varying levels of condoned usage. Additional insight can be gleaned from interviewing friends and family members, with the patient's permission. When it becomes clear that the substance use is interfering with the patient's ability to function, the diagnosis of a substance use disorder is warranted.

Medically Appropriate Use. This is not an issue in the assessment of alcohol or illicit drugs, but can be a consideration when there is suspicion of opiate analgesic or benzodiazepine abuse. Abuse of or dependence on these medications can lead to what is often derogatorily described as "drug seeking behavior." The implication is that to specifically request a potentially abuseable medication is, in fact, proof of the abuse. Caution is well advised here. The patient who is in severe pain may ask for pain medication with all the intensity of someone addicted to opiate analgesics, a reflection of the intense suffering that severe pain produces. The patient who has repeated episodes of severe pain, such as is experienced with sickle-cell anemia, might have learned which analgesics work and which ones do not through a difficult course of trial and error. This can be valuable information in the management of the pain and is another argument in favor of continuity of care for many chronic conditions. Obviously, some proportion of patients who request specific medications are abusing them and might already possess numerous prescriptions from multiple providers. Inquiring as to the number of different physicians the person has been seeing, if the patient gives permission to contact those physicians, or if the patient gives permission to contact pharmacies where the prescriptions have been filled can all become important pieces of what is typically a very confusing picture. Certainly, if the patient has been caught forging prescriptions, diagnosis of a substance use disorder is almost always warranted, though it might also be simply for the purpose of selling drugs on the street. All of these factors must be considered in attempting to determine whether a patient has been abusing prescription drugs.

Other Psychiatric Illness. When patients are acutely intoxicated or in withdrawal, they may exhibit symptoms of any of a variety of psychiatric illnesses. Patients actively abusing alcohol may appear depressed or those experiencing alcohol withdrawal may become psychotic. Patients who have been abusing cocaine or other stimulants can appear psychotic, agitated, or anxious while actively abusing these agents and may experience a withdrawal dysphoria that resembles major depressive disorder when they stop. These intense but often short-lived psychiatric side effects of substance intoxication and withdrawal must be separated from any preexisting psychiatric illness. However, this is often easier said than done. There are any number of young adults who have appeared to be in a first psychotic break or first manic episode only to later discover it was a symptom of intoxication with a designer drug such as Ecstasy that is not routinely detected in urine drug screens.

6.6 HISTORY OF TREATMENT

There are a wide variety of medications that have been used to treat substance use disorders. Although medication choices vary to some extent depending on the motivation of the patient and the substance being abused, there are a handful of theoretical bases that are common to all substance abuse treatment. We briefly review some of these theories.

Replacement Therapy. The idea of replacement therapy is to use a substance that is similar to, but less addictive than, the drug that has been abused. The replacement medication is typically derived from the same family as the abused drug and acts pharmacologically in much the same manner. However, a slower speed of onset and longer length of action usually renders the replacement medication less prone to abuse. In addition, its use is closely monitored in a controlled manner.

Replacement medications can help to reduce craving or to lessen withdrawal symptoms. They are frequently used in detoxification protocols and are usually tapered over several weeks and then discontinued. However, in some cases, such as methadone maintenance, the replacement therapy is continued indefinitely. The underlying rationale for maintenance therapy with a replacement medication is that the monitored use of a prescribed addictive medication is preferable to the uncontrolled use of a more highly addictive street drug. For example, the heroin addict in a methadone maintenance program is less prone to committing crimes to support his/her habit or contracting diseases such as HIV infection secondary to sharing needles. Replacement is the strategy implemented when using nicotine patches or gum to assist patients in smoking cessation. The nicotine replacement decreases craving and withdrawal while simultaneously avoiding the behavioral cues associated with the abused substance.

Reward Therapy. A similar (yet nonspecific) approach is to use a medication that stimulates the brain's reward centers. Reward medications usually do not work in quite the same way as the substance of abuse; however, the net effect in the final common pathway (i.e., the reward centers) may be the same. For the most part, these reward centers are activated by either dopamine or endogenous opioid agonists. One common feature of most abused drugs is that they stimulate these reward centers. This lies at the heart of their addictive potential. Some attempts have been made to use medications that activate these reward centers in place of the abused substance. The hypothesis is that the addict will have less intense craving for his/her preferred substance of abuse in the presence of these other agents. This is, of course, a relatively nonspecific approach that could theoretically be used to treat the abuse of many different substances. It has not yet, however, demonstrated any utility in the treatment of substance abuse.

Antikindling Therapy. This approach targets the problem of craving as well. One popular notion is that craving begins in one brain area and then spreads throughout the central nervous system, producing an intense desire to use. This same theory has been applied to both epilepsy and bipolar disorder with success. Consequently, some substance abuse researchers have suggested that the mood stabilizers and anticonvulsants may reduce craving by blocking kindling.

Interference Therapy. This is conceptually the opposite of the replacement and reward therapies. Whereas replacement medications substitute for the abused drug by stimulating the same brain receptors, interference therapies block these receptors. When the substance abuser uses his/her drug of choice, its effects are blocked by the interference medication. As a result, the drug does not produce the same intensity of pleasurable effects. By reducing the pleasurable effects of drug use, the incentive for repeated use should decrease as well.

Aversion Therapy. If interference medications make drug use less pleasurable, aversion medications make drug use extremely uncomfortable. In this approach, substance abusers routinely take a treatment medication. If and when they return to the drug of abuse, the combination of the aversion medication and the abused drug produces unpleasant effects. This can include headache, nausea and vomiting, or a number of other symptoms. Knowing that using the drug of abuse while taking the aversion medication will cause an uncomfortable reaction, repeated substance use is theoretically discouraged. Some substance abusers find comfort in this treatment approach. They will tell you that they are motivated and dedicated to remaining sober but have moments of weakness that they find difficult to resist. They say they can take the aversion medication when they are strong and thinking clearly and that knowing they will get sick will sustain them through moments of temptation. This approach is best exemplified by the treatment of alcoholism with disulfiram (Antabuse).

Dual Diagnosis Therapy. This approach is based on the theory that many addicts (in particular, alcoholics) are abusing drugs in an attempt to self-medicate other untreated psychiatric disorders. The main idea is that if you treat the other psychiatric illness, then you remove the primary incentive to continue drug abuse. Though we cannot say for sure how accurate this self-medication theory really is, patients with other psychiatric illnesses ranging from depression to bipolar disorder to schizophrenia to anxiety disorders are all at higher risk for abusing substances. As a rule, treating the psychiatric illness also tends to reduce the frequency and severity of substance use.

6.7 CURRENT APPROACHES TO TREATMENT

The first step in the treatment of substance use disorders is a comprehensive psychiatric evaluation as outlined earlier. Once the evaluation has been completed, the initial decision is where to provide treatment. The first stage of treatment may include detoxification, which if severe should be done in an inpatient setting for alcohol or opiate withdrawal. After detoxification is complete, most substance abuse treatment is conducted in the outpatient (i.e., not in a hospital) setting. This can include outpatient treatment, partial hospitalization, day treatment, or residential treatment. Residential treatment ranges from some degree of freedom to come and go to centers where patients are quite restricted in their movements and contacts with the outside world. One of the goals of residential treatment is to remove the patient from his/her typical environment to avoid habitual cues to substance use. Choosing the treatment setting depends in large part on the patient's ability to participate in his/her care and the need for additional structure and support. Those who have repeatedly failed treatment and those who are prone to frequent relapses may benefit from the increased structure of a residential program. Others may respond well to a brief course of partial hospitalization followed by routine outpatient care with weekly visits supplemented by support groups such as Alcoholics Anonymous.

Within any of these treatment settings, any of several specific psychiatric treatments can be applied. A comprehensive treatment plan that incorporates both medications, if indicated, and psychosocial treatments is generally believed to be most effective. The treatment plan should be customized to meet the patient's particular needs. Treatment planning should take into account not only the primary substance that is being abused but also family dynamics, the physical and social impact of the substance use disorder, and the presence of any complicating medical or psychiatric illnesses. Psychosocial treatments encompass several formats such as individual psychotherapy, support groups, and behavioral modification.

It is in this context, in which psychosocial treatments have been mobilized and an appropriate treatment setting has been chosen, that medications can be helpful. The use of psychiatric medications to treat substance use in isolation, apart from such a comprehensive treatment plan, sends the wrong message. The substance abuser typically already leans too heavily on substances to either escape or solve problems. We can quickly succumb to the temptation to join in this dependence on substances to resolve all problems. However, in the context of a comprehensive treatment plan, the substance abuser can benefit from psychiatric medication without unduly seeing it as a panacea. Just like the psychosocial treatments, the use of psychiatric medications should be tailored to the individual's specific treatment needs as well. This includes both medications to treat the substance use disorder by detoxification or craving reduction and medications to treat comorbid psychiatric and medical conditions that may be underlying much of the incentive for continued drug use.

Stage One: Detoxification. The treatment plan unfolds in a series of stages. The first stage is detoxification. For some substances, this can be a time of increased risk. Alcohol and benzodiazepine withdrawal can be quite dangerous if medical treatment is not provided. Withdrawal from opiates can be very unpleasant but is usually not life threatening. Withdrawal from other substances such as marijuana and cocaine is generally mild but can produce intense craving that makes it difficult to initiate a period of sobriety. Withdrawal phobia, the fear of having to go through withdrawal, is a known obstacle to successful treatment. During the detoxification phase of treatment, the primary goal is to provide medical care ensuring patient safety.

Stage Two: Rehabilitation. When the detoxification stage is complete, the treatment enters the rehabilitation phase in which the primary goal is to begin a period of sustained sobriety while learning new patterns of relating to others and coping with stress in order to minimize the chance of relapse. The rehabilitation phase has in the past been conducted on an inpatient basis, but it is now more typically done in the outpatient setting, which includes residential treatment programs. During this phase, medications can be helpful if indicated. In addition, compliance monitoring with drug testing helps to ensure continued sobriety.

Stage Three: Continuing Care. After the rehabilitation phase, the patient enters a period of continuing care. At this point, treatment often transitions to community resources such as self-help groups. In many cases, continuing care patients move beyond the need for intensive psychiatric treatment but continue to require the support of others as they move through the long-term recovery process.

In the event of relapse, patients often cycle through the detoxification (depending on the duration and intensity of the relapse) and rehabilitation phases of treatment. However, they should be advised that a relapse does not necessarily mean they are starting over and they need not feel too disheartened. Instead, a relapse can be viewed as a learning experience. The circumstances that led to the relapse can be reviewed, identified, and utilized for the development of better strategies to prevent subsequent relapses.

6.8 ALCOHOL USE DISORDERS

6.8.1 History of Treatment

Historically, the treatment of alcohol use disorders with medication has focused on the management of withdrawal from the alcohol. In recent years, medication has also been used in an attempt to prevent relapse in alcohol-dependent patients. The treatment of alcohol withdrawal, known as detoxification, by definition uses replacement medications that, like alcohol, act on the GABA receptor. These medications (i.e., barbiturates and benzodiazepines) are cross-tolerant with alcohol and therefore are useful for detoxification. By contrast, a wide variety of theoretical approaches have been used to reduce the likelihood of relapse. This includes aversion therapy and anticraving therapies using reward substitutes and interference approaches. Finally, medications to treat comorbid psychiatric illness, in particular, depression, have also been used in attempts to reduce the likelihood of relapse.

Barbiturates. The first barbiturate, barbital, was introduced at the turn of the 20th century. Hundreds of others, including phenobarbital and pentobarbital, were later developed. The barbiturates were a highly successful class of medications as it became clear that they treated not only alcohol withdrawal but seizure disorders, anxiety, and insomnia as well. By the 1960s, however, the barbiturates were largely surpassed by the benzodiazepines. The newer benzodiazepines act in a similar fashion and provide much the same therapeutic benefit but are significantly safer and easier to tolerate.

Currently, barbiturates are seldom used at all, including in the treatment of alcohol use disorders. Two exceptions are phenobarbital and pentobarbital, which are used solely during alcohol detoxification, though with a variety of safer and better tolerated medications now available the use of barbiturates becomes increasingly difficult to recommend and their use below is described primarily in the context of historical approaches to the problem of managing withdrawal. Pentobarbital's primary use is in determining, via a challenge test, the starting dose for detoxification. Remember, many substance abusers vastly underreport how much they are using. In this challenge test, 100 mg of pentobarbital is given every hour until the patient begins to appear drowsy or intoxicated. Once the beginning point for the detoxification is determined with the pentobarbital challenge test, then equivalent doses of phenobarbital are used for the actual detoxification procedure.

When used for detoxification, phenobarbital is given in equal doses four times a day. The maximum daily dose of phenobarbital is 600 mg, but much lower doses are usually sufficient. The phenobarbital dose is lowered (i.e., tapered) by about 20% per day. If the patient is too drowsy, then a dose should be skipped. If breakthrough withdrawal symptoms continue to occur, then the pace of the detoxification should be slowed. Before using phenobarbital, liver function tests should be obtained. All barbiturates depend greatly on the liver to be metabolized. Alcoholics with cirrhosis or other forms of liver impairment may have difficulty clearing phenobarbital. Phenobarbital should not be used in patients with poor liver function. In addition, the barbiturates can worsen a medical condition known as porphyria and should be avoided in those with this disorder. Phenobarbital, as noted, is seldom used today for alcohol detoxification.

Benzodiazepines. Like the barbiturates, benzodiazepines bind to the GABA receptor and are therefore cross-tolerant with alcohol. As a result, they also make suitable replacement medications for alcohol and are widely used for alcohol detoxification. Theoretically, any benzodiazepine can be used to treat alcohol withdrawal. However, short-acting benzodiazepines such as alprazolam (Xanax) are often avoided because breakthrough withdrawal may occur between doses. Intermediate to long-acting benzodiazepines including chlordiazepoxide (Librium), diazepam (Valium), oxazepam (Serax), lorazepam (Ativan), and clonazepam (Klonopin) are more commonly utilized.

When there is not a reliable history of just how much alcohol has been used or there are suspicions that use has been underreported or alcohol has been mixed with other sedatives or hypnotics, a challenge test can be performed to determine the starting point for the taper. Typically, the same benzodiazepine that will be used for the subsequent taper is used for the challenge test. In the presence of obvious signs and symptoms of withdrawal, many clinicians will make an educated guess of the initial dose, establish a set of parameters such as pulse rate, blood pressure, or agitation that will call for additional medication to be given, and then add up the total dose for the first 24 hours of detoxification, using this as the starting point from which decreases are made.

In the presence of cirrhosis or other liver impairment, lorazepam or oxazepam should be utilized for detoxification. These two benzodiazepines have no active hepatic metabolites and are generally considered safer choices for patients with liver damage. Once the starting point for the taper is determined, the dose is decreased by 10–20% per day. It is important to note that this rate of taper is much faster than that used for patients treated chronically with benzodiazepines who are discontinuing their anxiolytic in order to determine if it is still needed for control of symptoms. In that case, the rate of decrease is 10–20% per week. Should the patient display excessive drowsiness, then a dose should be skipped and the pace of the taper can be accelerated. If breakthrough withdrawal symptoms occur, then an extra dose may be needed and the pace of the taper reevaluated.

Side effects of benzodiazepines include drowsiness and reduced respiratory function. In patients who are severely medically ill, especially those with lung disease, this side effect can be problematic. However, benzodiazepines are much safer in this regard than their predecessors, the barbiturates, and untreated delirium tremens, the most severe form of alcohol withdrawal, can be fatal.

Dopamine-Stimulating Medications. Dopamine stimulates the reward centers in the brain. There is good evidence that alcohol in part produces its pleasant effects by acting on these dopamine systems. One theory of treatment has been to reduce alcohol craving by using a medication that stimulates these dopamine reward centers. To this end, several dopamine-stimulating medications that are more commonly used to treat Parkinson's disease have been tried in attempts to prolong sobriety in recovering alcoholics. This includes bromocriptine and L-DOPA. Although theoretically sound, this approach has not proved effective and has appropriately been abandoned.

Dopamine-Blocking Medications. Another approach to reducing craving in alcoholics has been to use medications that block the action of dopamine at one or more of its receptors in the reward centers as a form of interference therapy. By reducing the rewarding effects of alcohol, the incentive for its use might diminish or disappear altogether. To this end, haloperidol, pimozide, and other antipsychotic drugs have been tried. This approach to treatment has not proved successful and, in fact, has exposed the patients to the many unpleasant side effects commonly associated with conventional antipsychotic drugs. Consequently, the use of dopamine-blocking medications to treat alcohol abuse and alcohol dependence is inappropriate.

Serotonergic Medications. When we speak of serotonergic medications, this refers primarily to the SSRI antidepressants, including fluoxetine, citalopram, escitalopram, paroxetine, sertraline, and fluvoxamine. Of these, fluoxetine has been the most extensively studied. Such studies are based on the following rationale: First is the notion that many alcoholics use alcohol to self-medicate undiagnosed depression and anxiety. If their underlying psychiatric illness is treated, the primary incentive for continued alcohol use may be eliminated. Second, deficits in serotonin activity may contribute to the craving for alcohol. Therefore, increasing the availability of serotonin might directly reduce alcohol craving.

Although these medications have proved quite helpful in reducing alcohol use in depressed patients with comorbid alcoholism, they are not effective in treating nondepressed alcoholics. These antidepressants should only be used in alcohol-dependent patients with comorbid depression or anxiety.

Of course, there always exists some debate as to whether the depression is primary or secondary to the alcohol use. Making this distinction between an episode of major depression and a substance-induced depression can be difficult even for the most experienced clinician. So when should an antidepressant be considered? Many clinicians, ourselves included, recommend waiting about 7–10 days into a comprehensive alcohol treatment plan. While this will not make the distinction absolutely clear, many substance-induced depressions will have resolved or begun to resolve by this point. Should depressive symptoms persist at this time, then the addition of an antidepressant should be considered as a component of ongoing treatment for alcohol abuse and dependence.

Disulfiram (Antabuse). Disulfiram is the only medication specifically approved by the FDA as an aversion therapy for substance abuse, specifically alcohol abuse or dependence. Disulfiram's mechanism of action is quite simple; it is an inhibitor of alcohol dehydrogenase, the major enzyme responsible for the metabolism. Inhibiting this enzyme results in the accumulation of acetylaldehyde. Acetylaldehyde is primarily responsible for many of the unmistakable symptoms of a hangover, and when it accumulates in the presence of disulfiram, it produces a constellation of very uncomfortable physical symptoms.

Disulfiram is initiated at 50 mg/day for the first week. It can be continued indefinitely at 25 mg/day thereafter. Patients must be cautioned of the need to wait at least 1–2 weeks after their last dose before drinking. Otherwise, they risk the unpleasant effects of a disulfiram reaction. Disulfiram use should not be seen as a substitute for other ongoing therapies, but rather as an adjunct to outpatient follow-up and self-help groups.

Naltrexone (ReVia). Naltrexone is another medication that has specific FDA approval for the treatment of alcohol use disorders. It is used as an interference therapy. Naltrexone blocks opioid receptors in the brain and is believed to reduce alcohol-induced euphoria. The absence of pleasurable effects associated with alcohol consumption should plausibly lead to a decrease in the behavior of drinking alcohol. Evidence to date has demonstrated that recovering alcoholics treated with naltrexone have fewer days of drinking and longer periods of sobriety between relapses.

Naltrexone is prescribed at a dose of 50 mg once per day for at least 12 weeks as part of a comprehensive alcohol treatment program. Like all treatments for substance use disorders, it works only as well as the addict allows it to work. This is why it is important to use it as a component of an overall treatment plan. Otherwise, poorly motivated alcohol abusers will seldom remain adherent with naltrexone and it will have little chance of providing benefit. A long-acting depot formulation of naltrexone currently in development might improve these compliance problems.

The common side effects of naltrexone are nausea, headache, and dizziness. In addition, naltrexone has the potential for toxic effects on the liver and should not be used in an alcoholic with cirrhosis or other known liver disease. Because it blocks opiate receptors, patients treated with naltrexone are unable to benefit from the analgesic effects of opiates such as codeine or morphine. Naltrexone may increase serum levels of acamprosate in patients taking both medications.

Acamprosate (Campral). The most recent medication approved by the FDA for alcohol dependence, acamprosate—like alcohol, the benzodiazepines, and the barbiturates—acts by stimulating GABA receptors. Although its GABA effects are not sufficiently potent to be used for detoxification, it appears to promote abstinence by aiding in the reduction of alcohol craving. Supplied in 333 mg tablets, one or two tablets should be administered three times daily. Common side effects of acamprosate include nausea, diarrhea, dizziness, insomnia, and sweating. Serum levels of acamprosate can be increased by naltrexone if the two medicines are taken together.

Anticonvulsants. Antiseizure medications have long been used to treat alcohol use disorders. Historically, the focus has been on treating seizures that commonly occur during alcohol withdrawal or protecting against seizures in unstable patients prone to frequent withdrawal. Of course, we use the term antiseizure medication quite loosely here. The barbiturates and more recently the benzodiazepines were the most commonly used anticonvulsants in patients with alcohol withdrawal. Currently, benzodiazepines are the treatment of choice for alcohol withdrawal seizures, preferably by preventing their occurrence.

Anticonvulsants have also been used for relapse prevention based on their so-called antikindling action. Preliminary evidence suggests that the anticonvulsants carbamazepine, topiramate, and valproic acid may be helpful in reducing relapse in some alcoholics, but more study is needed before we can generally recommend this approach. Using anticonvulsants for relapse prevention does have the added benefit of guarding against alcohol withdrawal seizures should a patient relapse into an alcohol binge and then suddenly stop drinking again, but there are problems with their use as well. For example, anticonvulsants have the potential to produce adverse changes in liver function, which, while relatively rare, can be significant. The liver is, of course, a primary site of damage inflicted by alcohol. It is premature to use anticonvulsants in the treatment of alcohol dependence.

Vitamin and Mineral Supplements. Nutritional supplements do not reduce the frequency of drinking or treat alcohol withdrawal. However, alcohol dependence may lead to nutritional deficiencies. When the caloric intake during a prolonged alcoholic binge is largely restricted to alcohol itself, then the alcoholic often becomes depleted of several critical nutrients including magnesium, thiamine, folate, and sometimes potassium. These deficiencies can produce several significant medical problems. Low magnesium levels increase seizure risk; depressed folate levels predispose to birth defects, anemia, and depression; and decreased thiamine is associated with severe amnesia and other cognitive deficits.

When the alcoholic first presents for treatment, his/her nutritional status should be fully assessed. Vitamin supplementation should always be a component of this treatment. In the emergency room setting, the alcoholic patient usually receives intravenous fluids containing magnesium, thiamine, and multivitamin supplements. The yellow-colored fluid is commonly called a "banana bag" or "rally pack." A daily multivitamin and thiamine tablet should be a routine component of outpatient treatment to protect against the medical consequences of relapse.

6.8.2 Current Approach to Treatment

Medications can play a prominent role in the treatment of alcohol use disorders (see Table 6.4). As noted earlier, they are widely used during the initial detoxification phase of treatment. In recent years, psychiatric medications have taken on a more prominent role during the rehabilitation phase of treatment.

During the initial evaluation, providing for the safety of the patient is of paramount importance. The severity of intoxication and potential for withdrawal must be quickly and accurately determined. Extreme alcohol intoxication can be fatal either by the production of cardiac arrhythmias, aspiration (the inhalation of stomach contents that are vomited), or other causes. We have all seen reports of college students dying from alcohol poisoning. Likewise, up to 10% of patients in severe alcohol withdrawal can die without treatment. Fortunately, most patients do not experience the most severe forms of alcohol withdrawal such as the DTs. Mild withdrawal can be managed in the outpatient setting with appropriate support and patient adherence, but severe withdrawal requires an inpatient hospitalization. See Section 6.5 for further discussion of the initial evaluation.

When the patient is manifesting acute symptoms of withdrawal such as the "shakes," a rapid pulse, or increased blood pressure, then detoxification with a benzodiazepine should begin immediately. When the patient's liver function is unknown, we recommend lorazepam (1–2 mg) as the treatment of choice in the emergency room setting. The lorazepam can be repeated every hour until the patient's symptoms begin to resolve. Initial treatment should also include vitamin supplements as noted earlier, especially thiamine.

Following detoxification, alcohol treatment typically transitions to an outpatient setting. Largely gone are the 30 day inpatient programs of the 1970s and 1980s. Rehabilitation treatment is typically managed in outpatient clinics or, in severe cases, in residential treatment programs. At this stage of treatment, medications alone are not sufficient. Treatment with medications is used as an adjunct to self-help programs and other psychosocial interventions. The primary psychopharmacological treatment options include antidepressants, disulfiram, naltrexone, and acamprosate. In cases where alcoholism is clearly comorbid with depression, antidepressant therapy is indicated. We recommend using one of the newer generation antidepressants with a favorable side effect profile.

In the absence of depression, naltrexone, acamprosate, and disulfiram are the only options currently approved by the FDA for marketing. We prefer using acamprosate or naltrexone as a short-term treatment during rehabilitation. A physical examination focusing on signs of liver impairment and blood testing of liver enzymes must be performed before initiating naltrexone treatment. If there are no signs of liver damage, naltrexone can be started at 50 mg/day and continued for several months. In the future, nalmefene, another opioid receptor blocker, may provide the same benefits as naltrexone with less concern for liver impairment. Acamprosate avoids naltrexone's potential for liver toxicity but must be administered three times daily, potentially creating adherence problems with continued use.

Disulfiram can be very helpful in patients who are highly motivated yet find themselves vulnerable to brief repeated relapses into dangerous alcohol binges. Disulfiram offers the advantage of discouraging impulsive alcohol use, giving the alcoholic time to turn to alternative sources of support when faced with the temptation to drink.

The obvious question is whether combining naltrexone, acamprosate, and/or disulfiram is better than either medication alone. To our knowledge, this has not been systematically studied, but it may be a viable alternative in particularly severe cases when other treatment options have failed. The cornerstone of success in the treatment of alcoholism is clearly the behavioral intervention including Alcoholics Anonymous.

6.9 COCAINE USE DISORDERS

6.9.1 History of Treatment

Cocaine addicts uniformly report that the drug produces intense craving. Crack cocaine is particularly notorious in this regard. The medications used to treat cocaine dependence have focused on the reduction of craving. Although stopping cocaine use does produce a mild withdrawal syndrome, it is not life threatening. Therefore, there is no need for medications during detoxification from cocaine. Cocaine withdrawal can nonetheless be very unpleasant. Like amphetamine, withdrawing from cocaine produces a "crash" manifested by severe depression and lethargy. Fortunately, these typically resolve within 1–2 days.

Antidepressants. The tricyclic antidepressant desipramine has shown some small success in reducing cocaine craving, but the results are not overly impressive, and desipramine has many well-documented side effects and is dangerous in overdose (see Chapter 3 for more information). Cocaine-abusing patients who are not highly motivated will usually not remain adherent to the desipramine prescription. We do not recommend desipramine for the nondepressed cocaine addict.

Lithium. Lithium has also been used in an attempt to circumvent craving. Like alcohol dependence, cocaine-dependent craving is believed by some, based on limited data, to result from a kindling effect that begins in one area of the brain and spreads to induce an intense desire to use. Lithium's success in treating bipolar disorder, another purportedly kindling-dependent illness, led to its use for cocaine dependence. Unfortunately, lithium has not proved very helpful and has been abandoned in the treatment of cocaine dependence.

Anticonvulsants. Carbamazepine and, to a lesser extent, valproic acid have been tried in attempts to reduce craving by interfering with kindling as well. Initial pilot studies were positive but more recent results have been unimpressive.

Dopamine-Stimulating Medications. A variety of drugs that increase the availability of dopamine have been studied in cocaine addicts including L-DOPA, bupropion, amantadine, and methylphenidate. In small uncontrolled trials, these have shown some benefit, but definitive studies have yet to be performed. In addition, some dopamine-stimulating medications (in particular, the stimulants like methylphenidate or the amphetamines) are themselves subject to abuse, though, of note, this is typically not a problem when they are prescribed to patients who do not have a history of substance abuse such as, for example, in the treatment of attention deficit–hyperactivity disorder.

Buprenorphine. Buprenorphine has two major actions. It both stimulates and blocks opioid receptors and is therefore termed a mixed agonist/antagonist. In substance abusers, its net effect is to interfere with the pleasurable effects of an abused drug that would otherwise be mediated through the brain's opioid reward centers. Although cocaine's stimulating effects do not act directly through opioid receptors, many cocaine addicts also abuse opiates such as heroin. In these polysubstance-dependent patients, buprenorphine successfully reduces the addict's frequency of using both the opiate and the cocaine. However, there is no evidence that buprenorphine would be helpful for patients addicted to cocaine only.

6.9.2 Current Approach to Treatment

The cocaine addict most often presents during withdrawal after a binge of cocaine use. Cocaine withdrawal is not life threatening and does not require medical intervention in the same sense as alcohol or opiate withdrawal. It is, however, associated with a profound depression that can render the addict suicidal for 24–48 hours. The "crashing" cocaine addict should be assessed for suicide risk and, if indicated, the patient should be monitored in an emergency psychiatric setting or may require a brief 1–2 day inpatient psychiatric admission until the withdrawal resolves and the suicide risk is relieved.

Once the crash has abated, the patient should be reassessed and treatment recommendations made. Psychosocial treatments are the mainstay of treatment for cocaine addicts. Intensive outpatient programs and partial hospitalization programs are most effective during the initial phase of treatment. Psychotherapy and self-help treatment can help the patient devise means to manage craving and sustain sobriety.

Psychiatric medications do not currently play a prominent role in the treatment of cocaine-dependent patients (see Table 6.4). Although researchers have labored to find medications to treat cocaine addiction, there have not been any notable breakthroughs. As with other substance use disorders, the presence of a psychiatric disorder for which medication is indicated (i.e., depression, anxiety disorders, bipolar affective disorder, or schizophrenia) should prompt appropriate treatment. Similar to the presence of alcohol intoxication, deferring a diagnosis for a day or two in a new patient with no past history is often the more prudent course.

6.10 NICOTINE DEPENDENCE

6.10.1 History of Treatment

Tobacco and psychiatry have had an uneasy history. There is evidence that cigarette smoking (or more accurately, nicotine) is pleasurable in patients with schizophrenia and other chronic psychiatric disorders. Although tobacco abuse clearly provides some soothing benefit to the chronic mentally ill, should we encourage our severely mentally ill patients to continue smoking knowing that it might provide some degree of solace? In so doing, do we sacrifice their physical health in favor of their mental health? These are difficult ethical issues, and ones largely beyond the scope of our discussion. Nevertheless, we do well to remember that as dangerous and offensive as tobacco use may be, it is also highly addictive. As any smoker who has tried (successfully or unsuccessfully) to quit will tell you, it is very difficult to kick the habit.

Most patients who are addicted to cigarettes and other tobacco products at some time or another do seek treatment to help them stop. Perhaps they are faced with the crisis of medical illness (emphysema or lung cancer), or they have simply reached a point in life when they want to take better care of themselves. Whatever the motivation, smokers often seek professional help when trying to quit. We review the treatments for nicotine dependence.

Nicotine Replacement. These medications come in a wide variety of both prescription and nonprescription forms. They include patches applied to the skin, gum that is chewed, and even nasal sprays. They are used to treat or prevent the physical symptoms of nicotine withdrawal. Ideally, nicotine replacement treatments are gradually tapered over a period of weeks to months. They are generally well tolerated but can cause significant nausea, particularly if a patient has not completely stopped smoking. Nicotine replacement is targeted to reduce cravings, but it is not very effective as monotherapy.

Bupropion (Wellbutrin, Zyban). Bupropion is an antidepressant that is also FDA approved as a treatment for smoking cessation. It is marketed as an antidepressant as Wellbutrin and for the treatment of nicotine dependence as Zyban. Its mechanism of action in this regard is obscure, but it may act on dopamine and/or norepinephrine systems.

The sustained-release (SR) form of bupropion is prescribed at a dose of 150 mg/day for 3 days and then increased as tolerated to 150 mg twice a day. The XL form of bupropion is administered at a dose of 150 mg/day for 3 days and then increased as tolerated to 300 mg taken once daily. Bupropion should be taken for 12 weeks and can be used in conjunction with nicotine replacement. Patients should be advised to plan on total smoking cessation after the first week of treatment with bupropion.

Side effects of bupropion such as stomach upset are relatively mild. The immediate-release form of bupropion increases the risk of seizure in patients vulnerable to seizure. This is less true of the SR or XL forms. For more information on bupropion, please refer to Chapter 3.

Nortriptyline (Pamelor). A recent study suggested that the tricyclic antidepressant nortriptyline, like bupropion, is effective in the treatment of smoking cessation. Nortriptyline does not have any significant effect on dopamine reuptake activity, but it does increase norepinephrine availability. Like bupropion, nortriptyline may therefore reduce the physical symptoms of nicotine withdrawal. Because nortriptyline carries the danger of lethality in overdose and has the unfavorable side effect profile of the tricyclics, we do not recommend its use for smoking cessation. However, it does raise the question as to whether other newer antidepressants that increase norepinephrine activity (e.g., venlafaxine, mirtazapine, duloxetine) may also prove to be effective treatments for nicotine withdrawal.

6.10.2 Current Approach to Treatment

Smokers who quit are at especially high risk for relapse. A counseling program in lieu of or in addition to medical treatment can be especially helpful in sustaining the patient's success. Therefore, we highly recommend that this be incorporated into the treatment regimen.

Patients who are especially sensitive to the physical symptoms of nicotine withdrawal may benefit from the addition of a nicotine replacement that is eventually tapered over a period of time (see Table 6.4). It is very important for the patient to abstain from tobacco use (both smoked and chewed) during nicotine replacement therapy.

6.11 OPIATE USE DISORDERS

6.11.1 History of Treatment

The opiates have a variety of legitimate and important medical uses. They are potent pain relievers, suppress cough, and treat severe diarrhea. They are sometimes used in the ICU setting to reduce the uncomfortable sensations of "air hunger" in patients with severe lung disease. Opiates are available not only in prescription forms such as codeine, oxycodone, meperidine, and morphine but also in illicit street forms such as heroin. As a result, opiate misuse can arise in one of two ways. First, some patients begin using prescription opiate narcotics in a legitimate manner for the treatment of severe pain. A handful of these patients develop intense craving and begin an addictive pattern of use. They may resort to doctor-shopping to obtain multiple prescriptions for narcotics. In extreme cases, they may even resort to forging prescriptions. The second way that opiate abuse arises is through the use of "gateway" drugs such as alcohol and marijuana. A small percentage of abusers of alcohol, marijuana, and stimulants go on to abuse opiates as well. The most commonly used illicit opiate is heroin, though there has been an epidemic of Oxycontin

TABLE 6.4. Overview of Medication Treatments for Substance Abuse

	Medications Recommended During Each Treatment Stage		
Abused Substance	Stage 1 Detoxification	Stage 2 Rehabilitation	Stage 3 Continuing Care
Alcohol	Benzodiazepines Nutrient supplements[a]	Acamprosate Antidepressants[b] Disulfiram Naltrexone Nutrient supplements[a]	Acamprosate Antidepressants[b] Disulfiram Naltrexone Nutrient supplements[a]
Cocaine	None	Antidepressants[b] Buprenorphine[c]	Antidepressants[b] Buprenorphine[c]
Nicotine	Bupropion Nicotine gum/patch	Bupropion Nortriptyline	None
Opioid	Methadone[d] Naloxone[e]	Methadone[f] LAAM[f] Naltrexone[g] Buprenorphine[g]	Methadone[f] LAAM[f] Naltrexone[g] Buprenorphine[g]

[a] Nutrient supplementation during alcohol detoxification includes thiamine, magnesium sulfate, folic acid, and a multivitamin. During the rehabilitation and continuing care stages of treatment for alcohol dependence, nutrient supplementation includes thiamine and a multivitamin.
[b] Antidepressants are only recommended in the rehabilitation and continuing care stages of treatment for alcohol and cocaine dependence if the patient has a comorbid depressive or anxiety disorder.
[c] Buprenorphine is only recommended in the rehabilitation and continuing care stages of treatment for cocaine dependence if the patient is also addicted to an opioid.
[d] Methadone is typically used during opioid detoxification in conjunction with acetaminophen, promethazine, and/or clonidine.
[e] Naloxone is used for rapid opioid detoxification in conjunction with anesthetic agents for conscious sedation.
[f] Methadone and LAAM are used for maintenance therapy during the rehabilitation and continuing care stages of treatment for opioid dependence in those patients who are not seeking total abstinence.
[g] Naltrexone and buprenorphine are used for relapse prevention during the rehabilitation and continuing care stages of treatment for opioid dependence in those patients who are seeking total abstinence.

abuse recently. At epidemic proportions in the 1960s, heroin use subsided for about 20 years only to increase at an alarming rate in the 1990s. Heroin addicts and prescription narcotic addicts form two distinct populations, but the treatment is quite similar in both groups.

Opiate abuse and dependence can exact a tremendous social toll. Abusers have difficulty holding jobs, are often divorced, and sometimes resort to crime to obtain either the drug or the money to buy it. Opiate abuse also has severe health consequences. Sharing needles is a common source of transmitting HIV, hepatitis, and other infectious diseases. In addition, opiate abusers are prone to accidents and are often victims of crime.

Few patients with opiate dependence achieve long-term total abstinence. Instead, maintenance programs have become the mainstay of treatment. These replacement therapies sustain the opiate dependence but in a safer and more controlled manner. Using a slower and longer-acting and thus less addictive opiate such as methadone may be controversial but provides several benefits. Maintenance treatment can reduce craving for illegally obtained narcotic analgesics by increasing drug tolerance and as a result reducing the "high" that is experienced when a relapse occurs. Crime, disease, and other social consequences of uncontrolled opiate dependence are also avoided. When a component of a comprehensive treatment plan, replacement therapy provides an incentive to keep the patient in treatment, giving other psychosocial treatments a chance to work. Without maintenance therapy, many if not most opiate-dependent patients would be unable to sustain their motivation for sustained long-term treatment. We discuss next the medications used to treat opiate dependence.

Methadone (Dolophine). For over 30 years, methadone has been the mainstay of treatment for opiate dependence. A replacement therapy, methadone has been used both for detoxification and for long-term maintenance. It has a slower onset of action and is longer acting than other narcotic analgesics. It causes little of the euphoria produced by drugs such as heroin.

Methadone can be used for detoxification in either the inpatient or the outpatient setting. An inpatient methadone detoxification normally takes place over 1–2 weeks. Acetaminophen, promethazine (for nausea), and clonidine (to decrease some of the physical symptoms of withdrawal) are often given with the methadone to reduce the symptoms of withdrawal during the taper. During a taper, methadone is usually given in equal doses every 6 hours. It is easiest to the give the methadone in a liquid form mixed with the other medications in a cup of fruit juice. The starting dose for the methadone taper depends in large part on the magnitude of prior opiate use. An initial dose of 40 mg/day is reasonable, but some patients require over 100 mg/day to initiate their taper.

The methadone taper can also be conducted as an outpatient. In this case, the taper is done very slowly over a period of several months. Adjuvant medications such as acetaminophen are usually not needed for this slow detoxification. This outpatient taper is often best managed by a methadone clinic, the same clinic that provides methadone maintenance treatment.

Methadone maintenance is precisely what the name implies. Patients who will not or cannot tolerate being totally abstinent of opiates are maintained long-term on methadone replacement therapy. As noted previously, this continues the addiction but in a more controlled manner that averts the serious social and medical consequences of uncontrolled addiction. Daily doses for methadone maintenance range from 20 mg/day to over 100 mg/day.

Methadone is not without side effects. Although it is less addictive than other opiates, methadone can be abused and requires monitored use. Common side effects include sedation and constipation. Methadone is also safer than other opiates in overdose but does require careful monitoring of respiratory status when an overdose occurs.

LAAM (Levo-a-acetyl Methadol). LAAM is a synthetic analog of methadone that is even longer acting than methadone. Its extremely long duration of action make LAAM unsuitable for an inpatient taper, but it is approved for long-term maintenance treatment. Because of its long duration of action, LAAM need only be taken three times per week. The daily doses of LAAM range from 20 to 80 mg given three times weekly. The dose can gradually be incremented by 10 mg per dose at each weekly visit.

Buprenorphine. Buprenorphine differs from methadone and LAAM in that it is only a partial opioid agonist. As a result, buprenorphine is not a true replacement therapy but instead an interference therapy. When a patient taking buprenorphine uses an opiate, the buprenorphine, in effect, gets in the way. It interferes with opiate effects by blocking the drug's action at the brain's opioid receptors. As a result, it reduces craving and makes buprenorphine a suitable treatment for patients willing to abstain from opiates. It appears to be particularly helpful for patients who have been abusing both opiates and cocaine and has also been reported to be helpful in refractory depression.

Buprenorphine is initiated at 4 mg/day and can be increased up to 16 mg/day in a stepwise fashion.

Naltrexone (ReVia). Naltrexone is a very potent antagonist of the actions of opiates. It has been used to reduce the rewarding effects of not only opiates but alcohol as well. Like buprenorphine, naltrexone appears to reduce craving for opiates by blocking their pleasurable effects. Naltrexone is not useful for detoxification and in fact worsens withdrawal. Naltrexone can be useful for maintenance treatment in those patients motivated to achieve total abstinence. It is taken at a constant dose of 50 mg/day. A sustained-release depot formulation currently under development will likely help to overcome adherence issues that often undermine treatment for substance use disorders.

Potential side effects of naltrexone include anxiety, drowsiness, and nausea. In addition, it rarely causes a chemical hepatitis. For this reason, blood testing of liver enzymes should be conducted periodically. If any signs of naltrexone-induced hepatitis appear, it should be discontinued. Furthermore, patients should be advised that they must be totally abstinent from opiates for at least 2 weeks before using naltrexone or it can precipitate severe withdrawal symptoms.

Naloxone (Narcan). Naloxone, like naltrexone, is a potent opioid receptor blocker. Its primary use has been to reverse opiate toxicity after an overdose. However, some physicians have found it is also useful for a process known as *rapid opiate detoxification*. Although opiate withdrawal is not life threatening, it can be extremely unpleasant. Most opiate addicts are fearful of the withdrawal symptoms; therefore, it usually requires a slow, deliberate detoxification to keep the withdrawal symptoms in check. Rapid opiate detoxification is an alternative approach that keeps the taper and detoxification as brief as possible. In this approach, naloxone is used in conjunction with general anesthesia or a nonopiate sedative such as the benzodiazepine midazolam (Versed) to produce conscious sedation. This produces a very brief (less than 24 hours) but intense withdrawal that is counteracted by the anesthesia. This procedure is obviously reserved for the inpatient setting. It has the advantage of shortening the hospital stay but carries the inherent risks of anesthesia. Although popular with some physicians, rapid opiate detoxification has not received widespread use and remains in need of further research before its utility can be fully assessed.

6.11.2 Current Approach to Treatment

When beginning treatment for opiate dependence, it is imperative to assess the patient's long-term goals for treatment. The key variable is whether the patient desires to control his/her opiate use or whether the patient wants to achieve total abstinence. In both cases, the first stage of treatment is detoxification. The endpoint of detoxification differs, however. Detoxification is complete in a patient desiring abstinence when (s)he is entirely tapered from the opiate. Conversely, detoxification is complete in a patient desiring maintenance therapy when the withdrawal symptoms have abated.

The mainstay of opiate detoxification remains methadone (see Table 6.4). We prefer using a "single blind" approach to opiate detoxification so that the patient agrees not to ask how much methadone is in each day's dose. In this way, the patient can give you feedback on his/her withdrawal symptoms without being prejudiced by the knowledge of how much the dose was changed. By monitoring symptoms, the rate of decreasing the dose can be adjusted as needed.

Given a reasonable estimate of how much the patient was using, one can estimate the starting dose for the methadone taper using readily available charts that list the relative potencies between opiates. In the absence of this information, a starting dose of approximately 40 mg/day in divided doses given every 6 hours is usually reasonable. We find it helpful to use liquid methadone mixed in fruit juice with adjunctive acetaminophen (650 mg), promethazine (6.25–25 mg), and clonidine (0.05–0.1 mg) if necessary.

If the patient quickly becomes too drowsy, then the starting dose was too high and it should be reduced. If withdrawal symptoms persist, then the dose may be too low and should be increased at the next scheduled interval. We recommend against using nonscheduled "as-needed" doses during the detoxification process. This can set up a counterproductive battle over medication and even result in unduly increasing the patient's medication burden. Reassurance to the patient that the dose will be adjusted at the next interval to provide better relief is a better approach. An inpatient detoxification will usually take 1–2 weeks depending on the severity of abuse.

Once detoxification is complete, patients who desire to be totally abstinent may benefit from a trial of buprenorphine or naltrexone. Either medication can be used, but buprenorphine may be best for patients who are also abusing cocaine, whereas naltrexone may be best for patients who are also abusing alcohol.

For those patients who are not ready to attempt total abstinence, methadone or LAAM maintenance therapy is warranted. These maintenance treatments should be incorporated into a comprehensive treatment plan.

ADDITIONAL READING

Anton RF. Pharmacologic approaches to the management of alcoholism. *J Clin Psychiatry* 2001; 62(Supplement 20): 11–17.

Blondell RD. Ambulatory detoxification of patients with alcohol dependence. *Am Fam Physician* 2005; 71: 495–502, 509–510.

Boening JA, Lesch OM, Spanagel R, et al. Pharmacological relapse prevention in alcohol dependence: from animal models to clinical trials. *Alcoholism* 2001; 25(5 Supplement ISBRA): 127S–131S.

Carroll KM. Integrating psychotherapy and pharmacotherapy to improve drug abuse outcomes. *Addictive Behaviors* 1997; 22(2): 233–245.

De Lima MS, de Oliveira Soares BG, Reisser AA, et al. Pharmacological treatment of cocaine dependence: a systematic review. *Addiction* 2002; 97(8): 931–949.

Galanter M, Kleber HD. *The American Psychiatric Press Textbook of Substance Abuse Treatment, Second Edition*. Washington DC: American Psychiatric Press, 1999.

Garrett BE, Rose CA, Henningfield JE. Tobacco addiction and pharmacological interventions. *Expert Opin Pharmacother* 2001; 2(10): 1545–1555.

Henningfield JE, Fant RV, Gitchell J, et al. Tobacco dependence: global public health potential for new medications development and indications. *Ann NY Acad Sci* 2000; 909: 247–256.

Kosten TR. The pharmacotherapy of relapse prevention using anticonvulsants. *Am J Addictions* 1998; 7(3): 205–209.

Kranzler HR, Amin H, Modesto-Lowe V, et al. Pharmacologic treatments for drug and alcohol dependence. *Psychiatr Clin North Am* 1999; 22(2): 401–423.

Kreek MJ, LaForge KS, Butelman E. Pharmacotherapy of addictions. *Nature Reviews Drug Discovery* 2002; 1(9): 710–726.

Longo LP. Progress and issues in alcoholism pharmacotherapy. *Primary Psychiatry* 1999; 6(8): 65–73.

O'Connor PG, Fiellin DA. Pharmacologic treatment of heroin-dependent patients. *Ann Intern Med* 2000; 133(1): 40–54.

Rayburn WF, Bogenschutz MP. Pharmacotherapy for pregnant women with addictions. *Am J Obstet Gynecol* 2004; 191: 1885–1897.

Thase ME, Salloum IM, Cornelius JD. Comorbid alcoholism and depression: treatment issues. *J Clin Psychiatry* 2001; 62(Supplement 20): 32–41.

7

EATING DISORDERS

7.1 INTRODUCTION

Disturbances in appetite and eating behavior can complicate the course of many medical and psychiatric syndromes. Psychiatric disorders that are frequently associated with eating disturbances include major depression, bipolar disorder, social phobia, generalized anxiety disorder, schizophrenia, delusional disorder–somatic type, somatization disorder, undifferentiated somatoform disorder, conversion disorder, body dysmorphic disorder, and a variety of personality disorders. These changes in eating pattern can result from loss of appetite (anorexia), a voracious appetite, paranoid or bizarre ideas about food, intolerable psychosomatic gastrointestinal symptoms, or embarrassment at eating in front of others. If the change in eating is a symptom of a medical or psychiatric disorder, it typically resolves when the underlying illness is successfully treated. For example, the loss of appetite commonly occurring in major depression usually resolves when the depressive episode remits.

However, derangements in eating behavior requiring direct clinical intervention do occur both independent of and in association with other medical and psychiatric disorders. When the aberration in eating behavior leads to significant functional disruption and occurs in concert with a preoccupation with or distortions in the self-assessment of body weight or body shape, then the diagnosis of an eating

Principles of Psychopharmacology for Mental Health Professionals
By Jeffrey E. Kelsey, D. Jeffrey Newport, and Charles B. Nemeroff

disorder is warranted. Current diagnostic classification recognizes three eating disorders: anorexia nervosa (AN), bulimia nervosa (BN), and binge-eating disorder (BED). With careful collection of the history of eating behaviors and body image perceptions, these syndromes can readily be distinguished (see Table 7.1).

During the course of illness, most patients with one of the eating disorders experience the full range of aberrant eating behaviors. This includes the anorectic behaviors of restricting food intake and excessive exercising as well as the bulimic behaviors of binge-eating and associated purging. The latter includes self-induced vomiting and the abuse of laxatives, enemas, and diuretics. Patients with AN are distinguished from those with BN or BED not by the absence of bulimic behaviors, because a subset of AN patients frequently engage in binging and purging, but by the propensity to lower body weight to often dangerously low levels.

Perhaps more so than any category of psychiatric syndromes, the biopsychosocial model is readily applicable to the theoretical understanding of, and therapeutic approach to, the eating disorders. From the biological perspective, several neurotransmitters and neuromodulators involved in the regulation of appetite and feeding behavior have been identified. Consequently, dysregulation of these systems may plausibly play a role in precipitating or sustaining eating disorders. To date, the clinical focus of psychopharmacology for the eating disorders has been on the modulation of serotonergic neurotransmission in the brain. Newer research indicating a role in the control of satiety for other chemical messengers including cholecystokinin (CCK) and corticotropin-releasing factor (CRF), as well as the recently discovered leptins and orexins, may ultimately lead to a better understanding of these disorders and novel approaches to pharmacotherapy. Furthermore, a medical perspective of the eating disorders is essential because these syndromes often bear serious adverse medical consequences. The eating disorders, particularly AN, can lead to marked malfunctioning in essential organ systems including the cardiovascular, reproductive, and endocrine systems. The biological sequelae of eating disorders commonly require medical intervention and unfortunately sometimes result in death.

Clinical Vignette

Angela was a 28-year-old female with a longstanding history of anorexia. One weekend while vacationing with her family, she continued to be restrictive in her food intake but consumed large amounts of water. She became confused and was taken to a local emergency room for evaluation. Her serum sodium level was very low, and the emergency room staff attempted to correct this rapidly. Two days later, she was brought into the psychiatric emergency service of a large urban hospital because of her family's concern of her increasingly unsteady gait. A neurological examination indeed revealed a broad-based shuffling and uncoordinated gait. A CAT scan revealed cerebropontine myelinolysis, quite literally, the too rapid correction of her low sodium resulted in cells of her brainstem swelling and bursting. In other patients with severe anorexia in which the heart muscle has been broken down to provide fuel for the body, intravenous fluids have been known to precipitate congestive heart failure.

TABLE 7.1. Clinical Characteristics of Eating Disorders

Characteristic	Anorexia Nervosa	Bulimia Nervosa	Binge-Eating Disorder
Dieting/fasting	Always	Usually	Usually
Binge eating	Sometimes	Always	Always
Purging	Sometimes	Usually	Seldom
Weight preoccupation	Always	Always	Always
Body image distortion	Always	Sometimes	Sometimes
Body weight	Decreased	Normal	Increased
Amenorrhea	Always	Seldom	Seldom

Sociological factors also play a critical role in the pathogenesis of the eating disorders. In an era when food is plentiful in essentially all of the world's industrialized nations, being somewhat overweight is no longer a sign of wealth or social distinction. Instead, the maintenance of a thin physique connotes health, success, and a higher social status. Within a societal context that values thinness, pressure from friends and family in the form of teasing or unfavorable comparison can intensify the individual's preoccupation with the maintenance of a thin physique. Thus, the cultural premium that Western society places on a thin body creates a climate ripe for the development of body image distortions and consequent abnormalities in eating behavior.

Finally, psychological factors also impact the development of eating disorders. Although studies have shown that both healthy volunteers and patients with eating disorders exhibit some distortions in body image, the degree of distortion is greatly exaggerated in those with eating disorders. Additionally, the frequently low self-esteem of individuals with eating disorders renders them overly reliant on physical appearance as a vehicle to obtain acceptance or to attract potential mates. With the focus on physical attributes and presentation, the control or reduction of body weight provides an objective measure of success and a sense of personal mastery. These individuals may struggle with the complexities of social interaction; however, through the repetition of physically demanding but nonetheless simplistic behaviors such as fasting and purging, they can easily attain a readily measurable victory in their lives. The distortion of body image combined with the powerful objective reinforcement of weight reduction within a societal context in which "thin is in" sets the stage for the development of an eating disorder.

7.2 ANOREXIA NERVOSA

7.2.1 Brief Description and Diagnostic Criteria

Anorexia nervosa is a chronic and potentially life-threatening illness that has been recognized for over a century. Although appetite loss secondary to medical illness or depression may precipitate weight loss in the initial stages of AN, the avolitional loss of appetite (i.e., anorexia) is seldom a feature of AN. Instead, the measures

TABLE 7.2. Diagnostic Criteria for Anorexia Nervosa

A. Refuses to maintain normal body weight (85% of expected weight).
B. Despite being thin, feels afraid of being fat.
C. One of the following disturbances of body image:
   1. Misinterprets own body shape or weight
   2. Preoccupied with body shape or weight
   3. Denies seriousness of weight loss
D. In females, menstrual cycling stops for three full cycles.

Source: Adapted from DSM-IV.

taken by the patient with AN to achieve or sustain weight loss are usually willful and driven by an accompanying distortion in the self-assessment of body shape and size and a desire for emancipation from the expectations of parents and others.

The four key features of AN are universally recognized and include the refusal to maintain a minimally standard body weight relative to age and height, a concomitant distortion of body image, a persistent fear of gaining weight, and the cessation of menstrual cycling in females. The weight loss associated with AN is invariably severe and is ultimately complicated by a debilitating and potentially fatal compromise in cardiovascular and metabolic function.

One common misconception is that only patients with BN exhibit bulimic behaviors such as binge eating or laxative abuse. As previously noted, during the course of any eating disorder, most patients engage in the full spectrum of eating behavior derangements including dieting, binging, and purging. In accordance with DSM-IV nosology, each episode of AN is in fact subtyped by the presence or absence of bulimic behaviors (Table 7.2). In a restricting episode, the patient loses weight primarily through dieting, fasting, and exercising; whereas in a bulimic episode, the patient with AN also engages in regular binging or purging. The bulimic subtype of AN is distinguished from BN by its substantial weight loss and the cessation of menses.

7.2.2 Prevalence and Risk Factors

AN is a well-publicized yet rare disorder. The disproportionate media coverage given AN likely results from the strikingly emaciated appearance of those suffering from the disorder, the often tragic consequences of the illness, and the fact that those in highly visible occupations such as modeling and dancing are at increased risk for developing AN.

The onset of AN typically occurs in late adolescent or early adult females at a rate of 0.2–0.5% in that group. The average age at onset is approximately 17 years old; AN rarely begins prior to puberty or after 50 years of age. Contrary to reports in the popular media, there is no evidence that AN or other eating disorders have reached epidemic proportions; nevertheless, the prevalence of AN appears to have slowly increased and in conjunction with other eating disorders is among the most common psychiatric disorders affecting young women.

Numerous risk factors for the development of AN have been identified. The rate of AN among women is approximately ten times higher than that for males. Familial risk factors include the presence of a first degree relative with AN and a family environment in which weight control or weight reduction is emphasized. Cultural risk factors include being born into a Western, industrialized society or, among those immigrating to the West from other cultures, the degree of acculturation to Western ideals of body image. Dieting is also a major risk factor for the development of AN and other eating disorders. The risk of developing an eating disorder appears to rise with the increasing frequency or duration of dieting. Finally, certain personality traits including dependency, unquestioned compliance with authority, perfectionism, rigidity, and a lack of impulsivity are frequently observed among anorexia patients.

As noted earlier, AN is extremely rare in men. Little is known regarding the risk factors leading to AN in men.

7.2.3 Presentation and Clinical Course

The onset of AN frequently follows a stressful life event such as a severe medical illness, parental divorce, or leaving home for college. Patients with AN frequently minimize or hide their weight-reducing behaviors and may escape detection for some time. Because they commonly deny their illness and in fact embrace their symptoms as a statement of personal autonomy, patients with AN seldom present for medical care with complaints regarding weight loss. More often, the AN patient is reluctantly brought to medical attention by family members or friends understandably concerned by the marked weight loss. This poor insight into the illness is a hallmark of AN that complicates treatment compliance throughout the course of the illness. When a patient with AN does present for care without the urging of others, it is typically not to express concern regarding weight loss. Instead, AN patients usually complain of the unpleasant physical sequelae of starvation including abdominal pain and distension, constipation, cold intolerance, or fatigue.

The course of AN is highly variable. Some patients with anorexia experience a single episode of the disorder with full recovery. Others have recurrent exacerbations of AN interspersed with periods of remission during which they return to a normal weight. Finally, some AN patients experience a chronic, deteriorating course that results in frequent hospitalizations for medical stabilization. Of the chronic AN patients who are admitted to academic center hospitals for medical care, 10% ultimately die from AN due to starvation, suicide, or electrolyte imbalance.

7.2.4 Initial Evaluation and Differential Diagnosis

The differential diagnosis for AN includes the other eating disorders, other psychiatric disorders in which weight loss or eating disturbance may occur, and finally any undetected medical illness that may cause significant weight loss through either decreased appetite or excessive burning of calories (e.g., hyperthyroidism).

TABLE 7.3. Some Physical Signs of Anorexia Nervosa

Emaciation
Low blood pressure (<70 mm Hg)
Low pulse (<60 beats per minute)
Low body temperature
Dry skin
Yellow skin (hypercarotenemia)
Abundance of fine silky body hair (lanugo)
Swelling in extremities
Small red blotches on extremities (petechiae)

The prolonged starvation of AN produces a striking physical appearance. Most obvious is the pronounced emaciation in which the skin appears draped over the skeleton due to the loss of subcutaneous fat. Other physical signs of AN are listed in Table 7.3. It is this marked weight loss that primarily serves to distinguish AN from the other eating disorders. The key to diagnostic assessment is thus determining the cause of the patient's weight loss.

Because AN patients often hide their aberrant behaviors, the initial evaluation must include interviews with friends and family members who commonly provide a more reliable history of the eating patterns. Additionally, a thorough assessment of the patient's attitude toward food and weight including any evidence of preoccupation with or distortion of body image should be conducted. Finally, the initial evaluation must include a comprehensive medical evaluation. At this juncture, the medical examination serves two purposes. First, any occult medical causes for weight loss such as cancer, AIDS, hyperthyroidism, or gastrointestinal disease can be detected. Second, a prompt medical assessment can identify any dangerous medical complications of AN that require immediate intervention.

Appropriate management of AN also requires the early detection and treatment of any comorbid psychiatric disorders. The most common comorbid conditions associated with AN are major depressive disorder (MDD), obsessive–compulsive disorder (OCD), and substance use disorders. At the time of presentation, over 50% of AN patients also fulfill criteria for MDD; however, accurate diagnosis of depression in these patients is complicated by the fact that prolonged starvation often produces a mood disturbance and neurovegetative symptoms identical to MDD. If MDD appears to be comorbid with AN at the time of presentation, there is debate as to whether it is more prudent to withhold treatment of the depression until weight restoration has been initiated. If the depression persists despite refeeding, then treatment of the depression is likely warranted.

OCD is also frequently comorbid with AN; in fact, some researchers posit that the eating disorders are a modern variant of OCD peculiar to Western culture. In particular, the propensity for excessive exercise among some patients with AN may indicate the presence of comorbid OCD. Finally, the abuse of alcohol and other substances commonly complicates the presentation and course of AN. Comorbid substance abuse will likely undermine any progress in the treatment of AN and therefore must be detected and treated early if the treatment of AN is to be successful.

7.2.5 History of Pharmacological Treatment

The few controlled studies of pharmacotherapy for AN have largely been disappointing. No class of medication has consistently proved effective in the treatment of AN; consequently, pharmacotherapy plays a relatively minor role in the routine management of the disorder. Nevertheless, a review of the medications tested for the treatment of AN is informative. Medications used in the treatment of AN include appetite stimulants, antidepressants, antipsychotics, anxiolytics, trace mineral supplementation, prokinetics, and opiate antagonists.

Appetite Stimulants. A large body of neuroscience research indicates that serotonin plays a prominent role in the modulation of appetite. Increases in serotonin availability in certain brain regions confer a sense of satiety, and decreases of serotonin are associated with hunger. Consequently, agents that block the release or action of serotonin in the brain increase appetite and should theoretically be helpful in the treatment of AN.

Cyproheptadine (Periactin). Cyproheptadine is an antihistamine, commonly used to alleviate allergy symptoms, that also has serotonin-blocking properties. It has been successfully used to stimulate appetite in patients with medical illnesses such as cancer or AIDS. Cyproheptadine provides a small but measurable benefit in the rapidity of weight gain during the refeeding of patients with the restricting subtype of AN. However, bulimic subtype patients apparently fare worse with the addition of cyproheptadine.

Cyproheptadine is not an addictive or habit-forming substance. In the study referenced above, it was administered three times per day with a total daily dose from 12 to 32 mg/day. Common side effects of this medication include drowsiness, dry mouth, and drying of the nasal passages and airways. Caution should be exercised when administering cyproheptadine with other sedating medications.

Clonidine (Catapres). Clonidine, an antihypertensive medication that decreases serotonin availability through a mechanism distinct from cyproheptadine, has also been tested in the treatment of AN. Unfortunately, clonidine does not appear to promote weight gain in anorexia patients. In addition, clonidine may further exacerbate the low blood pressure that AN patients commonly experience. Consequently, clonidine has no role in the treatment of AN.

Tetrahydrocannabinol (Marinol). Finally, tetrahydrocannabinol, the psychoactive substance in marijuana, has also been used for its appetite stimulating effects. It is also ineffective in promoting weight gain in those with anorexia and has reportedly precipitated depression in a number of patients. It is also not used in the treatment of AN.

The use of appetite stimulants during the refeeding phase of AN treatment has not been particularly successful. This is likely due to the fact that AN is not a true disturbance of appetite. Instead, hunger is universally experienced by AN patients who gain a sense of achievement and personal mastery by overcoming hunger and resisting the urge to eat. With concomitant psychotherapeutic intervention to address the distortions of body image and personal achievement, the adjunctive use of cyproheptadine may be of limited help in some AN patients of the restricting subtype. In general, however, appetite stimulants are not useful in the treatment of AN.

Antidepressants. There are numerous reasons to expect that antidepressants may be helpful in the treatment of AN. First, depressed mood and other symptoms of depression such as anhedonia, decreased energy, poor concentration, and psychomotor retardation are common in cases of starvation from any cause. Second, AN patients and their family members have high rates of comorbid MDD and OCD, illnesses best treated with antidepressant medications. Finally, weight gain is a well-documented side effect of many antidepressants including the tricyclic antidepressants (TCAs) and mirtazapine.

TCAs. Two tricyclics, clomipramine (Anafranil) and amitriptyline (Elavil), have been studied in AN. The obsessive preoccupation with food and body image pathognomonic of AN led clinicians to study clomipramine first, recognizing its well-documented efficacy for the treatment of OCD. Unfortunately, clomipramine did not successfully improve weight gain. Amitriptyline has been evaluated in AN studies with mixed results.

Despite limited success with amitriptyline in some anorexia patients, using this class of antidepressants can be problematic in AN patients and therefore cannot be routinely recommended. TCAs slow gastrointestinal function and can therefore worsen the constipation and bloating that commonly plague AN patients during refeeding. In addition, TCAs can increase the likelihood of seizure or cardiac arrhythmia in patients already at risk due to electrolyte disturbances. Moreover, they are often lethal after overdose.

Monoamine Oxidase Inhibitors (MAOIs). There are no controlled studies of MAOIs for the treatment of AN. In addition, the dietary restrictions imposed on patients taking this class of antidepressant and their propensity for lowering blood pressure makes their use in AN inadvisable. In the future, the issue of using MAOIs may be reopened with the advent of the so-called reversible MAOIs such as moclobemide that apparently do not require a tyramine-restricted diet.

Specific Serotonin Reuptake Inhibitors (SSRIs). To date, the only SSRI studied in AN is fluoxetine (Prozac). During the acute refeeding phase of treatment, fluoxetine shows modest improvement in weight gain while a larger controlled study during the maintenance phase of treatment demonstrated effectiveness in the prevention of relapse. From the standpoint of side effects and toxicity, the SSRIs are clearly preferable to the older TCAs and MAOIs, particularly for medically compromised patients.

Atypical Antidepressants. None of the so-called atypical antidepressants have been tested in the treatment of AN. However, mianserin, an antidepressant available in Europe, has been found to increase body weight in patients with various depressive disorders. Although bupropion (Wellbutrin, Zyban) has not been tested in the treatment of AN, it is effective in the treatment of BN. However, immediate-release bupropion is associated with an especially high risk for seizures in these patients and is therefore contraindicated in those with eating disorders. The seizure risk associated with sustained-release bupropion remains unclear at this time, as the doses studied have not been as high as those for immediate-release bupropion.

Anxiolytics. The use of anxiety-reducing medications has not been systematically assessed in the treatment of AN. Nevertheless, many clinicians anecdotally report that the use of short-acting benzodiazepine such as lorazepam (Ativan) prior to mealtime diminishes anticipatory anxiety and thereby facilitates refeeding.

Zinc Replacement. Clinical similarities between the symptoms of zinc deficiency and the symptoms of AN have led some clinicians to institute zinc replacement therapy in the treatment of AN. The only controlled study of zinc therapy in AN demonstrated moderate efficacy of 100 mg/day of zinc gluconate during the acute refeeding phase of treatment. However, the use of zinc supplementation remains controversial. First, incontrovertible evidence for zinc deficiency in AN is lacking. Second, the psychological impact of a therapy that emphasizes a particular micronutrient constituent of food may undermine the overall goal of normalizing eating behavior.

Prokinetics. After prolonged fasting, it is natural for the gastrointestinal (GI) system to become quiescent. Consequently, if refeeding is started aggressively in the treatment of AN, delayed emptying of stomach contents may lead to bloating and abdominal distension. Prokinetic medications such as cisapride (Propulsid), metoclopramide (Reglan), and domperidone (Motilium) stimulate stomach contractility and therefore speed gastric emptying, which can in turn alleviate these early refeeding symptoms.

In most cases, however, a gradual stepwise increment in meal quantities during the initiation of refeeding naturally accelerates gastric emptying and sufficiently minimizes these unpleasant GI symptoms. Consequently, prokinetic medications are not recommended for routine use in the treatment of AN but may be helpful for a subset with severe or prolonged GI symptoms. Caution should be used with cisapride (no longer marketed in the United States) as it has recently been found to have the potential for producing cardiac conduction delay and a subsequent risk of sudden cardiac death much more frequently than was originally appreciated.

7.2.6 Current Approach to Treatment

The treatment of AN is divided into two distinct phases with unique treatment goals and approaches (see Table 7.4). The goals for the acute phase of AN treatment include the restoration of a minimally standard body weight and the correction of any adverse medical sequelae of prolonged starvation. As previously noted, AN patients should be referred promptly to a physician for thorough medical evaluation. Severely malnourished anorexia patients at less than 80% of normal body weight, patients with life-threatening metabolic abnormalities, patients with the binging–purging subtype of AN, and those who have been ill for 2 years or more usually require hospitalization during this phase of treatment. In addition, a nutritionist who exhibits empathy and a nonjudgmental attitude toward the AN patient can aid this stage of treatment through the promotion of healthy eating patterns and the development of a sound nutritional plan.

Critical to the success of the acute phase of treatment is implementation of an incremental diet that is coordinated with a behavioral plan. The diet should be initiated at 500 kilocalories/day in three balanced meals and two to three small snacks. Every 4–5 days the diet should be incremented by 500 kilocalories until reaching a maximum of 3500–4500 kilocalories/day. Once a safe and reasonable target weight is attained, the daily caloric intake can be reduced. Some degree of discomfort is expected during the refeeding phase, with bloating and constipation being the most common complaints. However, should the symptoms become severe or protracted, medical intervention may be necessary.

Medications may play an adjunctive role during this initial acute phase of treatment. For the restricting subtype of AN, cyproheptadine may provide some benefit

TABLE 7.4. Treatment Phases for Anorexia Nervosa

Acute Phase of Treatment

1. Medical evaluation
2. Nutritional assessment and counseling
3. Individual psychotherapy
4. Family psychotherapy
5. Substance abuse treatment (if indicated)
6. Adjunctive use of medication
   a. Consider antidepressant therapy (especially SSRI)
   b. Consider appetite stimulant (especially in restricting subtype)
   c. Consider anxiolytic (if significant premeal anxiety)
   d. Consider medical treatments for GI symptoms during refeeding

Maintenance Phase of Treatment

1. Continuation of psychotherapy
2. Consider maintenance antidepressant therapy
3. Periodic medical reassessment
4. Periodic nutritional reassessment

TABLE 7.5. Managing Gastrointestinal Symptoms During AN Refeeding

Mild-to-moderate GI symptoms
Continue diet increments
Constipation
Fiber supplement
Stool softener
Abdominal radiograph
Laxative (if x-ray confirms constipation)
Swelling of extremities
Low-sodium diet
Elevate feet
Delay diet increment until swelling resolves
Reflux
H2 blocker, proton pump inhibitor
If no improvement, endoscopy
Severe bloating
Prokinetic
If no improvement, endoscopy

in hastening weight gain. In addition, a short-acting benzodiazepine prior to meals may help patients with significant premeal anticipatory anxiety. Antidepressant therapy, preferably with a SSRI, may provide a modest benefit during the acute phase of treatment, particularly in patients with comorbid depression or OCD. Finally, management of any unpleasant symptoms during refeeding with fiber, stool softeners, or prokinetic agents can be helpful (see Table 7.5).

Treatment goals for AN during the maintenance phase of treatment include the gradual correction of body image distortions, which if unaddressed will eventually undermine the progress made during the initial phase of treatment, and the continuous monitoring for, and correction of, aberrant eating behaviors. Psychosocial interventions, including psychotherapy for the patient and family, and periodic nutritional assessment remain the nucleus of treatment.

There likely remains a role for pharmacotherapy for some AN patients during the maintenance phase of treatment. Appetite stimulants, prokinetics, and anxiolytics should be tapered and discontinued at the conclusion of the acute phase of treatment. However, early evidence suggests that continued antidepressant administration may help to sustain remission. The appropriate duration for maintenance pharmacotherapy in AN has not been well studied and remains open to debate.

7.3 BULIMIA NERVOSA

7.3.1 Brief Description and Diagnostic Criteria

Despite the fact that overeating has troubled humankind for centuries, an eating disorder whose chief feature is binge eating was not formally recognized in the psychiatric nosology until 1980. Bulimia nervosa (BN) is characterized by recurrent episodes of uncontrolled binge eating alternating with repeated compensatory behaviors such as fasting, excessive exercising, or purging, in order to prevent weight gain. Like anorexia nervosa (AN), BN is associated with a preoccupation with food, body shape, and weight. However, in contrast to AN, the patient with BN maintains a normal to slightly obese body weight.

Although binge eating is a conceptually meaningful term, the distinction between a binge and lesser degrees of overeating is not always apparent. Many consider the consumption of any quantity of calorie-laden "junk food" as a binge. From a diagnostic standpoint, a binge consists of the consumption of an amount of food over a particular period of time that is in excess of what most people would eat in a similar time frame. An accurate determination of the amount consumed during the typical binge is important. Binges are highly variable in size, sometimes ranging up to 10,000 kilocalories consumed in a single sitting. A binge is also characterized by a sense of being out of control. BN patients commonly report eating more rapidly than normal during a binge and being unable to stop eating until becoming uncomfortably full.

The subtyping of bulimia is predicated on the compensatory measures taken to counteract the often-massive caloric intake during binges. The nonpurging subtype of BN is characterized by fasting or excessive exercise to compensate for binging. The more common purging subtype is defined by frequent self-induced vomiting and less often by laxative or diuretic abuse. These patients induce vomiting by inserting a finger into the throat or rarely by ingesting ipecac. Most treatment studies of bulimia have focused on the purging subtype (see Table 7.6).

7.3.2 Prevalence and Risk Factors

Early reports that BN is epidemic among young women in the United States now appear overstated. Although many women occasionally binge or purge, the number of women who regularly engage in these behaviors remains small. Nevertheless, BN is more common than AN, affecting 2–3% of young women. Like AN, BN occurs ten times more often in women than men.

TABLE 7.6. Diagnostic Criteria for Bulimia Nervosa

A. Repeated binge eating characterized by both of the following:
   1. Eating excessive amounts of food in a short period of time
   2. Feeling unable to stop eating or control how much is eaten
B. Repeatedly tries to compensate for overeating by vomiting; abusing laxatives, diuretics, or enemas; fasting; or exercising excessively.
C. Both binge eating and attempts to compensate for overeating occur at least twice a week for 3 months.
D. Preoccupied with body shape or weight.
E. Does not fulfill criteria for anorexia nervosa.

Source: Adapted from DSM-IV.

Onset of the disorder typically occurs after puberty during late adolescence or early adulthood. The risk factors for the development of BN are similar to those for AN with a history of dieting being most important. A common scenario occurs in which a young woman diets in order to lose weight. After a period of success, the young woman then begins overeating. Concerned by her inability to control her eating and having heard from friends that purging is an effective means to control weight, she resorts to this more drastic method to preserve the earlier progress made by dieting. Gradually, the frequency of overeating and the amount consumed during these episodes increase and in turn require more frequent compensatory purging. A second commonly described scenario is binging in response to perceived stressors with the binge providing what is described as a temporary "emotional numbing." This numbing effect rarely persists for long after the conclusion of the binge.

Other risk factors common to BN and AN include shyness, perfectionism, and low self-esteem. Unique to BN is its apparent association with poor impulse control and reportedly higher rates among women with Cluster B personality disorders. Also distinguishing BN from AN is the greater vulnerability to obesity with higher rates of childhood obesity and family obesity among bulimia patients. Little is known regarding the risk factors for BN among men. Preliminary evidence suggests, however, that BN may be more common among homosexual and bisexual men compared with heterosexual men.

7.3.3 Presentation and Clinical Course

Patients with bulimia are typically embarrassed by their binging and purging behaviors and therefore seldom spontaneously report them. In addition, their weight is usually within the normal to slightly obese range. As a result, BN does not command the immediate clinic attention of AN and is often a secret, hidden illness for many years.

BN patients are dissatisfied with their body shape and preoccupied with food and weight control. In screening patients for BN and other eating disorders, patients should be asked their weight, what they wish to weigh, and how they have tried to control their weight. If this initial screening raises any concern for aberrant eating behavior, patients should be asked about fasting, binging, and purging. Specific questions should address self-induced vomiting, the use of diet pills, ipecac, diuretics, laxatives, and enemas. Despite having taken measures to hide their binging and purging for so long, many BN patients report a sense of relief in having finally revealed their secret.

Although those with bulimia usually maintain a relatively normal body weight, there are nonetheless telltale physical signs of their aberrant eating behavior (see Table 7.7). Specific to BN are dental erosion, "chubby cheeks" from enlargement of the parotid salivary glands, and abrasions on the back of one hand from repetitive self-induced vomiting.

The long-term course of BN remains unclear. In addition, reliable prognostic indicators are uncertain. It does appear, however, that for many patients the disorder

TABLE 7.7. Physical Signs of Bulimia Nervosa

Dental erosion
Chubby cheeks (enlargement of parotid salivary glands)
Abrasions on the back of one hand
Low blood pressure (systolic <70 mm Hg)
Low pulse (<60 beats per minute)

is chronic with periodic fluctuations in symptom severity. The mortality rate from BN is much lower than AN; however, the electrolyte disturbances from repeated purging can be hazardous. Of particular concern is the loss of potassium that primarily results from recurrent vomiting. Hypokalemia, or low serum potassium, can potentiate dangerous cardiac arrhythmias, which is an occasional cause of death in BN patients. A second potentially fatal, but fortunately rare, complication of bulimia is esophageal tearing caused by repeated self-induced vomiting that may in turn lead to sudden hemorrhage.

7.3.4 Initial Evaluation and Differential Diagnosis

When a thorough history of eating-related behaviors is obtained, BN is not difficult to diagnose. The bulimic subtype of AN shares the same behavioral characteristics but is invariably associated with a low body weight and in women the cessation of menstrual cycling. Binge-eating disorder also resembles BN but can be distinguished by the absence of routine compensatory measures to maintain weight.

The differential diagnosis of BN includes not only the other eating disorders but also major depressive disorder (MDD), particularly major depression with atypical features. Such patients overeat when depressed and often report significant weight gain during periods of depressed mood. The derangements in eating may simply be a symptom of the mood disorder and may not mandate the diagnosis of an eating disorder; however, if the overeating behavior meets the diagnostic criteria for binging and is accompanied by the aforementioned compensatory behaviors, then BN should be diagnosed in lieu of, or in addition to, a depressive disorder.

Finally, many persons experience nausea and involuntary vomiting in response to anxiety or stress. This is not always pathological. For example, it is commonplace for athletes to experience "butterflies" and occasionally vomiting prior to a game. They typically perform well during the game, are not bothered by these symptoms in other settings, and likely do not warrant a psychiatric diagnosis. However, when the nausea and vomiting are part of a more disabling complex of anxiety symptoms, then the diagnosis of an anxiety disorder such as panic disorder or social phobia should be considered. In instances in which the physical symptoms including nausea and vomiting are more pervasive and occur in a variety of social contexts, then the diagnosis of a somatoform disorder may be indicated. The key distinction between these syndromes and BN is the avolitional nature of the vomiting in the other disorders.

7.3.5 History of Pharmacological Treatment

Anticonvulsants. An early observation that BN patients may have abnormal electroencephalogram (EEG) results led to speculation that binge eating may represent an atypical behavioral presentation of seizure activity. Thus, the first controlled medication study for the treatment of BN evaluated the use of the antiseizure medication phenytoin (Dilantin). Phenytoin was not found to be significantly superior to placebo, and the earlier reports of EEG abnormalities were not confirmed. The results of a subsequent trial of carbamazepine (Tegretol), an anticonvulsant that has been reported to be effective in the treatment of bipolar disorder, were also disappointing. As a result, anticonvulsants are not routinely used in the treatment of BN.

Antidepressants. In the early 1980s, the recognition that depression is a frequent comorbid feature of BN coupled with the observation that appetite changes are a common feature of depression led researchers to evaluate antidepressant treatment for BN. Since that time, a series of controlled studies have demonstrated efficacy for a wide assortment of antidepressants including the TCAs imipramine (Tofranil) and desipramine (Norpramin), the MAOI phenelzine (Nardil), the SSRI fluoxetine (Prozac), and the atypical antidepressants trazodone (Desyrel) and bupropion (Wellbutrin). Overall, approximately two-thirds of antidepressant-treated patients with bulimia experience symptomatic improvement while nearly one-third achieves complete remission of binging and purging. In addition, the improvement in the symptoms of BN is not dependent on the presence of comorbid depression.

Although studies suggest that antidepressants of any class are efficacious for the treatment of BN, the favorable side effect profile and lower toxicity of the newer generation antidepressants make their use preferable. Of these, fluoxetine is the best studied and is the only antidepressant at this time with FDA approval for the treatment of BN.

Despite their efficacy, TCAs are not recommended as first-line medications in the treatment of BN for three reasons. First, this class of antidepressants has a potential for lowering blood pressure, a side effect not well tolerated by bulimia patients in a cycle of binging and purging. Second, the risk of dangerous cardiac arrhythmias or seizures while taking these medications is enhanced by common electrolyte disturbances resulting from recurrent vomiting in bulimia patients. Third, weight gain is a common side effect associated with TCA therapy that will often lead to noncompliance in the patient with BN.

MAOIs, although effective, are also problematic for routine use in the treatment of BN. First, like the TCAs, MAOIs have a propensity for lowering blood pressure. Additionally, bulimia patients, who are by definition prone to impulsive out of control eating, are not ideal candidates to maintain the strict tyramine-free diet restrictions imposed by MAOIs. Thus, they run a substantial risk of precipitating dangerous hypertensive crises through dietary noncompliance while taking MAOIs. It remains unclear whether the reversible MAOIs such as moclobemide will prove effective in the treatment of BN without the risks associated with other MAOIs.

Finally, although immediate-release bupropion is also effective in the treatment of BN, it is associated with a particularly high incidence of seizures in individuals with bulimia presumably due to electrolyte abnormalities and is now contraindicated for treatment of the disorder.

Appetite Suppressants. The evidence from laboratory animal studies that substances which increase serotonergic neurotransmission in the brain tend to decrease feeding in conjunction with the success of serotonin-modulating antidepressants in the treatment of BN encouraged the trials of serotonin-stimulating appetite suppressants. These include fenfluramine (Pondimin) and dexfenfluramine (Redux), which act primarily by increasing serotonin release and secondarily by blocking serotonin reuptake. The result is a potent increase in serotonergic neurotransmission in the brain.

Fenfluramine has not been systematically studied in the treatment of BN, but dexfenfluramine has been evaluated with disappointingly mixed results. Due to an association with the development of heart valve abnormalities and pulmonary hypertension, particularly when coadministered with phentermine (Ionamin) in the so-called Fen-Phen strategy, these medications have recently been removed from the U.S. market.

Conceptually, the use of appetite suppressants in the treatment of eating disorders is problematic. These agents are marketed not as eating disorder treatments but as antiobesity medications. A substantial portion of these agents is prescribed through weight loss clinics. Such clinics exist to treat obesity and do not always screen for the presence of eating disorders or offer the comprehensive treatment necessary to address these disorders. Unfortunately, this therapeutic rationale not only bypasses the significant psychodynamic issues of BN but may actually reinforce them. Appetite suppressants, instead of being an effective tool in the management of the eating disorder, can become yet another abused substance in the cycle of binging and purging. For more discussion of the role of antiobesity treatments in eating disorders, refer to the discussion of binge-eating disorder (Section 7.4).

Opiate Antagonists. The role of endogenous opioids such as endorphins in the rewarding aspects of satiation led to speculation that blocking their action may decrease the satisfaction experienced during binging episodes. It was hypothesized that binging could be extinguished by reducing the pleasurable sensations associated with it. Naltrexone (Revia) has been utilized in the treatment of BN, but with limited success. For additional information regarding naltrexone, please refer to the discussion in Chapter 6 Substance Use Disorders.

7.3.6 Current Approach to Treatment

The key symptoms of the disorder are for most patients with bulimia disgusting and distressful; therefore, once the secret of their illness has been uncovered, they are usually eager to accept help. This is in stark contrast to the treatment of individuals with anorexia whose symptoms are ego-syntonic and thus set up endless power struggles with care providers. Consequently, the treatment of BN is infrequently plagued by the deceptive, willful noncompliance seen in the treatment of AN. Nevertheless, the impulsive nature of the disorder does mandate vigilance for sporadic nonadherence with treatment.

The initial decision in treatment selection is the choice between psychotherapy, medication, or both. It appears that most structured, time-limited psychotherapies are beneficial, though cognitive-behavioral therapy (CBT) has been the best studied. In addition, the therapeutic gains from psychotherapy appear to be sustained after the therapy has concluded. Antidepressant medications are generally as effective as psychotherapy in reducing binging and purging behavior during short-term treatment; however, the evidence for long-term remission of bulimic symptoms after a single course of antidepressant treatment is lacking. As a result, short-term psychotherapy is recommended as the treatment of choice for most patients presenting with BN.

Some clinicians contend that the combination of psychotherapy with an antidepressant is more effective than either treatment alone. Although plausible, objective data to verify this assumption is not yet available. It is therefore recommended that patients with mild-to-moderate symptoms be treated with time-limited psychotherapy alone, while those with severe symptoms risking medical compromise and those with comorbid depression or OCD receive the combination of psychotherapy and antidepressant medication.

The first-line medication for the treatment of BN will usually be a SSRI of which fluoxetine is the best studied. Although most antidepressants effectively treat BN at doses comparable to those routinely used to treat depression, fluoxetine is considerably more effective at 60 mg/day than lower doses.

A primary concern, when administering any medication to a patient with bulimia, is the loss of medication through purging. In particular, vomiting within 1–2 hours after ingesting a dose can result in a significant loss of medication. When possible, it is recommended that medications be administered once daily at bedtime in order to minimize the likelihood of medication loss due to vomiting.

7.3.7 Patients with Refractory Disease

Patients with BN unresponsive to psychotherapy alone should likely receive a trial of antidepressant medication with continued psychotherapy. Switching to a different psychotherapeutic modality may be considered at this juncture as well.

When a patient does not improve with the combination of an antidepressant and psychotherapy, then a careful history regarding compliance and the timing of doses with respect to purging episodes should be collected. If nonadherence is an issue, then the reasons for the nonadherence should be explored. If vomiting is frequently occurring within 2 hours of medication administration, then changing the medication schedule can be attempted. If after obtaining a history it remains unclear whether significant amounts of medication are being omitted or lost through purging, then checking the serum level of the medication to ensure adherence can be helpful. For patients who are adherent with treatment and who are not losing the medication during purging episodes, yet who remain unresponsive after an adequate trial of medication, there may be benefit in trying alternative antidepressants. When switching antidepressants, choosing an agent with a different mechanism of action from its predecessor is generally recommended. For example, switching a patient who does not respond to fluoxetine to another SSRI is presumed less likely to afford a clinical advantage than switching to an antidepressant of another class.

Additional options for refractory disorders include the augmentation of antidepressant treatment with an opiate blocking agent such as naltrexone or consideration of partial or full hospitalization to provide a more structured environment for normalizing the aberrant eating behavior.

7.4 BINGE-EATING DISORDER

7.4.1 Brief Description and Diagnostic Criteria

Binge-eating disorder (BED) appears in DSM-IV without formal diagnostic recognition but as a diagnosis proposed for further study. Its relationship to milder forms of overeating and to other eating disorders, particularly bulimia nervosa (BN), remains unclear. BED may ultimately warrant classification as a subtype of BN, may remain a distinct diagnostic entity requiring independent consideration, or may simply exist on a continuum with other overeating behaviors not representing a psychiatric disorder.

Like BN, BED is characterized by recurrent binge eating; however, inappropriate compensatory behaviors such as fasting and purging are not a regular feature of BED. Consequently, the patient with BED is often obese. In addition, binge eaters exhibit a preoccupation with food and weight reminiscent of the other eating disorders and are commonly distressed by their inability to stop binging (see Table 7.8 for diagnostic criteria).

TABLE 7.8. Diagnostic Criteria for Binge-Eating Disorder

A. Repeated binge eating characterized by both of the following:
   1. Eating lots of food in a short period of time
   2. Feeling unable to stop eating or control how much is eaten
B. Plus at least three of the following occur during binges:
   1. Eats very rapidly
   2. Eats until uncomfortably full
   3. Eats lots of food even when not hungry
   4. Eats alone because embarrassed about binging
   5. Feels guilty, depressed, or disgusted with self after binging
C. Very upset about binging.
D. Binging occurs at least twice a week for 6 months.
E. No repeated attempts to compensate for overeating and does not fulfill criteria for bulimia nervosa or anorexia nervosa.

Soure: Adapted from DSM-IV.

7.4.2 Prevalence and Risk Factors

If formally recognized, BED would represent the most common of the eating disorders with a prevalence of 2–5% among adult women in the United States. In addition, BED is much more common among men than other eating disorders. The female/male ratio of BED is approximately 2 : 1 in contrast to the ratio of 10 : 1 for anorexia nervosa (AN) and BN.

The only comprehensive study of the risk factors for BED found that, like BN, BED is associated with risk factors both for general psychiatric disturbance and for obesity. The psychological risk factors include childhood physical or sexual abuse, parental depression, parental eating disorder, shyness, perfectionism, or low self-esteem. The obesity risk factors include childhood obesity, negative comments from family members regarding weight and eating, and a history of recurrent dieting. In comparison to BN, the association to psychological risk factors was predictably stronger for BN than BED. Surprisingly, the association to obesity risk factors was also stronger for BN than BED. This is surprising because obesity itself is much more common among patients with BED than those with BN. One plausible explanation is that the stronger association to obesity risk factors intensifies the bulimic patient's motivation to engage in compensatory behaviors that tend to normalize weight.

7.4.3 Presentation and Clinical Course

Although the majority of obese individuals do not exhibit BED, the disorder is common among those seeking obesity treatment. Evidence suggests that nearly one-third of weight loss program participants meet diagnostic criteria for BED. Definitive treatment for BED is not yet formulated; nevertheless, there are certain aspects of routine obesity treatment that may not be appropriate for patients with an eating disorder and there are aspects of eating disorder treatment that are not incorporated into most weight reduction programs.

The rising prevalence of obesity in developed nations, coupled with the evidence that a substantial number of obese individuals display BED, suggests that this is a significant public health problem. Unfortunately, the longitudinal course of the disorder is not well characterized. The disorder may arguably lead to progressive worsening of obesity or to the development of more debilitating eating disorders such as BN.

7.4.4 Initial Evaluation and Differential Diagnosis

Obesity, in the absence of an eating disorder, still carries significant health risks. Obese individuals exhibit higher rates of diabetes mellitus, hypertension, hyperlipidemia, gastrointestinal cancers, gallbladder disease, and heart disease. When assessing an obese patient for the presence of an eating disorder, the obesity should not be ignored or minimized for two key reasons. First, addressing the obesity can provide significant health benefit. Studies show that weight loss as small as 10% can significantly improve overall well-being even in morbidly obese individuals. Second, for many patients the motivating factor for treatment is not changing eating behaviors but losing weight. This motivation should not be discouraged but exploited during the early phases of treatment. If the patient's desire for weight loss is prematurely dismissed, then the development of a therapeutic alliance and continued adherence with treatment may ultimately suffer.

Assessment of obesity during the initial evaluation should minimally consist of the measurement of height and weight and calculation of the body mass index (BMI) (see Eq. 7.1). Treatment aimed at weight reduction is strongly recommended when the BMI is 30 kg/m^2 or greater. Risk factors for obesity should also be assessed including a history of childhood obesity, family history of obesity, and the lifetime history of weight fluctuations.

$$\text{BMI} = \frac{\text{Weight in kilograms}}{(\text{Height in meters})^2} \tag{7.1}$$

Although evaluation of obesity is important, the elucidation of patterns of eating behavior is the critical component in the assessment of eating-disordered obese patients. Unfortunately, it is just this aspect of the evaluation that is most often neglected in treatment programs that too narrowly focus on weight reduction. If a careful history is obtained, then BED is not difficult to diagnose.

The differential diagnosis of BED is very similar to that of BN. It primarily consists of BN and depressive disorders characterized by overeating instead of anorexia. BED can be distinguished from BN by the absence of regular compensatory behaviors in the former disorder. BED can usually be differentiated from hyperphagia (i.e., overeating) during depression by gathering a longitudinal history of eating behaviors and mood disturbance. If binging occurs exclusively in the context of a depression, then the diagnosis of BED may not be warranted. Conversely, obese patients with BED are at significant risk for depression; thus, the presence of depression does not exclude the coexistence of this eating disorder.

7.4.5 History of Pharmacological Treatment

As a relatively new diagnostic entity, the treatment of BED is in its infancy. Treatment offerings to date have been predicated on two key observations. First, BED is phenomenologically similar to BN; therefore, treatments known to be effective for patients with bulimia will likely benefit those with BED. Second, patients with BED tend to be overweight. The health and social consequences of obesity lead many patients with BED to seek out weight reduction treatments.

Antidepressants. Short-term studies of desipramine and fluoxetine indicate that both medications reduce binging in patients with BED. In addition, fluoxetine-treated patients may also experience a modest reduction in weight during short-term treatment. However, this early weight loss with fluoxetine may not be sustained despite continued treatment.

In summary, early evidence appears to confirm the assumption that antidepressants, which successfully effect behavioral change in those with bulimia, will also do so in patients with BED. After discontinuation of a brief course of an antidepressant, binging frequency and severity often resume at pretreatment levels. The long-term efficacy of continued antidepressant administration is unknown.

Weight Reduction Treatments. Obesity is simple to understand in theory, but often difficult to reverse in practice. Obesity occurs when energy intake exceeds energy expenditure for a sustained period of time. The surplus calories from this energy imbalance are stored for later use in the form of fat. Despite this simple equation, the potential causes for this imbalance are myriad and often difficult to determine in a given individual.

The pharmacological treatment of obesity can be targeted at four key points. First, appetite suppressants can be used to reduce the intake of calories. To date, most antiobesity medications utilize this approach. Second, digestion inhibitors in the form of medications or food additives can decrease caloric intake by reducing the absorption of fat from the intestines. A prominent example of this approach is olestra, a recently introduced fat substitute. Third, thermogenic substances can increase energy expenditure by stimulating the sympathetic nervous system and thereby increasing metabolic activity. Over-the-counter diet preparations of caffeine and ephedrine act in this manner. Finally, hormonal manipulation of the newly discovered leptin and orexin molecules may be used to modulate hunger. This avenue of treatment is in the preliminary stages of investigation and remains years away from producing treatment alternatives.

Treatment of obesity in patients with BED should optimally facilitate both weight reduction and changes in eating behavior. Thermogenic agents and digestive inhibitors bypass the behavioral aberration of binge eating and may theoretically enable continued binging by ameliorating its untoward consequences. Thus, there is no defensible rationale for prominent use of these agents in obese patients with BED. Although hormonal treatments offer promise, no medications are yet available.

Appetite suppressants have widely been used in the treatment of obesity. These medications reduce appetite by increasing the activity of serotonin, norepinephrine, or both. The first appetite suppressants, amphetamines, were quite effective in reducing appetite by increasing the brain activity of norepinephrine. Amphetamines were once a mainstay of weight reduction treatment; however, their euphoria-inducing properties, likely mediated through increases in dopamine availability, led to rampant abuse. As a result, amphetamines are no longer recommended for the treatment of obesity. One notable exception is phentermine (Ionamin), an amphetamine-derivative with less potential for abuse because it does not stimulate dopamine release like other amphetamines. At doses necessary to reduce appetite, phentermine produces unpleasant side effects including insomnia, headache, anxiety, irritability, palpitations, and elevated pulse and blood pressure. Consequently, phentermine is not used alone as an appetite suppressant; however, it does effectively augment the effects of serotonin-based appetite suppressants at lower, more tolerable doses. The typical role of phentermine in obesity treatment has thus been as an augmentation agent.

In recent years, the most widely used appetite suppressants were fenfluramine (Pondimin) and dexfenfluramine (Redux), which both act by stimulating the release of serotonin from nerve cells and subsequently blocking its reuptake. These medications have been used alone and in combination with phentermine in the so-called Fen-Phen approach. Fenfluramine and dexfenfluramine are demonstrably effective in helping obese patients lose weight; however, they have not been specifically studied in the treatment of BED. The most common side effects of these medications are similar to those experienced by patients treated with SSRIs, including nausea, diarrhea, drowsiness, dry mouth, and dizziness. In addition, these medications have been accused of inducing depression, theoretically by overstimulating and thus damaging serotonin-secreting neurons. Dexfenfluramine may also be associated with an increased risk for development of primary pulmonary hypertension, a serious and potentially lethal lung condition. The most ominous side effect of fenfluramine and dexfenfluramine is the development of heart valve abnormalities after prolonged coadministration with phentermine. This serious complication led the FDA to request the voluntary withdrawal of fenfluramine and dexfenfluramine from the U.S. market in the fall of 1997.

Since the withdrawal of fenfluramine and dexfenfluramine, some clinicians have begun coadministering fluoxetine and phentermine. Perhaps this combination will produce the clinical benefit of the Fen-Phen combination without the dangerous complications. Because the efficacy and long-term risk of this combination are unknown, augmentation of fluoxetine with phentermine cannot be recommended for routine practice.

The newest appetite suppressant, sibutramine (Meridia), works by blocking the reuptake of both serotonin and norepinephrine. It does not stimulate nerve cells to release serotonin, as do fenfluramine and dexfenfluramine. Administered at 20 mg/day, sibutramine effectively reduces weight in obese patients, but its use has not been assessed in eating disorder patients. The most common side effects of this medication are insomnia, dry mouth, and constipation. It has not been associated with the more serious heart and lung complications observed with fenfluramine and dexfenfluramine. Because sibutramine acts in part through modulation of norepinephrine, there is no rational basis for coadministering phentermine, which acts via this same mechanism.

7.4.6 Current Approach to Treatment

Like the other eating disorders, BED requires a comprehensive and well-coordinated treatment approach. The goals of acute treatment are the cessation of binging and, for most patients, weight reduction. Standard cognitive-behavioral therapy (CBT) and antidepressant medication are both effective in reducing binging and treating any comorbid depression. Combining these treatments may be superior to using either alone. However, with the possible exception of fluoxetine, these treatments do not reliably promote weight loss in BED patients.

During acute treatment, the institution of a behavioral weight program and dietary counseling can facilitate weight reduction. In difficult cases, appetite suppressants can be considered, but available data does not support the indiscriminate use of these medications in obese patients with BED. At present, a multimodal treatment, incorporating standard CBT, dietary counseling, and a behavioral weight program, and giving consideration to the use of an antidepressant, is the preferred method of treatment.

The goals of long-term treatment are to sustain the behavioral changes and weight loss that were accomplished during acute management. Brief courses of standard CBT or antidepressant monotherapy do not reliably achieve this goal. Patients commonly regain weight and increase binging frequency after medication or short-term psychotherapy has been discontinued. Supplementation of these treatments with the aforementioned behavioral weight program may offer the best hope for sustained remission.

ADDITIONAL READING

Attia E, Schroeder L. Pharmacologic treatment of anorexia nervosa. *Int J Eat Disord* 2005; 37(Supplement): S60–S63.

Bellini M, Merli M. Current drug treatment of patients with bulimia nervosa and binge-eating disorder: selective serotonin reuptake inhibitors versus mood stabilizers. *Int J Psychiatry Clin Pract* 2004; 8: 235–243.

Birmingham CL, Beumont PJV, Crawford R, et al. *Medical Management of Eating Disorders: A Practical Handbook for Healthcare Professionals.* Cambridge, UK: Cambridge University Press, 2004.

Casper RC. How useful are pharmacological treatments in eating disorders? *Psychopharmacol Bull* 2002; 36(2): 88–104.

Crow SJ, Mitchell JE. Pharmacologic treatments for eating disorders. In Thompson JK (ed.), *Body Image, Eating Disorders, and Obesity: An Integrative Guide for Assessment and Treatment.* Washington DC: American Psychological Association, 2003, pp 345–360.

De Castro JM, Plunkett S. A general model of intake regulation. *Neurosci Biobehav Rev* 2002; 26(5): 581–595.

Devlin MJ, Yanovski SZ, Wilson GT. Obesity: what mental health professionals need to know. *Am J Psychiatry* 2000; 157(6): 854–866.

Fernandez-Lopez JA, Remesar X, Foz M, et al. Pharmacological approaches for the treatment of obesity. *Drugs* 2002; 62(6): 915–944.

Glazer G. Long-term pharmacotherapy of obesity 2000: a review of efficacy and safety. *Arch Intern Med* 2001; 161(15): 1814–1824.

Husted DS, Shapira NA. Binge-eating disorder and new pharmacologic treatments. *Primary Psychiatry* 2005; 12: 46–51.

Phelan S, Wadden TA. Combining behavioral and pharmacological treatments for obesity. *Obes Res* 2002; 10(6): 560–574.

Roerig JL, Mitchell JE, Myers TC, et al. Pharmacotherapy and medical complications of eating disorders in children and adolescents. *Child Adolesc Psychiatr Clin North Am* 2002; 11(2): 365–385.

Strober M. The future of treatment research in anorexia nervosa. *Int J Eat Disord* 2005; 37(Supplement): S90–S94.

Zhu AJ, Walsh BT. Pharmacologic treatment of eating disorders. *Can J Psychiatry* 2002; 47(3): 227–234.

8

ATTENTION DEFICIT–HYPERACTIVITY DISORDER

8.1 BRIEF DESCRIPTION AND DIAGNOSTIC CRITERIA

In the past several years, attention deficit–hyperactivity disorder (ADHD) has received considerable attention from both the lay public and the medical and psychological communities. It has become one of the more controversial of the psychiatric disorders. There are several factors that contribute to this phenomenon.

Primarily, ADHD is a disorder with a childhood onset. This raises several issues related to the diagnostic process, which is unfortunately often based on incomplete information from the individual who is affected. Children typically cannot provide a reliable history of their own symptoms; therefore, parents, teachers, and other caregivers are needed to provide this information instead. Children also have difficulty understanding the treatment that is being offered. Consent for treatment must be provided not by the child but by his/her parents; however, this can become a sticky issue when the child's parents are divorced, separated, or have differing views on the advisability of any particular treatment, including pharmacological interventions. The child is able to provide assent for treatment, but ultimately the decision to treat resides with the parent or legal guardian of the child. Treating an illness

Principles of Psychopharmacology for Mental Health Professionals
By Jeffrey E. Kelsey, D. Jeffrey Newport, and Charles B. Nemeroff

during childhood is also complicated by the fact that one must consider not only the here and now but also the future implications of the illness. A worried parent may ask, "Does having ADHD mean my child will be labeled as a bad kid?" Thus, the discussion with the child and parents should involve the impact of ADHD in the classroom, on the playground, and at home, in addition to the potential long-term stigma of the ADHD diagnosis, as well as the benefits of its treatment on the child's ultimate intellectual, emotional, and social abilities as an adult.

A second factor that relates to the controversy is the fact that many, if not most, ADHD symptoms are not so much abnormal behaviors as they are an exaggeration of normal activity. By comparison, the person who hears voices, has panic attacks, or is suicidal is clearly having symptoms that are not normal. We would all agree that these people are in need of psychiatric treatment. Children are, of course, naturally more active and less attentive than adults. They are supposed to be this way. Why would we try to "treat" it? Therefore, some have argued that ADHD does not really exist. They believe that when we use medications to treat a child diagnosed with ADHD, we are actually treating our own shortcomings as parents and teachers. The argument posed is that if we were able to better cope with our children, we would not unnecessarily resort to using medication. Furthermore, the question is often asked, "Doesn't the dramatic increase in the number of children diagnosed with ADHD show that we are all too quickly labeling these kids?"

Probably the greatest controversy surrounding ADHD stems from the fact that the mainstays of treatment, and until very recently the only FDA-approved treatments for ADHD, were the psychostimulant drugs. This of course raises even more concerns. First, some say that we as a society are prescribing our children drugs of abuse, and in so doing, we are condemning our children to a life of drug abuse as adults. Certainly, stimulant drugs can be abused. But is it true that we are getting our kids hooked on drugs just so they will behave for us? Are we truly setting them up to become alcoholics and drug addicts when they grow up? The data suggest that stimulant medications, though they have the potential for abuse, tend not to be abused by the individual for whom they are prescribed.

Others have said that we are just giving our children performance-enhancing drugs. Let us compare taking a stimulant to taking an antidepressant. When a person who is depressed takes an antidepressant, his/her mood improves, assuming successful treatment; however, if a person who is not depressed takes an antidepressant, it does not make that person happier or euphoric. Antidepressants are not "pep pills" that perk everyone up but medications that are believed to reverse the chemical abnormalities and relieve the clinical symptoms of depression. In this way, antidepressants help depressed patients recover from their illness, but they do not further elevate an already normal mood. The effects of stimulants are different. As a rule, a stimulant will help anyone to be more focused and to concentrate better, at least temporarily. Whether you have ADHD or not, stimulants do improve these abilities. This confounds the treatment of children for whom the treatment approach is reversed; namely, a diagnosis of ADHD may be entertained with the notion that a positive response to a stimulant means the child has the disorder. This is analogous to diagnosing hypertension in the absence of a blood-pressure cuff by saying that those who do not get dizzy if prescribed an antihypertensive must by definition have high blood pressure.

Although some groups have used the controversy surrounding ADHD as a platform to attack the use of psychiatric medications as a whole, we should not in our haste to dismiss such perspectives overlook the fact that these are fair and reasonable questions. For that reason, we will try in this chapter to address these questions as we discuss the diagnosis, the long-term course, and the treatment of ADHD. The treatment options have recently expanded with the FDA approval of atomoxetine (Strattera), a selective norepinephrine reuptake inhibitor that is not a psychostimulant, for the treatment of ADHD.

The diagnostic criteria for ADHD have undergone considerable evolution. What we now call ADHD was once known as minimal brain dysfunction (MBD) or hyperkinetic syndrome. These terms gave the mistaken impression that we had some clear notion of the underlying cause of the illness. In 1980, the name for the disorder was changed to the more meaningful term ADHD in DSM-III. At that time, the symptoms of ADHD were organized into three domains: inattention, hyperactivity, and impulsivity. When the manual was revised in 1987 (DSM-III-R), this distinction between symptom clusters was removed. This eliminated the inattentive subtype and in practice resulted in a greater emphasis on the hyperactivity symptoms. In DSM-IV, the core symptoms of ADHD were again divided into symptom clusters. The DSM-IV symptom list thus falls into two domains: inattention and hyperactivity/impulsivity (see Table 8.1).

These symptom clusters deserve closer examination. Inattention can be manifested in several ways. The child or adult with ADHD may appear bored, disorganized, forgetful, or distractible. Hyperactivity can also take several forms including being fidgety, loud and talkative, or "on the go." Blurting out answers, temper tantrums, and going out of turn are common examples of impulsivity. Working from these two symptom clusters, there are three subtypes of ADHD defined in DSM-IV. The subtypes of ADHD include Predominantly Inattentive Type, Predominantly Hyperactive/Impulsive Type, and Combined Type.

In addition to having a certain number of these symptoms, DSM-IV also requires that the illness be evident before age 7 and that it be seen in at least two settings (usually school, work, or home). The age of onset is important. Many adults, for example, with major depressive disorder will have symptoms of ADHD, and perhaps even score high on standardized ADHD scales. One does not, however, develop ADHD at 20, 30, or 40 years of age.

8.2 PREVALENCE AND RISK FACTORS

ADHD is surprisingly common. In fact, it is one of the most common psychiatric disorders affecting children. In the United States, somewhere between 3% and 5% of elementary school children have ADHD. This translates into an average of one or two children with ADHD in every classroom.

TABLE 8.1. Diagnostic Criteria for ADHD[a]

A. Six-month history of problems due to six or more symptoms of poor attention or six or more symptoms of hyperactivity impulsivity.

Symptoms of Poor Attention
1. Makes careless mistakes while doing schoolwork.
2. Has a hard time paying attention for very long.
3. Doesn't seem to listen.
4. Doesn't finish chores or schoolwork.
5. Cannot organize things.
6. Avoids tasks that require paying attention for a long time.
7. Loses things.
8. Is distracted.
9. Is forgetful.

Symptoms of Hyperactivity Impulsivity
1. Fidgets and squirms.
2. Cannot stay in seat.
3. Runs around or climbs at inappropriate times.
4. Can't play quietly.
5. Always on the go.
6. Talks excessively.
7. Blurts out answers.
8. Can't wait his/her turn.
9. Interrupts others.

B. Symptoms were present before age 7.
C. Symptoms are present in at least two places (school, home, work, etc.).
D. Symptoms clearly make it hard to get work done or get along with others.
E. Symptoms are not due to another disorder.

[a] A diagnosis of ADHD requires not only the presence of symptoms with an onset in childhood, but also a degree of distress and/or dysfunction associated with them.

The rate of diagnosing ADHD has risen substantially in the past 10 years. As mentioned earlier, this has led some to say that it is overdiagnosed. But there are, in fact, other rational explanations for this increase. First, there is greater public awareness of ADHD and its treatment. As a result, teachers are more likely to recommend treatment, and parents are more likely to seek it. Second, DSM-IV reinstituted the inattentive subtype of ADHD. Under the older DSM-III-R criteria, children who weren't especially hyperactive or impulsive but yet were still having difficulties with poor attention were too often being overlooked. These children were struggling at school and at home but were not getting treatment. They now appropriately meet the diagnostic criteria for ADHD.

A wide variety of risk factors and causes for ADHD have been proposed. Cultural factors such as low socioeconomic status do not increase the risk for having ADHD. Although the rate of ADHD is higher in some countries (including the United States) than others, this is most likely due to greater public awareness of ADHD in some countries than any true difference in the rate of illness based on cultural factors.

There are occasional reports of specific causes of ADHD such as allergies to certain foods or exposure to toxins such as lead. But to date, there is no solid evidence to support these hypotheses. It would be helpful if a single cause of ADHD could be found, but this is unlikely. Although we do not want to unnecessarily discourage anyone from searching for contributory factors that may worsen the problem, our concern is that tried and true treatments are too often neglected in a fruitless quest for a simple remedy.

One obvious risk factor for ADHD is having a close relative with the disorder. ADHD clearly runs in families, suggesting that there is a genetic basis for the illness, though the mechanism or the genes involved are not yet determined.

We do not yet understand the role that gender plays in ADHD. In elementary school children, ADHD is at least twice as common in boys as girls. Some even estimate the ratio is closer to 10:1. However, by adolescence the rate of ADHD is equal in the two genders. These trends then reverse in early adulthood. ADHD appears to be about twice as common in young adult women as in men. There certainly may be inherent biases in the way boys and girls are evaluated and who is brought to treatment. These biases may in part explain the differences, but we must recognize the fact that we have much to learn about gender differences in this disorder.

8.3 PRESENTATION AND CLINICAL COURSE

By definition, ADHD must appear before age 7. ADHD has been diagnosed in preschool children as early as age 3, but it is very difficult to diagnose the disorder reliably at this young age. Many preschoolers are called hyperactive by their parents, but they do not have the symptoms of ADHD when they begin school. Only children with the most severe cases of ADHD can be diagnosed accurately during the preschool years.

Most children are initially diagnosed with ADHD during first grade. First grade and beyond mandates a more structured environment than preschool or kindergarten. It requires more sustained attention and better impulse control. School-age children have to work together with others, obey rules, remain seated, pay attention, and organize their work. At home, chores become more demanding. The child is now expected to complete his/her work with a greater degree of independence.

Placing these increased expectations on the school-age child makes it considerably easier to recognize ADHD. In school, children with ADHD often disrupt class by getting out of their seat and impulsively yelling out answers. They are unable to finish their schoolwork, and what is completed is often sloppy and littered with careless mistakes. They may meet people easily, but find it difficult to sustain friendships. On the playground, they can be bossy and aggressive, going out of turn and breaking rules. Soon, they find themselves with few friends and often play alone because no one else wants to play with them.

What happens to children with ADHD as they grow up has become a hot topic. Not long ago, many believed that children outgrew ADHD. Nowadays, we know that this is often not the case. ADHD is not necessarily a childhood illness; it is an illness that *begins* in childhood, but many children with ADHD continue to have problems not only as teenagers but also going on into adulthood. Nevertheless, the clinical picture does change over time. The child with ADHD differs from a teenager with ADHD, and a teenager with ADHD in turn differs from an adult with the disorder.

The teenager with ADHD usually continues to be plagued by poor school performance, though very bright children can sometimes "get by" to an extent simply on the basis of their sheer intelligence. Poor school performance is usually why parents bring their teenagers with ADHD for an evaluation. However, these children and adolescents also have problems with irritability, getting along with their peers, excessive risk-taking, and even legal difficulties. In fact, children with ADHD are at a much higher risk for developing conduct disorder and bipolar disorder as they age.

ADHD may continue into adulthood. This issue has been debated not only in medical journals but on TV talk shows and in news magazines as well. However, adult ADHD is no trivial matter. Certainly, the physical hyperactivity of the 6 year old with ADHD is not so readily evident in the 26 or 36 year old. Nevertheless, some individuals with ADHD continue to be plagued by impulsive outbursts of anger and poor concentration even after they reach adulthood. This continues to take a toll as it often leads to marital strife and problems holding a job. Like the child and adolescent with ADHD, adults with the disorder are often considered underachievers and may even be dismissed as lazy.

It is still unclear how many children with ADHD continue to have the disorder as adults. Estimates range from as few as 10% to as many as 60%. In any case, there is no doubt that a certain number of children with ADHD will continue to have the disorder as adults.

8.4 INITIAL EVALUATION AND DIFFERENTIAL DIAGNOSIS

Evaluating a Child. Parents will often bring their children with the expectation that someone can "test them" for ADHD. It is true that certain tests can help in the initial assessment; however, no single test or even battery of tests can alone make the diagnosis. Instead, this diagnosis is made only after collecting a thorough database of information from the child, his/her parents, and teachers.

We say "the child" because the onset of ADHD is by definition before age 7. However, we acknowledge that there will be occasions when a patient first seeks treatment for ADHD as a teenager and sometimes even as an adult.

During the initial evaluation, the database of valuable information is comprised of several key components (see Table 8.2), the most important of which is the psychiatric interview. In evaluating a child, it is imperative that the child and at least one parent be interviewed. These interviews should be conducted separately to avoid

TABLE 8.2. ADHD Evaluation

Interview: child, parents, and teachers
Direct observation
Rating scales
Psychological testing

the awkward (and potentially harmful) moment of having an exhausted parent complaining vehemently about the child's problems while the child sits nearby listening to the complaints.

Direct observation is another important component of the evaluation. Remember that the office is not a natural setting for a child. The child with ADHD may be able for a short period of time to control his/her symptoms. Because the child may be on his/her best behavior when visiting the office, observing the child with ADHD during structured activities (such as a structured playroom) can provide a clearer picture of his/her symptoms.

Another set of tools that could be utilized are brief rating scales. DSM-IV mandates that ADHD symptoms must be present in at least two settings. For children and adolescents, school is invariably one of the two settings. To get a sense of the comparative problems in school versus those at home, psychiatrists often use rating scales that can be completed by both parents and one or more teachers. The Conners Teacher Rating Scale, Conners Parent Rating Scale, and the Child Behavior Checklist are the most commonly used scales to evaluate the symptoms of ADHD.

Finally, psychological testing is sometimes used to complete evaluation. This testing not only provides feedback regarding the child's attention and ability to process information but can also identify other problems such as learning disabilities (e.g., dyslexia) that can complicate the picture.

Evaluating an Adult. Evaluating an adult for ADHD carries its own dilemmas and is no less difficult. Although the diagnostic criteria remain the same, ADHD in an adult does look somewhat different from the way it does in a 6-year-old child. In addition, one must also determine that the illness was present before age 7. Without parents and elementary school teachers there to help, it can certainly tax the memory of an adult patient when asking about any problems experienced in the first grade. However, the task is not impossible.

Several features from the patient's childhood and early adult history can be helpful. Patients with ADHD are more likely to report a history of poor grades, learning disabilities, being placed in special education classes, dropping out of school, reading and spelling difficulties, and receiving grades that were poorer than would be expected on the basis of intelligence alone. They often have tempestuous relationships that are difficult to sustain and frequent job changes.

In an adult, hyperactivity usually takes the form of being restless and fidgety when being seated for long periods of time in the office, church, or meeting place.

Impulsivity is manifested by a hot temper or quick decision making that is later regretted. Finally, adults with ADHD often have significant problems with alcohol or illicit substance abuse. They may also heavily use caffeine or cigarettes. This pattern of substance use is likely, in part, an attempt to medicate the illness.

Differential Diagnosis. With a careful assessment and a dependable history, one can reliably diagnose ADHD (even in an adult who was never diagnosed as a child). However, the broad array of symptoms results in a rather wide differential diagnosis. Please consider each of the following when trying to determine if a patient has ADHD.

Active Child. Children are, almost by definition, active. Sometimes we lose sight of the fact that behavior that we as adults find distracting may be entirely appropriate for a child of 5, 6, or 7 years of age. In these cases parents generally need reassurance that their child is doing well. They may also need a referral for parenting skills training to refine their ability to deal with their active child.

Mental Retardation. Children with low IQ understandably struggle when they are placed in classes that are poorly suited to their abilities. They become inattentive and at times disruptive. In many respects, there is a similarity to the child with ADHD. Placing them in an appropriate setting generally improves these behaviors to some degree. When the distinction between mental retardation and ADHD is unclear, psychological testing can assist in clarifying between the two.

Other Childhood Disruptive Disorders. The child with ADHD typically avoids schoolwork that taxes his/her attention. Difficulty completing work can quickly become a frustrating experience independent of one's age. A child with ADHD who complains about an assignment in many respects resembles the defiant refusal of a child with oppositional defiant disorder or conduct disorder. These disorders must be carefully distinguished from ADHD, but it is entirely possible that a child with ADHD may also have a comorbid disruptive behavior disorder.

Pervasive Developmental Disorders. Children with autism or one of the other pervasive developmental disorders can be impulsive and inattentive much like those with ADHD. However, the severe social disability and language problems of children with an autistic disorder usually far exceed that of ADHD. These differences are usually sufficient to clarify the diagnosis. When one is unsure, neuropsychological testing can help clarify matters.

Depression. Depressed children and adolescents are often irritable and argumentative. They may also be inattentive and easily distracted. A depressed child therefore potentially looks and behaves much like a child with ADHD. In such cases, one should not immediately make both diagnoses. First, treat the child for depression. If the symptoms of ADHD remain after the depression has resolved, then and only then does it make sense to diagnose and treat ADHD as well.

Bipolar Disorder. Not too long ago, this was a moot point. We have long known that ADHD starts in childhood. Bipolar disorder was believed to have an onset in adulthood, not during childhood or adolescence. There is now a growing awareness that bipolar disorder not uncommonly begins during childhood. We can therefore no longer cavalierly dismiss bipolar disorder from the differential diagnosis of ADHD.

During a manic episode, a bipolar patient is impulsive, hyperverbal, hyperactive, inattentive, and distracted, which can, of course, be very similar to the presentation of ADHD. So how do you distinguish between the two? Three features are potentially helpful. First, the symptoms are relatively continuous in someone with ADHD and are more episodic in bipolar disorder. For the child with bipolar disorder, this represents a clear departure from his/her usual behavior, though this can be difficult to differentiate in rapid cycling bipolar disorder. Second, the child with bipolar disorder is often grandiose, not so with ADHD. Finally, family history can also be helpful. Usually, childhood onset bipolar disorder is accompanied by a strong family history of the illness, whereas ADHD is often accompanied by a family history of that disorder. This is but one example of the importance of collecting a thorough family history when performing a psychiatric evaluation. The differentiation between ADHD and bipolar disorder is important. Experts remain divided as to how often bipolar disorder and ADHD occur together as comorbid illnesses.

Absence Seizures. Most seizure disorders cause abnormal jerking movements called clonus. But absence (petit mal) seizures cause little or no abnormal movements. During an absence seizure, the patient does not fall to the ground, have obvious jerking movements, or lose control of bowel or bladder. Instead, a patient with absence seizures typically has a blank stare while becoming unaware of the surroundings for no more than a few seconds. When the seizure is over, alertness is restored.

It is easy to see why no one may realize that the patient is having a seizure. At first, the individual experiencing absence seizures usually is unaware of them as well. But when absence seizures happen frequently, much of what is occurring around the person is missed and can be mistaken for the inattentiveness of ADHD. An evaluation by a neurologist, including an electroencephalogram (EEG), can clarify this issue.

8.5 HISTORY OF PHARMACOLOGICAL TREATMENT

The most successful treatments for ADHD have been those that increase the activity of the neurotransmitters dopamine and norepinephrine. It has been known for some time that our brains use these two substances to focus attention during response to challenging or stressful situations. The theory that medications that increase the activity of either dopamine and/or norepinephrine would be good treatments for ADHD has largely proved true, and we now have medications that can help children and adults with ADHD tremendously.

But there are patients with ADHD who continue to have problems with impulsivity despite these treatments. This has led to several innovative approaches to help address these residual symptoms with medications ranging from antidepressants to mood stabilizers, antipsychotics, and even medicines that are more commonly used to treat high blood pressure. The problem here is finding a medication that will alleviate the remaining impulsivity without worsening the problems with attention. There has been modest success with these more difficult cases, but there remains room for improvement.

Stimulants. From coca leaves chewed by native laborers in South America to brewed teas and coffees used across the globe, stimulants have been used since antiquity. In these essentially naturally occurring forms, coca and caffeine were long known to provide a boost of energy, focus attention, and decrease appetite. However, compared to today's refined stimulants, the effects were relatively mild. There is no clear evidence that these substances were used to treat the ancient antecedents of psychiatric illness in past cultures. The isolation of cocaine in the mid-1700s and the synthesis of amphetamine in the late 1800s dramatically increased stimulant use (and abuse) in society.

Amphetamine (Benzedrine). Amphetamine was synthesized in 1887. It was quickly found to be a potent stimulant with effects similar to cocaine, which had been discovered over 100 years before. In the subsequent years, amphetamine found a variety of uses. It was used to treat narcolepsy, Parkinson's disease, barbiturate overdose, bed wetting (enuresis), and obesity. It was also used to counteract the sedating effects of other drugs and medications including antiseizure medications and alcohol.

As early as the 1940s it became clear that amphetamine could also produce a calming effect in adults prone to aggression and agitation. Later, this so-called paradoxical effect was also seen in children with hyperkinetic syndrome, the precursor to ADHD.

In the aftermath of World War II, problems with amphetamine abuse began to arise. An epidemic of amphetamine abuse and related cases of amphetamine-induced psychosis arose first in Japan and later in the United States. Since that time, use of amphetamines and other stimulants has been greatly curtailed and as a class are more tightly regulated than virtually any other psychotropic agents, with the exception of narcotic analgesics.

Methylphenidate (Ritalin). Methylphenidate was developed in the late 1950s and its first use was the treatment of what we now call ADHD. Since that time, it has also been approved for the treatment of narcolepsy. Its only other use is the treatment of severe refractory depression either in medically ill patients who need rapid clinical improvement or as an augmentation agent when added to other antidepressants. In the treatment of ADHD, methylphenidate not only improves attention but also reduces hyperactivity and impulsivity. Verbal and physical aggression typically decreases as well.

Methylphenidate is now the most widely used of the stimulants. It has a well-established record of safety and tolerability and has been used in children throughout the school years and in adults as well. In preschool children, the effects of methylphenidate can vary.

Methylphenidate is typically initiated at a dose of 5 mg given twice a day. At each weekly visit, the dose can be increased by 2.5–5 mg. Usually 20–30 mg/day is sufficient, though as much as 60 mg per dose is occasionally needed. Many children with ADHD experience rebound hyperactivity at night when the daytime dose of medication has worn off. When this occurs, an after-school dose that is usually 25–50% of the earlier doses is helpful. The benefit of methylphenidate is often apparent within the first few days or so, and the dose can be increased weekly as needed.

The side effects of methylphenidate are very similar to the amphetamines, but because it is somewhat less potent they may be a little milder. The common side effects of methylphenidate are appetite loss, weight loss, insomnia, and nausea. Taking methylphenidate with meals and no later than 6 PM can control most of these. On rare occasions, methylphenidate can cause headache, dizziness, nervousness, increased heart rate, increased blood pressure, tics, and, in extremely rare cases, paranoia.

The prescribing physician should be notified immediately if tics or psychosis (usually paranoia) develop. The medication should always be stopped when psychosis occurs. We once said the same about tics, but recent research suggests that stimulants may not worsen tics. Methylphenidate is now available in a controlled-release preparation (Concerta), which can be prescribed once daily. One key advantage to once-daily dosing is not pharmacological, but rather that it avoids the stigma children may experience when they need to go to the school nurse's office to receive their afternoon dose. Focalin is the active isomer of methylphenidate.

Dextroamphetamine (Dexedrine). Dextroamphetamine is the second most widely used stimulant and the most commonly used amphetamine in the United States. It is about twice as potent as methylphenidate and should be initiated in the treatment of ADHD at 2.5 mg taken twice daily with breakfast and lunch. Like other stimulants, the benefits of dextroamphetamine can be seen almost immediately. With weekly visits while starting treatment, the dose can be increased in 2.5–5 mg increments until the effective dose is found. Because dextroamphetamine is also slightly longer acting than methylphenidate, patients may be less likely to need an evening dose. If an after-school dose is used, then like methylphenidate it should be 25–50% of the daytime dose.

The side effects of dextroamphetamine are comparable to other stimulants. Patients may experience insomnia, poor appetite, weight loss, and occasional nausea and diarrhea. Taking the medication just before meals helps to minimize the nausea and diarrhea. To avoid insomnia, dextroamphetamine should rarely be taken any later than 6 PM.

Infrequent side effects of dextroamphetamine include euphoria, nervousness, irritability, headache, involuntary movements (tics), increased heart rate, and paranoia. If paranoia develops, the patient's doctor should be notified immediately, and the medication should be stopped. As noted earlier, there remains some debate as to whether dextroamphetamine and the other stimulants should be discontinued when tics develop.

Amphetamine/Dextroamphetamine (Adderall). Adderall is the newest of the stimulants. It is actually a combination of four stimulants consisting of two forms of amphetamine and two forms of dextroamphetamine. Its potency is similar to that of dextroamphetamine and therefore the doses are generally similar. Likewise, its duration of action is about the same as dextroamphetamine, though some believe its effects can last as long as 10 hours. Despite these claims, we have generally found that it still requires at least two doses given with breakfast and lunch. However, an after-school dose is less often needed than with methylphenidate. An extended-release formulation of Adderall (Adderall XR) is available and typically results in single daily dosing in the morning.

The side effects and potential for abuse with Adderall are essentially the same as for dextroamphetamine. We recommend starting Adderall at 2.5 mg twice a day or 5 mg each morning and then adding the second dose after a week or so. Using the extended-release formulation allows for the titration of the single dose with weekly adjustments as needed.

Pemoline (Cylert). Pemoline was introduced as an alternative stimulant. Its two key advantages are that it can be taken once a day, though with the extended-release versions of methylphenidate and Adderall this is less of an issue, and it may be less prone to abuse. It was generally believed that pemoline has a gradual onset of action, taking several weeks to reach full therapeutic benefit, but some researchers discount this assumption.

Pemoline is less potent than the other available stimulants. It is started at 18.75 mg each morning and is increased in increments of 18.75 mg every week or two. The maximum dose is 112.5 mg/day, though some patients do require higher doses. Because pemoline is less potent than other stimulants, it is more likely to be ineffective even at its higher doses. When pemoline does not relieve the symptoms of ADHD, patients should be changed to a different stimulant.

One benefit of pemoline's milder effects and slower onset of action is that it appears to possess less abuse potential than other stimulants. The abuse potential, however, is usually a concern not for patients who are prescribed the stimulant, but for others who may want to buy it "on the street" or steal the pills from someone else. Although pemoline does have some potential for abuse, it is limited.

The side effects of pemoline are similar to other stimulants but milder. The most common side effects are loss of appetite, nausea, and insomnia. Infrequent side effects include headache, dizziness, changes in mood, increases in blood pressure or pulse, and psychosis.

The greatest concern is that pemoline on rare occasions causes a chemical hepatitis (liver malfunction). For this reason, patients with known liver disease should never take pemoline. Patients should have a baseline laboratory assessment of liver function before initiating pemoline therapy. The liver function tests should then be repeated periodically. If abnormalities are detected, the pemoline must be stopped. The incidence of liver dysfunction in recent years has markedly diminished the prescribing of pemoline and at this time the other stimulants have largely supplanted its use.

Methamphetamine (Desoxyn). Methamphetamine is a relatively long-acting stimulant. Lasting up to 12 hours, it can often be taken only once a day and is just as effective at treating ADHD as other stimulants. However, methamphetamine is seldom used today. For one thing, it is much more expensive than other stimulants. For another, this variant of amphetamine is the form often produced in illicit "speed" labs for street use. Many families and physicians are understandably reluctant to use a medication with this reputation for abuse.

Modafinil (Provigil). The newest stimulant, modafinil, is not, pharmacologically, a true stimulant. Nevertheless, it is an effective treatment for narcolepsy at doses from 200 to 400 mg/day. Several studies indicate that modafinil has little potential for abuse and is easier to tolerate than other stimulants. Modafinil has been studied in the treatment of ADHD. Though not approved for marketing by the FDA at the time of this writing, it may gain the indication in the near future.

Atomoxetine (Strattera). Atomoxetine has recently been approved as a treatment for ADHD. Atomoxetine, similar to some of the antidepressants discussed later, is a preferential inhibitor of norepinephrine reuptake. Because nerve terminals in the cerebral cortex have no dopamine reuptake sites, dopamine is taken up at nearby norepinephrine reuptake sites. Consequently, all norepinephrine reuptake inhibitors increase the availability of dopamine in the prefrontal cortex, likely the primary mechanism of atomoxetine action in ADHD.

Tablet sizes of atomoxetine are 10, 18, 25, 40, and 60 mg. Initial dosing is at 0.4 mg per kg of body weight for children up to 70 kg and then increased to the target dose of 1.2 mg/kg, with a maximal dose of 100 mg/day (or 1.4 mg/kg, whichever is less) administered as once daily in the morning or split between morning and late afternoon/early evening. In adults and children or adolescents over 70 kg of body weight, the starting dose is 40 mg/day, which can then be raised to 80 mg after a minimum of 3 days. The maximal recommended dose is 100 mg/day. In general, atomoxetine is well tolerated with side effects that are associated with sympathetic nervous system activation given its mechanism of action as a norepinephrine reuptake inhibitor. These include dry mouth, nausea, constipation, urinary hesitancy, decreased appetite, and insomnia. Atomoxetine is not a schedule II compound so, unlike the stimulants, it does not require a written prescription and samples can be dispensed.

Antidepressants. A wide variety of antidepressants have been used to treat ADHD. These include the older tricyclic antidepressants (TCAs) and monoamine oxidase inhibitors (MAOIs) as well as the newer selective serotonin reuptake inhibitors (SSRIs) and atypical antidepressants. Antidepressants are not in this case simply used to treat depression when it occurs in a patient with ADHD (although ADHD patients often have depression), but are effective in alleviating one or more of the symptoms of ADHD itself. The usefulness of any particular antidepressant for treating ADHD depends in large part on its mechanism of action. Although some antidepressants can be quite helpful in the treatment of ADHD, others do not appear to provide much benefit at all.

Tricyclic Antidepressants (TCAs). The TCAs have been used to treat ADHD for 30 or more years. Most often used are imipramine (Tofranil) and desipramine (Norpramin), mainly because they are the TCAs that most specifically increase norepinephrine activity. Remember, boosting norepinephrine activity in the brain should improve attention. Other TCAs, namely, amitriptyline (Elavil, Endep) and nortriptyline (Pamelor), have been used, though they also increase norepinephrine activity. TCAs do offer a modest benefit for both the inattention and the hyperactivity of ADHD. In addition, they are often effective at doses much lower than those required to treat depression. However, their effectiveness usually falls short of the stimulant medications. In addition, TCAs have considerable side effects including dry mouth, constipation, drowsiness, weight gain, and adverse cardiac effects.

Finally, there have been a handful of sudden deaths occurring in children with ADHD who were taking the TCA desipramine. Checking blood levels of the medications and electrocardiogram (EKG) results gave no warning that these children were in danger. It appears that this risk is limited to desipramine, but it bears noting that all TCAs can interfere with heart function. We must advise extreme caution before prescribing TCAs to children, and as a rule, desipramine should be avoided in this age group.

For more information regarding the use of TCAs please refer to Chapter 3 (Mood Disorders) and Chapter 9 (Sleep Disorders).

Monoamine Oxidase Inhibitors (MAOIs). MAOI antidepressants were derived from drugs developed in the early 1950s to treat tuberculosis. They act by interfering with the MAO enzymes that metabolize and thus eliminate dopamine, norepinephrine, serotonin, and other related substances. The MAO enzyme comes in two varieties, MAO-A and MAO-B. It is the MAO-B enzyme that metabolizes dopamine.

There are currently three approved MAOI antidepressants in the United States: phenelzine (Nardil), tranylcypromine (Parnate), and isocarboxizide (Marplan). These antidepressants block both the MAO-A and MAO-B subtypes. These MAOIs are also irreversible; that is, they deactivate the enzyme permanently.

MAOIs have the potential to cause numerous side effects including dizziness, drowsiness, insomnia, palpitations, rapid heart rate, and sexual dysfunction. Phenelzine also often produces weight gain and fluid retention. Of greater concern are the potentially dangerous interactions of the MAOIs with certain foods and both prescription and over-the-counter medications. Because the MAOIs permanently inactivate MAO enzymes (until your body over about 3 weeks replaces its supply of the enzymes upon discontinuation of the MAOI), eating food or taking medication that contains one of the substances eliminated by MAO, such as tyramine, can result in its toxic accumulation. This can lead to a so-called hypertensive crisis in which blood pressure is uncontrollably elevated, risking heart attack, stroke, or death. As a result, patients taking these MAOIs must maintain a strict diet devoid of tyramine (a substance metabolized by MAO and typically found in aged or fermented foods) and must avoid several medications including decongestants such as pseudoephedrine (Sudafed), meperidine (Demerol), and epinephrine-containing local anesthetics.

Moclobemide, a reversible MAOI, is available in Europe and Canada. Because it is reversible, moclobemide has little risk of diet or medication interactions.

Yet another MAOI is selegiline (Eldepryl). Unlike the other MAOIs, selegiline is seldom used to treat depression. At low doses, selegiline only inhibits the MAO-B enzyme. Therefore, it increases dopamine activity but does not have any pronounced effect on norepinephrine or serotonin. For this reason, it has been less useful as an antidepressant; however, its primary use has been to treat Parkinson's disease. Of course, this selectivity for dopamine suggests that it may be helpful for ADHD as well.

Although selegiline has not been extensively used or tested in ADHD, it has been shown to improve attention in patients including those with Alzheimer's disease. Because selegiline has little effect on the MAO-A enzyme at low doses, the dietary restrictions are unnecessary. Therefore, selegiline may help improve attention in patients with ADHD without the risk of other MAOIs. It should be noted, however, that at higher doses selegiline acts much like the other MAOIs, with the same dietary risks. The dose at which inhibition of serotonin metabolism occurs can vary from patient to patient, so selegiline should not be combined with the SSRIs. The most common side effects of selegiline are nausea, dizziness, dry mouth, and indigestion. Some care should still be taken to avoid taking selegiline with medications known to interact with the other MAOIs.

Although selegiline is by no means a first-line treatment for ADHD, it does provide an alternative for those who cannot tolerate other drugs or who are at risk for stimulant abuse. Selegiline can safely be given with clonidine, another medication commonly prescribed to patients with ADHD. We would, however, suggest that giving selegiline together with a stimulant should be avoided because this may increase the risk for a hypertensive crisis.

For more information regarding the use of MAOIs please refer to Chapter 3 (Mood Disorders) and Chapter 5 (Anxiety Disorders).

Bupropion (Wellbutrin, Zyban). Bupropion is a newer "atypical antidepressant" that was initially suggested to increase both norepinephrine and dopamine activity in the brain, though controversy surrounds this hypothesis. Although bupropion has not been studied extensively in ADHD, early evidence does indeed indicate that it may be effective for both inattention and hyperactivity/impulsivity. Its effectiveness for ADHD does not appear to rival the stimulant medications, though a recent controlled study for adult ADHD showed that bupropion outperformed placebo.

Bupropion is generally easy to tolerate but can cause insomnia, restlessness, upset stomach, poor appetite, and dizziness. Of greater concern is the fact that at higher doses (greater than 150 mg per dose or greater than 450 mg/day), bupropion, in its original immediate-release form, can increase the risk of seizures. Children or adults with known risk factors for seizure, such as a history of a serious head injury, an eating disorder, or a known seizure disorder, are at higher risk for seizure when taking bupropion. This risk of seizure is extremely small except in individuals previously vulnerable to seizures. The new extended-release preparations of bupropion (Wellbutrin SR, Wellbutrin XL) decrease this risk.

Bupropion treatment should be initiated at 50 mg taken once or twice a day and then increased in a stepwise fashion over a few weeks to a dose of 100–150 mg taken twice to three times daily. The total daily dose should never exceed 450 mg. One form of extended-release bupropion, Wellbutrin SR, can be started at 100 mg taken once a day and can be increased to a maximum of 400 mg/day, though no single dose should exceed 200 mg. Wellbutrin XL is started at 150 mg taken once a day and can be administered in single daily doses as high as 450 mg.

Bupropion is also effective both in the treatment of depression and in smoking cessation. For more information, refer to Chapter 3 (Mood Disorders) and Chapter 6 (Substance Use Disorders).

Serotonin-Boosting Antidepressants. Antidepressants that enhance serotonin activity in the brain have also been studied in ADHD. In particular, fluoxetine (Prozac) and the serotonin-selective TCA clomipramine (Anafranil) have been the most extensively evaluated, with mixed success. They provide some benefit for aggression and impulsivity but don't significantly improve the poor attention of ADHD. As a result, the SSRIs and other serotonin-boosting antidepressants do not appear to be effective first-line treatments for ADHD. Conversely, depressed patients without ADHD often show improvements in symptoms of concentration and attention when treated with a SSRI. Although SSRIs are not widely used in the treatment of ADHD, they may be worthy of consideration in ADHD patients whose impulsivity is not controlled by stimulants alone. Those with comorbid conduct disorder or ODD who are prone to agitation and at times violent outbursts may be helped by the addition of a SSRI.

Venlafaxine (Effexor, Effexor XR). Venlafaxine, a dual serotonin–norepinephrine reuptake inhibitor, has only recently been used to treat ADHD with a few case reports suggesting it may provide modest benefit for both inattention and impulsivity. Effexor XR is generally well tolerated, though it can elevate blood pressure somewhat at higher doses. This should be monitored especially when venlafaxine is coadministered with a stimulant. Controlled trials are needed.

Norepinephrine-Blocking Medications. Medications that enhance dopamine activity and to a lesser extent those that enhance norepinephrine activity are believed to be the most successful treatments for ADHD. It may seem counterintuitive to try a medication that reduces norepinephrine turnover. The other ADHD medications do not always reduce impulsivity and hyperactivity, but norepinephrine-blocking medications have been shown to produce a calming effect in other disorders associated with agitation and aggression.

Clonidine (Catapres). Clonidine is largely used to treat high blood pressure. Although we don't fully understand how clonidine acts, it appears to reduce norepinephrine activity by stimulating a norepinephrine receptor known as the alpha-2 receptor. When clonidine binds to alpha-2 receptors on norepinephrine neurons, so-called autoreceptors, the cells are "tricked" into believing that there is already sufficient norepinephrine released and thus decrease any additional release of norepinephrine. As one might anticipate, clonidine is somewhat effective at reducing the hyperactivity and impulsivity of ADHD. It does not, however, provide nearly as much benefit for the inattention of ADHD.

In contrast to the stimulants that act in a relatively rapid manner, the effects of clonidine are delayed by several weeks. It must be taken regularly and should be started at a dose of 0.05 mg at bedtime for children or 0.1 mg at bedtime for adults. Over several weeks the dose can be increased to a total of 0.3 mg/day in three divided doses.

The most common side effect of clonidine is drowsiness. This can begin with the very first dose and usually goes away after a few weeks. Clonidine's sedating effects can actually be useful when it's taken at bedtime. Insomnia is a common problem for patients with ADHD either as a side effect of stimulants or as a consequence of rebound hyperactivity at night when the daytime dose of stimulant has worn off. Clonidine can help the ADHD patient with insomnia to go to sleep. Other side effects of clonidine include low blood pressure, dizziness, depression, dry mouth, nausea, and slowed heart rate. One important point to remember is that not only does clonidine not cause tics, it can, in fact, relieve tics when they appear in patients with ADHD.

Similar to the TCAs, there have been reports of sudden deaths reported in children with ADHD who were taking both clonidine and a psychostimulant. For this reason, precautionary measures should be taken before starting a patient (particularly a child) on clonidine. A baseline EKG should be obtained before starting the medication. If the EKG shows any problems in the heart's electrical conduction system, then clonidine should not be used. In addition, if the patient has any history of known heart problems, fainting spells, slow heart rate (i.e., less than 60 beats per minute), or low blood pressure, we would recommend avoiding clonidine. When clonidine is used, the patient's blood pressure and pulse rate should be measured at each office visit, and an EKG should be periodically repeated.

Finally, clonidine should only be used by patients who can be counted on to take their medication reliably. Clonidine is first and foremost a medication used to treat high blood pressure. Clonidine lowers blood pressure and can slow the pulse rate. However, when clonidine is suddenly stopped, dramatic rebound effects can occur, including a rapid rise in blood pressure that can be dangerous. Patients who suddenly stop taking clonidine or who routinely forget to take their clonidine run the risk of severe side effects. These risks must be discussed with the patient prior to initiating clonidine therapy. In addition, medication compliance should be evaluated at each visit (e.g., "How many doses did you miss since the last visit?"), and especially for medications such as clonidine for which poor compliance can be hazardous.

Besides the tablet form, clonidine is also available in a patch that is worn on the arm and changed once every 5–7 days. Once the appropriate dose has been found using oral clonidine, both children and adults can be switched to the patch. The patch provides more consistent levels of the medication and obviously minimizes the potential for rebound effects due to poor compliance. This patch does sometimes cause local skin irritation. Rotating the application site from arm to arm each week can minimize this.

Guanfacine. Guanfacine is another antihypertensive medication that works in much the same way as clonidine, that is, by stimulating the alpha-2 norepinephrine receptors that decrease norepinephrine activity in the brain. It has not been as widely used to treat ADHD as clonidine, but limited evidence suggests that it may work just as well. In fact, recent evidence suggests that guanfacine may provide some benefit in improving memory and attention that clonidine does not provide. Guanfacine can be started at a 0.5 mg dose administered once a day. The dose can gradually be increased every week or two to a maximum of 1 mg given up to three times per day.

Because it has not been used extensively to treat ADHD, not as much is known about its safety in children. It appears to cause less sedation than clonidine and fewer untoward effects on blood pressure as well. Because of its similarity to clonidine, the same precautions should be taken when prescribing guanfacine. EKGs should be performed periodically, and blood pressure and pulse should be checked at each office visit.

Mood Stabilizers. Lithium (Eskalith, Lithobid), valproic acid (Depakene), sodium valproate (Depakote), and carbamazepine (Tegretol) are most often used by psychiatrists to treat the bipolar disorders. These so-called mood stabilizers are also used to treat impulsivity and agitation in a variety of psychiatric disorders including dementia, certain personality disorders, and the disruptive behavior disorders of childhood.

Unfortunately, the mood stabilizers have not proved very helpful in the treatment of uncomplicated ADHD. They can, however, help the child or adolescent who has ADHD complicated by severely disruptive behavior. For example, a child with ADHD or ODD who is prone to outbursts of rage that are not controlled by other medications such as antidepressants or clonidine may require a mood stabilizer.

Mood stabilizers are not, in general, as easy to manage as other medications. Most require periodic laboratory monitoring including drug levels. Mood stabilizers are typically not used except in severe cases of ADHD when several other medications have failed.

Recently, other medications have been evaluated as mood stabilizers. This includes gabapentin (Neurontin), lamotrigine (Lamictal), and topiramate (Topamax). Only lamotrigine has been shown in controlled trials to be effective in the treatment of bipolar disorder; neither gabapentin nor topiramate is effective in mania as a monotherapy. They may be effective as adjuncts in bipolar disorder. To our knowledge, these mood stabilizers have not yet been tested in the treatment of ADHD; however, they may in the future be added to the list of medicines to consider. For more information on the mood stabilizers, please refer to Chapter 3 (Mood Disorders).

Typical Antipsychotics. The high potency antipsychotic haloperidol (Haldol) and low potency antipsychotics chlorpromazine (Thorazine) and thioridazine (Mellaril) have also been used to treat ADHD. Although they provide a tranquilizing effect (they are in fact sometimes called "major tranquilizers") that can reduce hyperactivity and impulsivity, antipsychotics remain markedly less effective than stimulants. Antipsychotics do not noticeably improve attention in patients with ADHD, and at this time the typical antipsychotics cannot be considered a reasonable monotherapy in uncomplicated ADHD.

Antipsychotics also have a troublesome side effect burden that includes an often-irreversible movement disorder known as tardive dyskinesia (TD). Other side effects include so-called parkinsonism, dystonic reactions (i.e., abrupt onset of muscle spasms), akathisia (an uncomfortable sense of motoric restlessness), sedation, weight gain, dizziness, dry mouth, and constipation among others. These side effects, in particular the risk for TD, limit the usefulness of antipsychotics in the treatment of ADHD, and at this time the typical antipsychotics cannot be considered a reasonable monotherapy in uncomplicated ADHD.

One exception is the patient with both ADHD and tic disorders such as Tourette's syndrome. High potency antipsychotics have proved quite effective in treating both vocal and motor tics.

Atypical Antipsychotics. The so-called atypical antipsychotics are not well studied in the treatment of ADHD. However, a few case reports have indicated that risperidone (Risperdal) may reduce the impulsivity and hyperactivity of ADHD. There is also preliminary evidence that risperidone may be effective in treating tics. Although the usefulness of risperidone and other atypical antipsychotics in treating ADHD needs more study, this may prove another viable treatment alternative for patients with ADHD and tics or agitation.

8.6 CURRENT APPROACH TO TREATMENT

Starting Treatment in Children. The importance of an accurate diagnosis confirmed by obtaining information from multiple sources cannot be overstated. The mainstay of treatment for ADHD, psychostimulants, are less helpful for the other disruptive behavior disorders of childhood and may worsen the course of bipolar disorder in patients misdiagnosed with ADHD.

We also want to warn against the tendency to rely solely on medication when treating ADHD. Although psychosocial treatments alone are usually insufficient for ADHD, they are an important component of a comprehensive treatment plan. For example, all ADHD patients can be helped by age-appropriate behavioral modification techniques. Parental skills training can teach parents to use constructive techniques that aid their child with ADHD rather than counterproductive measures that sometimes add to his/her frustration. Family therapy can also aid in this process. Finally, direct observation of the child with ADHD in the classroom will often help to identify adaptations that will help the child in school. In some cases, this means placing the child in a special class that is tailored to his/her needs.

All these approaches can be helpful, but stimulants remain the mainstay treatment for children with ADHD. Before starting stimulant therapy, the child's height, weight, blood pressure, and pulse should be checked and recorded. Height and weight should be plotted on a standardized growth chart and followed longitudinally during the course of treatment.

First-line pharmacotherapy treatments include methylphenidate, dextroamphetamine, the mixed amphetamine salts (Adderall), and atomoxetine (see Table 8.3). When an early evening dose is indicated (e.g., completion of homework) it is typically at 25–50% of the doses prescribed earlier in the day.

When they work, stimulants often work quickly. They do not act in a delayed fashion like many other psychiatric medications. With feedback from parents and teachers, it is often evident within a few days how well the medication is working. The child should be seen each week when starting stimulant therapy so that the dose can quickly be adjusted to maximize its benefit. Once the effective dose has been reached, it can be maintained indefinitely.

Close to 70% of children with ADHD will respond to a stimulant. When the child is not helped by the first stimulant that is prescribed, there is still a good chance of responding to a different one. If an initial trial of methylphenidate isn't successful, then switching to dextroamphetamine or Adderall is a reasonable strategy. If dextroamphetamine or Adderall was used first and did not work well, then we recommend switching to methylphenidate. Because dextroamphetamine and Adderall are more similar, it makes less sense to switch between these two. We do not recommend pemoline as a first-line treatment.

Starting Treatment in Adults with ADHD. Beginning treatment of an adult is not significantly different from doing so in a child. The stimulants and atomoxetine remain the most effective medications. Methylphenidate, dextroamphetamine, and Adderall appear to be equally effective in group trials, but individuals may respond preferentially to one medication or the other.

Obviously, the need for input from parents and teachers does not exist when treating an adult with ADHD. Nevertheless, patients may be poor judges of the effectiveness of their own treatment. A patient, for example, may record little or no improvement, but his/her spouse may have noted significant positive changes. Therefore, visits with a significant other can be especially important during the start-up phase of treatment. Patients may also have unrealistic expectations about what successful pharmacotherapy entails. This is yet another reason to include psychotherapy and, at times, approaches that acknowledge and address organizational skills deficits that may exist.

TABLE 8.3. Medications Commonly Used to Treat ADHD

Medication Class	Generic Name	Trade Name	Improves Attention[a]	Improves Impulsivity[a]	Starting Dose	Maximum Daily Dose
Stimulants	Amphetamine/ dextroamphetamine	Adderall	Y	Y	2.5 mg twice a day	40 mg
	Dextroamphetamine	Dexedrine	Y	Y	2.5 mg twice a day	40 mg
	Methylphenidate	Ritalin	Y	Y	5 mg twice a day	60 mg
	Pemoline	Cylert	Y	Y	18.75 mg	112.5 mg
Antidepressants	Bupropion	Wellbutrin XL	?	?	150 mg	450 mg
	Desipramine[b]	Norpramin	Y	?	10 mg	200 mg
	Fluoxetine	Prozac	N	Y	10 mg	80 mg
	Imipramine[b]	Tofranil	Y	?	10 mg	200 mg
	Venlafaxine	Effexor XR	?	?	37.5 mg	225 mg
Other	Atomoxetine	Strattera	Y	Y	0.5 mg/kg	100 mg
	Clonidine	Catapres	N	Y	0.05 mg at bedtime	0.3 mg
	Guanfacine		Y	Y	0.5 mg	3 mg
	Selegiline	Eldepryl	Y	?	5 mg	10 mg

[a] Y—yes; N—no.

[b] Avoid desipramine in children.

In children, stimulants are the "gold standard" of treatment and, in the absence of MDD, are generally first-line medication selections. In the presence of MDD, antidepressants may be used, but the antidepressants are not as well studied as are the stimulants for the treatment of ADHD. There is a divided opinion on the choice of medications in adults with ADHD. One view advocates the use of noradrenergic antidepressants such as venlafaxine or certain TCAs as a first-line approach due to the often high rates of comorbid depression and the complications that can arise in trying to make an accurate diagnosis. The higher rates of substance abuse that are often seen in this population are also cited in support of trying something other than stimulants initially. If antidepressants do not work after a period of time, then stimulants are tried next. No antidepressants have FDA indications for the treatment of ADHD, but they can be somewhat less complicated to prescribe because they are not schedule II substances. The opposing view is that stimulants are the "gold standard" of treatment in children, so even though stimulants do not have a FDA indication for adults with ADHD, with the exception of Adderall, they should still have the benefit of their use. Clinically it is often quite easy to find patients for whom one perspective seems more relevant than the other.

Continuing Treatment. Once the effective dose has been found, it can usually be maintained indefinitely. Children with ADHD almost never develop tolerance to the therapeutic effects of the medication. The key issues when continuing treatment are (1) monitoring for long-term side effects, (2) simplifying the stimulant regimen, (3) adding adjunctive medications to treat any remaining symptoms that the stimulants have not addressed, and (4) replacing the stimulant with another medication if the patient cannot tolerate a stimulant. A number of sustained-release preparations are either available or currently undergoing clinical trials. Sometimes switching to a sustained-release preparation is helpful from an adherence point of view, though there are patients who do not do as well as they did with the immediate-release preparation.

Monitoring Side Effects. The patient's blood pressure, pulse, and weight should be monitored on a regular basis. For growing children and adolescents, height should also be measured and recorded on a growth chart along with body weight. When any of these measurements significantly deviates from their growth curve, it may be an indication to consider changing dose or switching medications.

Insomnia, irritability, and appetite in addition to rebound hyperactivity between doses should be scrutinized at visits. The dose may occasionally need to be lowered to alleviate a side effect or raised to provide better treatment. Increasing the dose in a child is sometimes needed not because of tolerance to the medication but because the child has outgrown the previous dose, as body weight increases over time.

Simplifying the Regimen. Another issue that arises is the desire to switch to a longer-acting form of the medication that can be taken once a day. Taking medication once a day is preferable for two reasons. First, it's easier and less likely to be forgotten than medication taken two or more times per day. Second, the school-age child avoids the potential embarrassment of leaving the classroom to visit the school nurse each day to take his/her medicine.

Methylphenidate and Adderall are available in sustained-release forms. When switching to the longer-acting form, the prescribed dose should approximate the sum of the short-acting doses that are being replaced. For example, if a child is taking 10 mg of methylphenidate twice a day, this should be replaced by about 20 mg of the sustained-release formulation. Earlier sustained-release preparations triggered some debate as to whether they worked as well as the short-acting forms. Current formulations seem to have solved this problem for most patients. Of the controlled-released forms, we believe Concerta is the most reliable in terms of bioavailability. On occasion, it is necessary to supplement the longer-acting form with doses of the short-acting form. For example, an after-school dose of short-acting methylphenidate may still be necessary when taking the extended-release form in the morning.

Adjunctive Medications. Addition of a second medication should be considered after at least two stimulants have been tried. When treatment with a stimulant alone is not sufficient, a second medication can be utilized for augmentation. Because stimulants work fairly well for attention and other medications offer little benefit there, the need for augmentation usually arises because the impulsivity and hyperactivity persist.

Antidepressants and clonidine are the most commonly used augmentation strategies for ADHD. If the patient has tics or is troubled by insomnia, clonidine is a reasonable choice. After collecting a baseline EKG, clonidine should be started at 0.05 mg at bedtime for children and adolescents and 0.1 mg at bedtime for adults. The dose can be increased every 2 weeks or so while monitoring the patient's blood pressure and pulse. Although it has not been studied as well, guanfacine may work in much the same manner as clonidine.

If depression is a problem, many clinicians prefer an antidepressant as an augmentation strategy. Because of the problems mentioned earlier, most now avoid using TCAs to treat ADHD. Bupropion, SSRIs, and venlafaxine are viable alternatives, and may add to the effect of the stimulant. Bupropion and venlafaxine are believed to offer some additional improvement in attention. SSRIs may be more likely to improve impulsivity. Each should be started at a low dose and increased gradually. None of these are approved for use in children however.

When these measures have failed and impulsivity and aggression remain a problem, additional strategies are available. First, reconsider the diagnosis. Does the patient have bipolar disorder rather than ADHD? Is there another disruptive behavior disorder in addition to or instead of ADHD? Does (s)he have an impulse control disorder? In these more severe cases, other medications such as atypical antipsychotics or mood stabilizers are often helpful.

Replacing the Stimulant. Unfortunately, there are patients who are unable to continue taking any of the stimulants. The stimulants may render them irritable, may cause intractable insomnia, may interfere with appetite and slow growth, or may cause tics. In addition, some teenagers or adults with ADHD also have a history of abusing substances. These are all reasons that have been reported for stopping stimulant treatment. Before the decision is made to discontinue stimulant treatment, one should remember that the success of all other treatments to date pale by comparison. It therefore makes sense to try first to remedy the side effect without stopping the stimulant.

For example, stimulants can cause irritability. However, irritability can also result from depression. So it is always important to rule out comorbid depression in the patient with ADHD before discontinuing the stimulant medication. If the irritability does result from depression, then the obvious solution is to add an antidepressant to the stimulant. Conversely, irritability can also be a symptom of emerging hypomania or mania.

Stimulants can also cause insomnia. However, insomnia can also result from rebound hyperactivity when the daytime dose of stimulant has worn off. In either case, before stopping the stimulant, it is prudent to consider a bedtime dose of clonidine. Clonidine may relieve not only nighttime hyperactivity but insomnia as well.

Poor appetite and slow growth have also been reported in children taking stimulants. Although the impact of stimulants on final adult height is unnoticeable, children with ADHD do often lag behind their peers in growth. While this may be attributable at least in part to treatment with stimulants, recent research suggests that children with ADHD who are NOT taking stimulants often exhibit delayed growth. Growth deficits may be a symptom of the illness itself. In any case, the growth charts for both height and weight should be followed when treating children with stimulants. If a child deviates below the normal growth curve, then medication changes may be needed. First, if stopping the medication during school holidays or on weekends is a viable alternative, this should be tried. These brief times off medication may be enough to counteract any effect of the stimulant on the child's growth. If this does not prove successful or taking holidays from the medication is impossible (due to the severity of the illness), then one should try switching to another stimulant before concluding that stimulant therapy is contraindicated.

A subset of children with ADHD also display tics. Stimulants have been said to either cause tics or worsen them when they are already present. Until recently, the presence of tics was considered reason enough to stop stimulants. However, recent research has shown that children with ADHD and tics can indeed continue to take stimulants, and, moreover, stimulants do not appear to worsen tics over time.

Yet another concern is the potential for stimulant abuse. Granted, this is a valid concern when the patient has a history of substance abuse. There should be concern when a child on stimulants has a family member with a history of substance abuse who has access to the child's medication. For these reasons, it is always important to document carefully each prescription that is written, keeping an account of how much medication has been prescribed. Repeatedly lost medication with requests for additional prescriptions should arouse suspicion that someone may be abusing the stimulant. When stimulant abuse is a legitimate concern, one may consider atomoxetine.

Despite these alternatives, there are a few patients who cannot tolerate stimulants or who may be susceptible to abusing them. In such cases, the alternatives are limited. The best treatments for poor attention (in lieu of the stimulants) are antidepressants that boost norepinephrine and/or dopamine activity in the brain. Currently, this includes the TCAs, MAOIs, and possibly venlafaxine or duloxetine.

When stimulants cannot be used, clonidine or antidepressants are the best initial treatments for impulsivity. As noted earlier, more aggressive measures including antipsychotics and mood stabilizers may be needed in severe cases.

ADDITIONAL READING

Castellanos FX. Stimulants and tic disorders: from dogma to data. *Arch Gen Psychiatry* 1999; 56(4): 337–338.

Croft HA. Physician handling of prescription stimulants. *Psychiatr Ann* 2005; 35: 221–226.

Dodson WW. Pharmacotherapy of adult ADHD. *J Clin Psychol* 2005; 61: 589–606.

Elia J, Ambrosini PJ, Rapoport JL. Drug therapy: treatment of attention-deficit–hyperactivity disorder. *New Engl J Med* 1999; 340(10): 780–788.

Greenhill LL, Ford RE. Childhood attention-deficit–hyperactivity disorder: pharmacological treatments. In Nathan PE, Gorman JM (eds), *A Guide to Treatments that Work, 2nd Edition*. London: Oxford University Press, 2002, pp 25–55.

Jensen P. Longer term effects of stimulant treatments for attention-deficit/hyperactivity disorder. *J Attention Disord* 2002; 6(Supplement 1): S17–S30.

Kent L, Craddock N. Is there a relationship between attention deficit hyperactivity disorder and bipolar disorder? *J Affect Disord* 2003; 73(3): 211–221.

Maidment ID. The use of antidepressants to treat attention deficit hyperactivity disorder in adults. *J Psychopharmacol* 2003; 17(3): 332–336.

Rubia K, Smith A. Attention deficit–hyperactivity disorder: current findings and treatment. *Curr Opin Psychiatry* 2001; 14(4): 309–316.

Santosh PJ, Taylor E. Stimulant drugs. *Eur Child Adolesc Psychiatry* 2000; 9(Supplement 5): 127–143.

Spencer TJ, Biederman J, Wilens TE, Faraone SV. Novel treatments for attention-deficit/hyperactivity disorder in children. *J Clin Psychiatry* 2002; 62(Supplement 12): 16–22.

Steer CR. Managing attention deficit/hyperactivity disorder: unmet needs and future directions. *Arch Dis Child* 2005; 90(Supplement 1): 19–25.

Wilens TE, Spencer TJ, Biederman J. A review of the pharmacotherapy of adults with attention-deficit/hyperactivity disorder. *J Attention Disord* 2002; 5(4): 189–202.

9

SLEEP DISORDERS

9.1 INTRODUCTION

Psychiatrists and psychologists have long possessed a keen interest in sleep, including the function of sleep, the role of dreams as the gateway to the unconscious, and the variety of disorders that can disrupt sleep. A good night's sleep, one that leaves the person feeling refreshed upon awakening and without daytime drowsiness, is often taken for granted. Perturbations of sleep take many forms including difficulty falling asleep, difficulty staying asleep, waking too early, sleep apnea, and restless legs syndrome to name a few. Changes in sleep often accompany a number of psychiatric disorders including depression, bipolar disorder, anxiety disorders, and substance use disorder. Furthermore, primary sleep disorders are distinct from psychiatric illnesses, though they are often associated with comorbid psychiatric symptoms. Unfortunately, few mental health professionals have received any formal training in the diagnosis and treatment of sleep disorders. As a result, our patients with sleep problems often receive inadequate diagnostic evaluation and ineffective, and sometimes potentially dangerous, treatment for sleep disorders.

To address this shortcoming, the new discipline of sleep disorders medicine has arisen in recent years. These specialists are dedicated to caring for all patients who

Principles of Psychopharmacology for Mental Health Professionals
By Jeffrey E. Kelsey, D. Jeffrey Newport, and Charles B. Nemeroff

are having problems with their sleep. The primary diagnostic tools of a sleep specialist are collecting a careful history and performing an inpatient sleep study. During a sleep study, a patient is videotaped overnight in a sleep laboratory while brain activity is recorded using electroencephalography (EEG). This technique, called polysomnography, allows the sleep specialist to diagnose many sleep problems with great accuracy. Some investigators in the field believe that sleep should be monitored over two to three consecutive nights in a sleep laboratory because of the effects of novelty on sleep during the first night.

9.1.1 Normal Sleep

Circadian Sleep Rhythm. Sleep can be conceptualized as a pair of cycles each regulated by a biological clock. The larger cycle is the rhythm of sleep and wakefulness that operates according to a 24 hour (circadian) biological clock. The sleep–wake cycle is not our only circadian rhythm. Body temperature and certain hormones fluctuate in accordance with this same biological rhythm.

This 24 hour circadian clock is regulated largely by the daily changes in light intensity at sunrise and sunset. However, in laboratory conditions removed from time cues such as light changes and clocks, most people drift to a sleep–wake cycle of about 25 hours. The classic demonstration of this is when people agree to live in a sleep laboratory for extended periods of time and receive no cues as to the time of day. This implies, of course, that in addition to the effect of light and dark, we have an internal biological rhythm that regulates the timing of our sleep.

Purpose of Sleep. Why do we sleep? The answer to this question remains obscure. At the risk of appearing obtuse, the simple answer is "because we are sleepy." The longer one is awake, the more likely one is to feel sleepy.

How much sleep is enough? Your mother probably insisted that you get at least 8 hours of sleep per night. In fact, there is no specific number of hours that equals "enough sleep." In addition, there is no medical test to determine if one is getting "enough sleep." A useful rule of thumb is to ask if the individual awakens feeling refreshed and is able to function during the day without getting drowsy during quiet or monotonous activities. An adequate amount of sleep should also translate to requiring 15–20 minutes each night to fall asleep after the head hits the pillow. Falling asleep less than 5 minutes after getting in bed is often a sign of sleep deprivation or not getting enough sleep. For many adults, 7–9 hours of sleep are needed each night, but this can vary from as few as 3–4 to as many as 10 hours or more per night.

Ultradian Sleep Rhythm. As we previously noted, there are two biological clocks that regulate sleep. In addition to the 24 hour (circadian) rhythm that manages the sleep–wake cycle, another clock, operating on a shorter (ultradian) rhythm, regulates the timing of the well-ordered phases and stages of sleep.

Thanks to the technique of polysomnography, many of the mysteries of sleep are now becoming better understood. First, sleep is divided into two main phases: rapid eye movement (REM) sleep and non-rapid eye movement (NREM) sleep. During REM sleep, the brain is quite active; this is when dreaming occurs. One can easily be awakened during REM sleep, and if awakened, many are able to recall the dream they were having at the time. NREM is the phase of sleep during which the brain activity is slowest. The NREM sleep phase is comprised of four distinct stages. Stages I and II of NREM are relatively light sleep; stages III and IV are deeper sleep. It is hardest to wake someone during the deeper stages of NREM sleep, and if they do awaken, they are typically confused and disoriented for a brief time immediately upon awakening.

An ultradian biological clock regulates these phases of sleep. There is, in fact, a typical pattern to sleep termed "sleep architecture." When someone falls asleep, sleep quickly progresses from stage I of NREM to stage IV of NREM sleep. This initial phase of NREM sleep lasts close to 90 minutes from the time someone falls asleep (stage I NREM) before giving way to REM sleep. NREM and REM then alternate throughout the remainder of the night. The most efficient rest occurs during stage IV of NREM, but REM sleep is also a necessary part of a good night's sleep.

Aging and Sleep. Age has a pronounced effect on sleep. Newborns may sleep as many as 16 hours per day and spend half that time in REM sleep. Sleep patterns change dramatically between infancy and adolescence. As a child ages, daytime napping is gradually eliminated as nighttime sleep becomes more efficient with longer periods of deep stage III and IV NREM sleep. By adolescence, an adult pattern of sleep is usually attained and remains rather stable for many years.

As we enter old age, our sleep again enters a period of change. We tend to spend more time in bed but spend less of that time actually sleeping. This is often referred to as a decrease in sleep efficiency. Sleep efficiency is simply the ratio of time asleep to time in bed. The more time in bed that is spent sleeping, as opposed to being awake, the greater the sleep efficiency. With aging, sleep becomes lighter with shorter periods of stage III and IV sleep, and the night is often punctuated with frequent awakenings. Daytime naps appear again, most likely resulting from decreased efficiency of nighttime sleep.

9.1.2 Overview of Sleep Disorders

The sleep disorders fall into four main categories: (1) insomnia, (2) hypersomnia, (3) parasomnias, and (4) sleep schedule disorders. Insomnia is the most common sleep problem. It is simply defined as "poor sleep" and can be manifested by difficulty falling asleep, difficulty staying asleep, waking up too early, or waking up in the morning without feeling refreshed.

Hypersomnia is the opposite of insomnia; it is excessive sleepiness. This can be dangerous when driving or operating heavy equipment. It can be a hindrance in school or at work and additionally can be a source of great embarrassment. In reality, it can be difficult to distinguish a patient who is suffering from hypersomnia from one who is suffering from insomnia. This may seem odd, but in fact the most common complaint in both cases is feeling tired and sleepy during the day. The distinction lies in the underlying cause of the daytime drowsiness.

Parasomnias are abnormal behaviors that occur during sleep. These abnormal behaviors may or may not disturb the quality and duration of sleep. Many parasomnias, such as sleepwalking (somnambulism), bed wetting (enuresis), teeth grinding (bruxism), and night terrors, are common during childhood but are often outgrown before adolescence. Some parasomnias, however, such as periodic limb movement (PLM) and nightmares, can continue to plague adults.

The final category is termed the sleep–wake schedule disorders. These are seen in people who "get their days and nights turned around." The most common examples are shift workers and travelers with jet lag. Additionally, in the elderly, especially those with dementia, a malfunction in the circadian biological rhythm that regulates sleep can leave them awake and alert at night but drowsy and sleeping during the day.

Although we are focusing on the primary sleep disorders, sleep disturbance quite often occurs as a symptom of another illness. Depression, anxiety, and substance abuse can impair the quality of sleep, though in the setting of chronic insomnia, other psychiatric disorders account for less than 50% of cases. Nightmares are a frequent complication of post-traumatic stress disorder (PTSD), and pain, endocrine conditions, and a host of medical illnesses can produce sleep problems. Thus, when discussing insomnia or hypersomnia, we are well advised to remember that these can be either a symptom of a psychiatric syndrome, a medical illness, or a sleep disorder.

In this chapter, we will not attempt to provide an exhaustive description of every sleep disorder. Medication therapy plays a minimal role in the treatment of many sleep disorders. In fact, we contend that medication, apart from being an integral component of a comprehensive multimodal treatment program, is seldom an effective treatment for any sleep problem with the possible exception of acute insomnia due to an identifiable and short-lived stressor. Nevertheless, medications do play a part in the treatment of some sleep disorders.

The discussion that follows will be limited to those sleep disorders that are common in adults and that frequently require medication as part of the usual treatment. Specifically, we will discuss insomnia and narcolepsy (the most common hypersomnia). We will briefly mention treatments for the nighttime limb movement disorders.

9.2 INSOMNIA

9.2.1 Brief Description and Diagnostic Criteria

Insomnia is not so much a diagnosable illness as a symptom. Simply put, insomnia is poor sleep, and there are a number of ways that the quality of sleep can be diminished. Although it may be tempting to identify insomnia by counting the number of hours spent sleeping, insomnia is much more than that. Insomnia is the experience of a poor quality sleep characterized by any of the following: having difficulty falling asleep (initial insomnia), staying asleep (middle insomnia), or waking too early (terminal insomnia). The poor quality sleep of insomnia is nonrefreshing and leads to distress and/or impairment. Insomnia can increase the vulnerability to motor vehicle accidents, decrease productivity on the job or in the classroom, and lead to increased irritability. Approximately one-third of Americans complain of insomnia, and half of these individuals exhibit poor quality sleep by polysomnography.

When making the diagnosis of insomnia, counting the absolute number of hours of sleep is not very helpful. Some people routinely require little sleep, but they wake feeling rested and refreshed. They don't have insomnia. Others may get 8–10 hours of poor quality sleep, leaving them listless and drained. These people probably do have insomnia. Again, the key is not the number of hours of sleep. The main problem is that poor sleep leaves the patient feeling tired and less able to function during normal waking hours.

A variety of factors can trigger insomnia. Medications, medical illness, pain, stress, schedule changes, depression, anxiety, and nighttime breathing problems all can produce insomnia. When insomnia has no clear cause, that is, it is not secondary to another condition, it is termed primary insomnia. The diagnostic criteria for primary insomnia are shown in Table 9.1.

9.2.2 Prevalence and Risk Factors

Insomnia is often subdivided into acute or chronic types. Acute insomnia lasts from one night to a few weeks and is thought to afflict perhaps as many as 30% of the adult population during the course of a single year. Chronic insomnia, in contrast, is more longstanding, occurring at least three nights per week for one month or more, and is experienced by 10–15% of the adult population in any given year.

The elderly have even more trouble with insomnia. In a given year, about half of those over 65 years of age will experience a period of insomnia. Although normal aging causes the elderly to sleep less soundly and leaves them vulnerable to insom-

TABLE 9.1. Diagnostic Criteria for Primary Insomnia

A. The predominant complaint is difficulty initiating or maintaining sleep, or nonrestorative sleep, for at least 1 month.
B. The sleep disturbance (or associated daytime fatigue) causes clinically significant distress or impairment in social, occupational, or other important areas of functioning.
C. The sleep disturbance does not occur exclusively during the course of narcolepsy, breathing-related sleep disorder, circadian rhythm sleep disorder, or a parasomnia.
D. The disturbance does not occur exclusively during the course of another mental disorder (e.g., major depressive disorder, generalized anxiety disorder, a delirium).
E. The disturbance is not due to the direct physiological effects of a substance (e.g., a drug of abuse, a medication) or a general medical condition.

Source: Adapted from DSM-IV.

nia, suffering from insomnia is not an expected or normal result of getting older. Nevertheless, insomnia is a major problem for the elderly and can be triggered by medications, illness, or pain (all of which are far more common in the elderly).

For reasons that are not entirely clear, insomnia is also more common in women than men. There are particular times when a woman is especially vulnerable to insomnia, including pregnancy, the transition into menopause, and the premenstrual phase of the menstrual cycle. This, of course, suggests that it is changes in the female reproductive system that somehow alter sleep. Depression and anxiety are also more common in women at these times, and insomnia is a common symptom of these psychiatric illnesses.

9.2.3 Presentation and Clinical Course

Everyone has experienced a sleepless night at one time or another. Typical triggers include the night before an important presentation, a test at school, or after some stress like a dispute with a loved one. Insomnia usually has an abrupt onset during a period of stress or illness. Most insomniacs were sleeping well just before the stress and usually return to normal sleep when the stress subsides. During this brief period, most do not seek professional help. They simply "tough it out" or use home remedies (e.g., warm milk, hot bath, and unfortunately sometimes alcohol) or over-the-counter medications (e.g., Sleep-Eze, Benadryl, Tylenol PM) to hasten the onset of sleep.

Sometimes bad sleep habits develop during the period of stress. This is termed "poor sleep hygiene" and it may consist of taking daytime naps, drinking a nightcap, or engaging in other behaviors that ultimately interfere with quality nighttime sleep. When such bad sleep habits persist after the initial stress has passed, then a vicious cycle of anxious anticipation and ever-poorer sleep may arise.

Instead of going to bed relaxed and drifting off to sleep, individuals with insomnia go to bed worrying whether they will be able to fall asleep, how long it will take to do so, or whether they will be too tired to wake up on time the next day. They try hard to fall asleep, but trying so hard actually increases their level of arousal, making it ever more difficult to sleep. They become increasingly frustrated and develop a conditioned dread of bedtime.

Once chronic insomnia has developed, it hardly ever spontaneously resolves without treatment or intervention. The toll of chronic insomnia can be very high and the frustration it produces may precipitate a clinical depression or an anxiety disorder. Insomnia is also associated with decreased productivity in the workplace and more frequent use of medical services. Finally, substance abuse problems may result from the inappropriate use of alcohol or sedatives to induce sleep or caffeine and other stimulants to maintain alertness during the day.

9.2.4 Initial Evaluation and Differential Diagnosis

The cause for short-term insomnia is usually clear and requires little diagnostic assessment. As we previously noted, these brief disturbances of sleep seldom come to professional attention anyway. In contrast, the causes and patterns of chronic insomnia are very complex. Even when it is triggered by a single easily recognizable event, many factors contribute to the maintenance of chronic insomnia. Because there are no simple solutions to the problem of chronic insomnia, a careful clinical evaluation is required. The initial evaluation of chronic insomnia should include several key components:

- Careful history from the patient *and* partner (if applicable)
- Complete inventory of all medications, alcohol, caffeine, and other substances
- Completion of a sleep log by the patient
- Consideration of a referral for a sleep study

The duration and pattern of the sleep problems are assessed when collecting the history. If the problem is primarily difficulty falling asleep, then the patient may have an underlying anxiety or mood disorder. Early-morning awakening after falling asleep is also suggestive of depression, particularly the melancholic subtype. If patients describe suddenly waking at night fearful or short of breath, they may be experiencing nocturnal panic attacks. The patient's partner can be a helpful source of information as well. Be sure to ask the partner about snoring and frequent tossing, turning, jerking movements (particularly of the arms and legs) in bed, or whether or not the sheets are a mess in the morning. These can suggest sleep apnea or a nighttime movement disorder.

A complaint of persistent insomnia usually should not be taken at face value. This is not to diminish the distress that it produces, but rather to acknowledge that several psychiatric and medical conditions can either cause insomnia or masquerade as insomnia. In the next few paragraphs, we will review the differential diagnoses of chronic insomnia.

Primary Insomnia. Primary insomnia is a sleep disturbance lasting at least a month with no clear cause. However, many well-recognized psychological and physical factors contribute to prolonging the insomnia. For this reason, some call this condition psychophysiological insomnia.

Pseudoinsomnia. Some patients report chronic insomnia, but no abnormality can be detected during a sleep study. This condition is also called "sleep-state misperception" because these patients appear to have some difficulty distinguishing wakefulness from sleep. Such patients are not malingering; nor are they "faking" it. They are truly convinced that they are not sleeping. In extreme cases, sufferers with pseudoinsomnia may even report going months or years without sleeping. Sleep state misperception can be diagnosed reliably by EEG recording during a sleep study. Of the individuals who complain of insomnia, one-half show no evidence of sleep disturbance when studied in a sleep laboratory.

Nighttime Movement Disorders. There are two disorders that are characterized by involuntary movements at night. These are periodic limb movement disorder (PLMD) and restless legs syndrome (RLS). The PLMD patient is usually unaware of the movements, but the disorder results in frequent arousals to a lighter sleep stage. The result is a patient who complains of fatigue despite a full night's sleep. Asking the patient's partner about nighttime movements can help to clarify the diagnosis. A definitive diagnosis of PLMD can be made with a sleep study.

RLS is not a true sleep disorder. It actually occurs prior to sleep. RLS patients describe unpleasant "pins and needles" sensations in their legs, which are usually worse in the evening. These nagging sensations are temporarily relieved by movement, hence the name "restless legs." Unlike PLMD, patients with RLS are aware of their nighttime movements; however, many of those suffering from RLS also prove to have PLMD. Whereas PLMD causes a restless, fitful sleep, RLS essentially makes it difficult to fall asleep.

Breathing-Related Sleep Disorders. The breathing-related sleep disorders include obstructive sleep apnea, central sleep apnea, and alveolar hypoventilation. Of these three, obstructive sleep apnea is by far the most common. The patient with sleep apnea usually breathes normally when awake and only stops breathing while asleep. Occasional episodes of apnea are normal, but five or more episodes of apnea per hour are usually considered diagnostic of the disorder.

In obstructive sleep apnea, the muscles of the throat relax during sleep and collapse inward to close the upper airway, producing an obstruction to air flow. In central sleep apnea, the brain center that controls the drive to breathe malfunctions during sleep. In both cases, the body becomes oxygen starved during the period of apnea. As a result, the patient partially awakens to a lighter level of sleep, gasping for air. A period of normal breathing follows until the next episode of apnea occurs.

Patients with apnea rarely fully awaken and are thus unaware of their problem. They may occasionally awaken with a sense of suffocation, but this can just as easily be a nighttime panic attack or asthma attack.

Sleep apnea is no trivial condition. Short-term, it causes daytime drowsiness that interferes with work and increases the risk of accidents. Long-term, sleep apnea worsens blood pressure control and may even shorten life expectancy.

The syndrome is most common in obese males and should be considered when such patients complain of persistent drowsiness. However, the patient's partner provides the key to diagnosis. If the patient's partner reports frequent snoring and gasping for air or has even noticed episodes of apnea, then one should suspect sleep apnea. The final diagnosis is made during a sleep study in which the episodes of apnea can be observed directly. Although obese individuals have an elevated risk for obstructive sleep apnea, there are clearly individuals with sleep apnea who would be considered normal weight.

It is important that the breathing-related sleep disorders be distinguished from other forms of insomnia. The key reason is that many of the most common medications used to treat insomnia worsen the breathing-related sleep disorders. For example, benzodiazepines, the most commonly used class of "sleeping pills," can worsen obstructive sleep apnea by further relaxing the muscles surrounding the throat.

Substance-Induced Insomnia. A variety of substances can cause or worsen sleep problems (see Table 9.2). Patients often miss the connection between the ingestion of a medication or caffeine and the onset of their insomnia, and they rarely spontaneously volunteer this information.

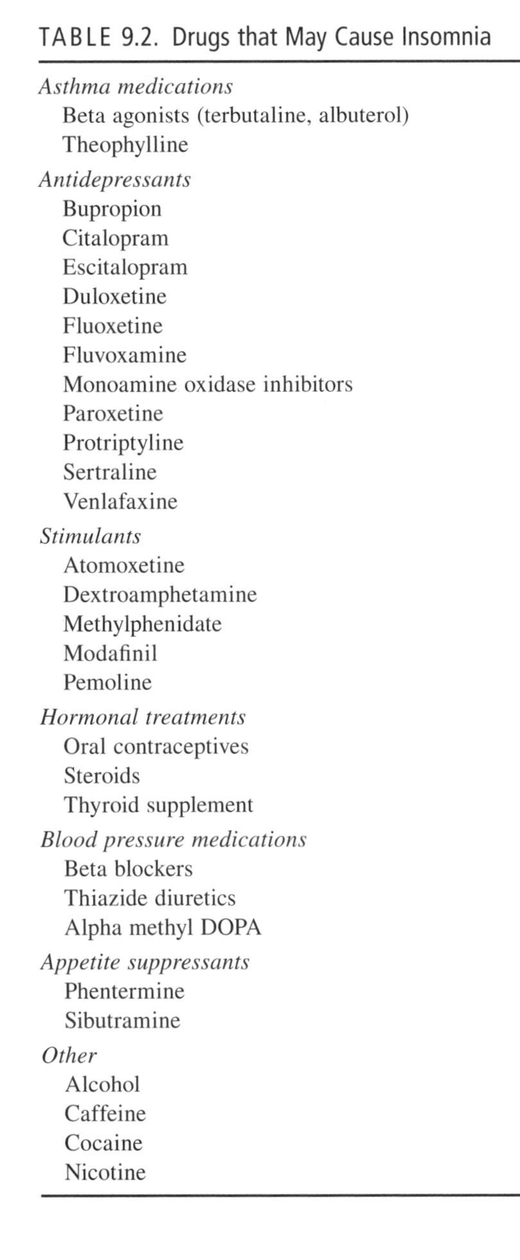

TABLE 9.2. Drugs that May Cause Insomnia

Asthma medications
Beta agonists (terbutaline, albuterol)
Theophylline
Antidepressants
Bupropion
Citalopram
Escitalopram
Duloxetine
Fluoxetine
Fluvoxamine
Monoamine oxidase inhibitors
Paroxetine
Protriptyline
Sertraline
Venlafaxine
Stimulants
Atomoxetine
Dextroamphetamine
Methylphenidate
Modafinil
Pemoline
Hormonal treatments
Oral contraceptives
Steroids
Thyroid supplement
Blood pressure medications
Beta blockers
Thiazide diuretics
Alpha methyl DOPA
Appetite suppressants
Phentermine
Sibutramine
Other
Alcohol
Caffeine
Cocaine
Nicotine

Other important substances that patients should be asked about include all prescription and over-the-counter medications, herbs, and substances of abuse. Any that are known to cause insomnia and any that were initiated just prior to the onset of insomnia should be considered suspect and discontinued if it is safe for the patient to do so.

Insomnia Due to Another Psychiatric Illness. Insomnia is often a symptom of mood and anxiety disorders. Depression is classically associated with early-morning awakening of the melancholic type, whereas so-called atypical depression leads to hypersomnia. Anxiety commonly leads to problems falling asleep. These patterns are not invariable. One should therefore always perform a thorough assessment for anxiety or depression in patients complaining of insomnia.

During episodes of mania or hypomania, patients also have difficulty sleeping. This usually does not represent true insomnia but a decreased need for sleep. During episodes of hypomania or mania, patients may go days with little or no sleep; nevertheless, they feel refreshed and energetic during the day. The key to evaluating these patients is to focus less on the number of hours of sleep, and more on the degree of sleepiness during the day. Remember that insomnia is characterized by the consequences of poor sleep such as daytime sleepiness; the decreased need for sleep seen in mania or hypomania is not insomnia.

Insomnia Due to a Medical Illness. Medically ill patients often have trouble with insomnia. Acute insomnia is frequently precipitated by anxiety regarding the prognosis of the illness, pending test results, or the anticipation of unpleasant treatments or diagnostic procedures. These situations can at times be the trigger that ultimately produces a chronic course of insomnia independent of the medical illness.

Sometimes, a medical illness produces insomnia in a more immediate fashion. Pain, shortness of breath, cough, and the urge to urinate or defecate are just a few of the medical symptoms that can interfere with sleep. Fibromyalgia and several neurological conditions can directly interfere with sleep quality (see Table 9.3).

The key to helping the medically ill patient with insomnia is first to recognize and then optimize the treatment of the underlying medical illness. If the insomnia remains problematic, it can then be treated.

9.2.5 History of Pharmacological Treatment

Dating back to the 1800s, some of the earliest successful psychiatric medications were those used to promote sleep. Sleep-promoting medications, called sedative-hypnotics, have remained an important component of our pharmacological armamentarium. Over the past 100-plus years, as we have learned more about both pharmacology and sleep physiology, a series of refinements have improved the safety and effectiveness of sleep medications.

It is easy to imagine the ideal sleeping pill. It would help you to fall asleep quickly and remain asleep through the night. There would be no hangover effect the next

TABLE 9.3. Medical Illnesses that May Cause Insomnia

Alzheimer's disease
Asthma
Cancer
Chronic
obstructive pulmonary disease (emphysema/bronchitis)
Chronic pain
Congestive heart failure
Coronary artery disease
Diabetes mellitus
Fibromyalgia
Gastroesophageal reflux disease
Huntington's disease
Parkinson's disease
Peptic ulcer disease
Rheumatoid arthritis

morning, and one would still be able to awaken during the night to the sound of a ringing telephone or a crying baby. The sleeping pill would not be addictive nor would one develop tolerance to its effect. It would not alter normal sleep architecture. Finally, the ideal sleeping pill would have no unpleasant or dangerous side effects, and it would be safe if taken in overdose. It may be easy to imagine the perfect sleeping pill, but unfortunately, it does not exist. All the substances used to treat insomnia represent a series of compromises between various favorable and unfavorable characteristics.

Alcohol. It may seem odd to list alcohol among the treatments for insomnia, but it has long been among the most common self-administered treatments for insomnia. Alcohol usually does help the person fall asleep, but it is otherwise an extremely poor treatment for insomnia. It can lead to fragmented sleep later in the night, not to mention the potential for hangover and tolerance. In fact, with repeated use, alcohol itself can *produce* insomnia. Even without taking the social and medical consequences of frequent alcohol use into account, alcohol has no place in the treatment of insomnia.

Alcohol-like Medications. The earliest sleep medications were chemically related to alcohol. These include chloral hydrate and ethchlorvynol, which were introduced in the 1800s and are still occasionally used today. These medications effectively induce sleep, decrease sleep fragmentation during the night, and do not interfere with sleep architecture. However, they can cause dizziness and impair coordination. In addition, tolerance can develop after as little as a week of treatment, and these medications can be dangerous in overdose, especially ethchlorvynol. Chloral hydrate (Aquachloral, Welldorm) is taken in nightly doses of 500–1500 mg. Ethchlorvynol (Placidyl) is taken in 500–1600 mg doses per night.

Barbiturates. The next advance in treatment was the introduction of the barbiturates in the early 1900s. These medications are not only effective sleep inducers, but they also treat epilepsy and alcohol withdrawal; at higher doses they produce anesthesia. The barbiturates can help one to fall asleep and to sleep soundly through the night. However, they markedly alter sleep architecture, reducing REM sleep.

Barbiturates have several serious drawbacks. They are extremely dangerous in overdose. In addition, barbiturates can cause dangerous suppression of breathing in patients with undiagnosed sleep apnea or other respiratory disorders. The side effects of barbiturates include a groggy hangover effect and poor physical coordination. Barbiturates also potentiate the effects of alcohol. With repeated use, physical dependence on and tolerance to their beneficial effects develop. Barbiturates, including phenobarbital (Luminal), secobarbital (Seconal), and pentobarbital (Nembutal), are seldom used to treat insomnia any longer but continue to be used to treat epilepsy and acute alcohol withdrawal.

Thalidomide. Thalidomide is a chemically unique sleep medication that was introduced in the 1950s. It is not clear how thalidomide works, but in contrast to most sleep agents, it has beneficial effects on sleep architecture.

Unfortunately, thalidomide had to be quickly withdrawn from the worldwide market when it was discovered to cause severe limb malformations in the offspring of women who ingested the drug during pregnancy. The thalidomide tragedy served as a major impetus for the refinement of FDA drug development protocols, and it therefore has a prominent place in U.S. medical history. Thalidomide has recently been reintroduced on a limited basis for the treatment of leprosy, but it is no longer used to treat insomnia.

Benzodiazepines. Safer than the barbiturates but acting in a similar manner, the benzodiazepines have largely replaced barbiturates since their introduction in the 1960s. Other uses of benzodiazepines include treatment for epilepsy, alcohol withdrawal, several anxiety disorders, agitation, and impulsivity, as muscle relaxants, and as "conscious sedation" during certain medical procedures.

Like the barbiturates, the benzodiazepines make it easier to fall asleep and to stay asleep through the night. However, they also suppress REM sleep, which can lead to "REM rebound" when they are discontinued. Tolerance to their sleep-promoting effects often develops after chronic use. Some long-acting benzodiazepines, such as flurazepam (Dalmane), are associated with pronounced hangover effects in the morning and are therefore problematic as sedative-hypnotics. Others, with a short-to-intermediate duration of action, are more desirable as hypnotics.

The potential side effects of benzodiazepines include dizziness, lack of coordination, and, at higher doses, amnesia. Benzodiazepines also increase the effects of alcohol; drinking alcohol should therefore be avoided. Benzodiazepines can also worsen the breathing problems of patients with sleep apnea and other respiratory disorders such as emphysema. Like the barbiturates, long-term use of benzodiazepines can lead to physical dependence. The major advance of benzodiazepines (besides their many uses) is that they are much safer in overdose than barbiturates.

The benzodiazepines that have been most commonly marketed as sedative-hypnotics include temazepam (Restoril), estazolam (ProSom), flurazepam (Dalmane), quazepam (Doral), and triazolam (Halcion). Of these five, temazepam is the most easily metabolized and eliminated. Therefore, temazepam is preferred for elderly and medically ill patients to minimize the risk of drug accumulation.

Ultimately, it is a drug's half-life combined with its potency that dictates its utility as a sedative-hypnotic. Like other benzodiazepines, clonazepam (Klonopin) can be used to treat insomnia, but its long duration of action renders it prone to hangover effects at doses needed to treat insomnia. Nevertheless, low doses of clonazepam (0.25–2 mg) are a treatment for PLMD and are also used to treat RLS. When hangover effects of even low doses of clonazepam are a problem, other benzodiazepines can be used.

The development of tolerance is a major drawback to the use of benzodiazepines in the long-term treatment of insomnia. Whereas tolerance to the hypnotic effects of benzodiazepines permits them to be used without excessive sedation when treating anxiety disorders, this is counterproductive when attempting to treat insomnia. Patients often find themselves requiring higher doses to obtain the same sedative-hypnotic effect initially accomplished by lower doses. For this reason, careful consideration must be given before benzodiazepines are used to treat chronic insomnia.

Antihistamines. After alcohol, antihistamines are the most commonly self-administered sleep medications. Foremost among these is diphenhydramine (Benadryl), which is also available as a component in a variety of over-the-counter nighttime medications including Tylenol PM and Excedrin PM. Prescription antihistamines like hydroxyzine (Vistaril, Atarax) are also occasionally used to treat insomnia. Finally, it is the antihistamine effect of some antidepressants and antipsychotics that contribute to their utility as sedative-hypnotics.

Antihistamines help to initiate sleep and, depending on their half-life, may produce little hangover. They are not addictive and therefore may be preferred for patients with a history of substance abuse. Diphenhydramine is usually an effective hypnotic at 25–50 mg at bedtime. The same dose tends to be effective for hydroxyzine.

With long-term use, the most problematic side effect is weight gain. However, many antihistamines including diphenhydramine also possess potent anticholinergic effects. This can cause dry mouth, blurred vision, constipation, confusion, and urinary retention. Because anticholinergic effects are especially problematic for the elderly, we advise against the routine use of antihistamines to treat elderly patients with insomnia.

Antidepressants. For three apparent reasons, antidepressants have long been used to treat insomnia. First, some of them are quite sedating. In particular, doxepin (Sinequan), amitriptyline (Elavil), and trazodone (Desyrel) have been used to treat insomnia. Second, insomnia is often a core component of depression. Some physicians prefer to use a sedating antidepressant to treat depressed patients with insomnia, because one medication can be used to treat both conditions. Of course, the problem with this approach is that the insomnia usually resolves when the depression is treated, regardless of the antidepressant prescribed. In that case, patients are left with the now unwelcome burden of a sedating medication when they no longer have insomnia. In addition, the dose of the antidepressant effective in relieving insomnia is often insufficient to treat depression. Finally, some physicians prefer sedating antidepressants for their patients who have a history of substance abuse because the antidepressants are not habit forming.

When treating insomnia without depression, doxepin and amitriptyline (both tricyclic antidepressants) can be administered in low doses (25–100 mg) at bedtime. These antidepressants, however, do have troublesome anticholinergic side effects (dry mouth, constipation, blurred vision, dizziness) and adverse effects on the heart, and they can be lethal if taken in overdose. Because of their effect on heart function, these antidepressants should be avoided in patients with heart problems and administered cautiously, if at all, to those who are already receiving one of any number of newer antidepressants that inhibit the metabolism of the TCAs.

Trazodone can be administered at 25–200 mg at bedtime for insomnia. It is much safer in overdose but has some troublesome side effects as well, the most common of which is dizziness. Another (extremely rare) side effect of trazodone is priapism. Priapism is a painful and persistent erection of the penis that may require surgical intervention. An advantage to trazodone is in the treatment of late insomnia (waking 1–2 hours too early). Trazodone has a sufficiently long half-life that it often remains in the system long enough to get the patient through the last one or two hours of sleep. The drawback of course is the potential for a morning hangover effect, but this is true for most, if not all, of the sedative-hypnotics that remain active throughout the night. See Chapter 3 for more information regarding the antidepressants.

Antipsychotics. Low potency classical antipsychotics like chlorpromazine (Thorazine) and thioridazine (Mellaril) can be quite sedating. They have on occasion been used to treat insomnia. Like the older antidepressants, the low potency antipsychotics can cause constipation, blurred vision, dry mouth, and dizziness. In addition, they can cause extrapyramidal effects including stiffness and shuffling gait, and with extended use can cause involuntary oral, facial, and limb movements termed tardive dyskinesia (TD). TD is often irreversible, even when the antipsychotic drug is discontinued. Because of these potentially permanent side effects, we strongly recommend against the use of classical antipsychotics to treat insomnia. One potential exception is the patient with chronic psychotic illness who has insomnia. For this patient, adding a low potency antipsychotic for insomnia to the antipsychotic regimen will not appreciably increase the risk of extrapyramidal side effects. Low doses of atypical antipsychotic drugs, such as quetiapine (Seroquel) or olanzapine (Zyprexa), are increasingly being used to treat insomnia and to augment the antidepressant action of the SSRIs. Although the newer generation atypical antipsychotics are safer and better tolerated than the older typical antipsychotics, there are other agents better suited as first-line treatments for insomnia.

Benzodiazepine-like Agents. There are currently three nonbenzodiazepine sedative-hypnotics available in the United States: zolpidem (Ambien), zaleplon (Sonata), and eszopiclone (Lunesta). All three display an identical mechanism of action by binding to the omega-1 receptor subunit of the benzodiazepine receptor complex. They are termed "nonbenzodiazepines" as they are structurally unrelated to the benzodiazepines and do not possess the muscle relaxation properties of the benzodiazepines. Perhaps due to their lack of muscle relaxant properties or their receptor selectivity, they are thought to possess markedly lower abuse potential. This does not mean that they can be prescribed without any concern for abuse, because if dosed high enough, their effects become benzodiazepine-like. Each of these medications, like the benzodiazepines, is considered to be a controlled substance by the federal Drug Enforcement Agency (DEA).

One principal difference between the medications is half-life, that is, the time required to metabolize 50% of the compound present in the body. Zolpidem has a half-life of 1.4–4.5 hours, zaleplon has a half-life of 0.9–1.1 hours, and eszopiclone has a half-life of about 6 hours. The key is the markedly shorter half-lives that are displayed by many other sedative-hypnotics, as shown in Figure 9.1. Only eszopiclone has been shown effective for the long-term (up to 6 months) treatment of chronic insomnia.

Zolpidem is often effective at doses of 5 or 10 mg per night. Similarly, zaleplon is usually dosed at 10 mg just before bedtime (5 mg for medically ill or geriatric patients). Due to the short half-life of zaleplon, some clinicians use it to treat the occasional middle of the night awakening if there is at least 4 hours remaining until awakening. Eszopiclone is administered at doses of 2 or 3 mg at bedtime (1 or 2 mg for elderly patients). These agents have fewer effects on sleep architecture than the benzodiazepines and little hangover effect.

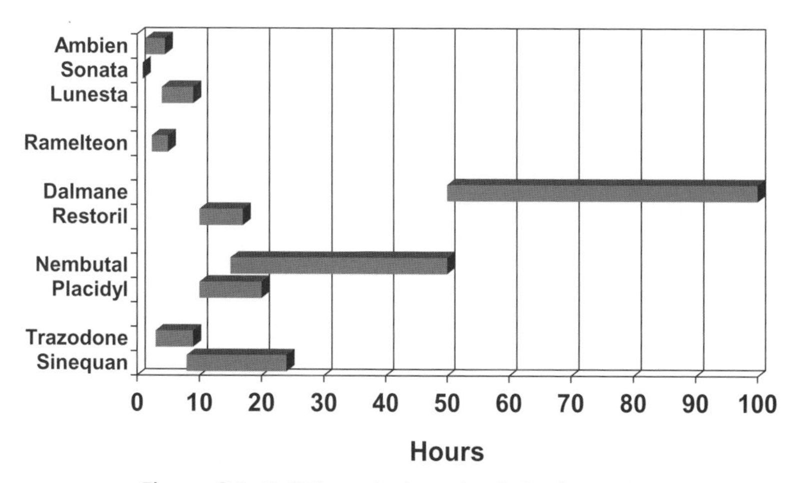

Figure 9.1. Half-lives of selected sedative-hypnotics.

Gabapentin (Neurontin). Like the benzodiazepines, gabapentin also works by increasing GABA neurotransmission in the brain. However, because it has little, if any, potential for abuse, gabapentin has been recommended for those with insomnia and a history of substance abuse. When used to treat insomnia, gabapentin should be initiated at 300 mg at bedtime and titrated as needed. The usual effective dose is 600–1500 mg at bedtime.

In addition to treating insomnia, gabapentin has been used to treat epilepsy, anxiety disorders, and bipolar disorder. It is generally well tolerated with sedation and headaches being the only prominent side effects. Because gabapentin is excreted unchanged in urine, it does not require metabolism by the liver. It is therefore easily eliminated by elderly patients and those with liver disease, although it should be used with caution in those with poor renal (kidney) function.

Dietary Supplements. In the past 10 years, melatonin, available as a dietary supplement from health food stores or over the Internet, has become a popular sleep agent. Melatonin is a hormone produced by the pineal gland at peak levels during the night. It is believed to help regulate the 24 hour circadian sleep–wake cycle.

Melatonin does appear to initiate sleep effectively, but its extremely short duration of action raises questions about its ability to sustain sleep through the night. The effective dose of melatonin is not known. It has not yet been well studied in controlled clinical trials, and inaccuracies in the reported dosage of many dietary supplements remain a problem.

Valerian root, an over-the-counter herbal supplement, has also been used for insomnia. Thought to act, like the benzodiazepines, by increasing the activity of the neurotransmitter GABA, preliminary studies indicate that 400 mg of valerian root decreases sleep latency and enhances sleep quality.

Dopamine-Boosting Medications. Levodopa/carbidopa (Sinemet), bromocriptine (Parlodel), pramipexole (Mirapex), and ropinirole (Requip) increase dopamine neurotransmission in the brain by one or another mechanism. These medications do not reliably induce sleep, and in some patients are activating. They are certainly not true sedative-hypnotics. They are most often used by neurologists to treat Parkinson's disease.

However, these dopaminergic medications are very effective treatments for the nighttime movement disorders, PLMD and RLS. L-DOPA effectively relieves the symptoms of RLS and PLMD, and unlike the benzodiazepines, patients do not develop tolerance to its effects.

L-DOPA can be initiated at 50 mg taken at bedtime and increased stepwise over a few weeks until the symptoms are relieved. Bromocriptine can be initiated at 7.5 mg at bedtime, pramipexole is often dosed at 0.125–0.375 mg at night, and ropinirole, which has an indication for RLS, is typically administered at 0.25–3 mg at bedtime. These medications are not without side effects. They may cause nausea and, over time, insomnia. Less commonly, these medications can cause hallucinations or involuntary movements called dyskinesias. These side effects usually resolve rapidly upon discontinuing the medication.

Magnesium. Recent research suggests that magnesium supplementation may also be a helpful treatment for RLS and PLMD. More study is needed, however, before we can recommend its routine use.

Ramelteon (Rozerem). Recently approved by the FDA for treatment of insomnia in the US, ramelteon acts via a completely novel mechanism of action, that is, stimulating so-called melatonin T_1 and T_2 receptors in the brain's suprachiasmatic nucleus (SCN). The SCN is regarded as the body's "master clock" that regulates the sleep–wake cycle and other circadian rhythms. The effects of ramelteon in some respects mimic those of melatonin. Ramelteon, in clinical trials, administered at bedtime doses of 8 mg, outperformed placebo with respect to several indices of sleep disturbance (see Table 9.4).

9.2.6 Current Approach to Treatment

Identify Other Causes. As has already been stressed, the first step in developing a treatment plan is to identify and treat any underlying problem that may be triggering the sleep disturbance.

Patients suspected of having sleep apnea should undergo a sleep study. If sleep apnea is diagnosed, these patients should be treated with weight reduction, a continuous positive airway pressure (CPAP) machine, and, in extreme cases, surgery. Sleep apnea patients in general should not be prescribed sedative-hypnotics.

Patients suspected of a nighttime movement disorder should also undergo a sleep study. This will help not only to document the movements but also to determine

TABLE 9.4. Sleep-Promoting Medications

Class	Generic Name	Brand Name	Daily Dosage
Alcohol-related	Chloral hydrate	Aquachloral	500–1500 mg
	Ethchlorvynol	Placidyl	500–1600 mg
Antidepressants	Amitriptyline	Elavil	25–100 mg
	Doxepin	Sinequan	25–100 mg
	Trazodone	Desyrel	50–100 mg
Antihistamines	Diphenhydramine	Benadryl	25–50 mg
Benzodiazepines	Estazolam	ProSom	0.5–2 mg
	Flurazepam	Dalmane	15–30 mg
	Quazepam	Doral	7.5–15 mg
	Temazepam	Restoril	15–30 mg
	Triazolam	Halcion	0.125–0.5 mg
Benzodiazepine-like	Eszopiclone	Lunesta	1–3 mg
	Zaleplon	Sonata	5–10 mg
	Zolpidem	Ambien	5–10 mg
Melatonin-like	Ramelteon	Rozerem	8 mg
Other	Gabapentin	Neurontin	300–1500 mg

how much they interfere with sleep. Once the diagnosis of PLMD or RLS is confirmed, then a trial of clonazepam or one of the dopaminergic agents should be initiated. If it is believed that a long-term course of treatment is likely to be needed, many clinicians will opt for a dopaminergic agent to avoid the tolerance that may occur with clonazepam. For short-term use, clonazepam is an equally good first choice.

Other medical conditions, drugs, or psychiatric disorders that may be causing the insomnia should also be identified. Once these conditions have been ruled out or treated, treatment for the remaining insomnia can be initiated.

Acute Phase Treatment. Hypnotic medications are useful for short-term treatment of insomnia, but they should always be accompanied by behavioral and psychoeducational treatments, including a review of good sleep hygiene practices. It may also include more aggressive measures such as relaxation training, sleep restriction therapy, and stimulus control therapy.

Nevertheless, sedative-hypnotic agents often play a useful role in treatment. In particular, by providing a "successful" night's sleep, these medications can break the cycle of anxious anticipation and dread that afflicts the insomnia sufferer during the night. We generally prefer using zolpidem or zaleplon as a first-line treatment for early-to-middle insomnia. Late insomnia often responds well to trazodone or eszopiclone, and trazodone often is a first choice in the presence of substance abuse for all insomnias.

Whichever sedative-hypnotic agent is selected, the following guidelines can help ensure a safe and effective treatment. Use the minimal therapeutic dose at first to decrease possible hangover effects. Consider using the medication on an "as-needed" basis if the insomnia is intermittent, and after 2–4 weeks attempt a trial off medication to see if it is still required. Many individuals with chronic insomnia will relapse after a 14–28 day trial of treatment, but this time frame also affords an opportunity to implement sleep hygiene improvements.

Long-Term Treatment. When sleep medications are used on a long-term basis, they are potentially not helping the problem but contributing to it. Unfortunately, this all too commonly results when a hypnotic medication is started without giving any thought to changing the behaviors that sustain the insomnia.

What to do with the patient who is a long-time user of sedative-hypnotics is often a difficult clinical decision. The most successful treatment approaches seem to be those that are gradual and address the insomnia from a multimodal perspective. Many of the sedative-hypnotics with moderate or longer half-lives will display rebound insomnia on discontinuation and this only complicates the treatment picture. At some point, one has to ask if discontinuing the chronic use of a sedative-hypnotic, in the absence of any harmful effects, is treating the patient or the prescriber.

Though this book focuses on pharmacotherapy, we would be remiss if there was not some mention of sleep hygiene. The goal of sleep hygiene is to provide an environment that is maximally conducive to the onset and sustaining of sleep for the desired time period in bed. General principles include:

- Use the bed only for sleep or sex. Read, eat, work, and watch television elsewhere.
- Keep the bedroom a cool temperature, ideally 65–70°F.
- Awaken at the same time every morning.
- Do not take naps during the day.

9.3 NARCOLEPSY

9.3.1 Brief Description and Diagnostic Criteria

Whereas insomnia consists of too little sleep or poor quality sleep, hypersomnia is just the opposite. Hypersomnia is literally "too much sleep." This may mean either persistent drowsiness or an irresistible urge to sleep despite a good night's sleep. There are several variants of hypersomnia, but most are extremely rare with the notable exception of narcolepsy. For this reason, we will confine our discussion to the treatment of narcolepsy, by far the most common of the hypersomnias.

Narcolepsy is sometimes termed a "dyssomnia," but whatever classification is used, it essentially represents an intrusion of REM sleep into wakefulness. Narcolepsy is comprised of a quartet of potential symptoms, but only a few individuals exhibit all four narcolepsy symptoms. The most common symptom of narcolepsy is the sleep attack. Sleep attacks consist of an irresistible urge to fall asleep and can occur several times each day. Patients with narcolepsy usually feel refreshed and energized after a 10–20 minute nap; however, their sleepiness returns after just a few hours.

Sleep architecture in narcolepsy is distinctly abnormal. Recall that sleep normally begins in a NREM phase and that the first phase of REM does not occur until about 90 minutes after falling asleep. The patient with narcolepsy, in sharp contrast, experiences REM onset within 15 minutes of falling asleep.

The second most common symptom of narcolepsy is cataplexy, which occurs in about 60% of patients. Cataplexy is a sudden but usually brief loss of muscle tone. It can be as mild as a drop of the jaw or as severe as falling to the ground. The person remains fully alert during an attack of cataplexy, and this helps distinguish cataplexy from fainting or seizures. Cataplexy most often occurs after the experience of strong emotions such as laughter, crying, or excitement.

A third symptom of narcolepsy is sleep paralysis. Sleep paralysis is an inability to move while falling asleep or shortly after waking. Normal people may occasionally and briefly experience sleep paralysis when waking, but sleep paralysis at the beginning of sleep is unique to narcolepsy.

Finally, patients with narcolepsy may experience very vivid visual or auditory hallucinations, called hypnagogic hallucinations, while falling asleep. Similar to sleep paralysis, hypnagogic hallucinations occasionally occur in the absence of narcolepsy, but the patient with narcolepsy may experience them several times a week.

To fulfill the diagnostic criteria for narcolepsy, a person must have sleep attacks occurring at least daily for 3 months. In addition, at least one of the so-called

TABLE 9.5. Diagnostic Criteria for Narcolepsy

A. Irresistible attacks of refreshing sleep that occur daily over at least 3 months.
B. The presence of one or both of the following:
   1. Cataplexy (i.e., brief episodes of sudden bilateral loss of muscle tone, most often in association with intense emotion)
   2. Recurrent intrusions of elements of rapid eye movement (REM) sleep into the transition between sleep and wakefulness, as manifested by either hypnopompic or hypnagogic hallucinations or sleep paralysis at the beginning or end of sleep episodes
C. The disturbance is not due to the direct physiological effects of a substance (e.g., a drug of abuse, a medication) or another general medical condition.

Source: Adapted from DSM-IV.

auxiliary symptoms of cataplexy, sleep paralysis, or hypnagogic hallucinations must also be present (see Table 9.5).

9.3.2 Prevalence and Risk Factors

Narcolepsy does not receive much media attention, but it is a surprisingly common condition. It is estimated that about one in every one to two thousand people has narcolepsy.

The main risk factor appears to be a genetic susceptibility to the illness. The majority of narcolepsy patients, particularly those with cataplexy, have a genetic marker known as HLA-DQB1*0602. Recent evidence indicates that the key dysfunction in narcolepsy is diminished activity of a newly discovered neurotransmitter known as hypocretin. This new evidence has led to the development of a new diagnostic test for narcolepsy and may ultimately lead to new treatments that act directly on hypocretin systems in the brain.

9.3.3 Presentation and Clinical Course

The first symptoms of narcolepsy usually begin during childhood or in the early teen years and commonly involve excessive drowsiness and sleep attacks. Several years later, one or more of the auxiliary symptoms arise.

Many years often pass before the disorder comes to clinical attention. In its milder forms, friends and co-workers of undiagnosed narcolepsy sufferers may view the daytime sleepiness as a sign of laziness, poor motivation, or overt hostility. They may also suspect the person of abusing alcohol or other substances. In these cases, narcolepsy patients may seek an initial mental health consultation at the insistence of others.

Occasionally, the presentation is more dramatic. Narcolepsy, for example, can sometimes first come to attention after a work or automobile accident.

Once diagnosed, narcolepsy should be considered a lifelong condition. There may be fluctuations in the severity of the illness, but there are hardly ever any periods of complete remission. Untreated and/or unrecognized, narcolepsy exacts a tremendous toll. Friends can become alienated, and jobs are often lost. Fortunately, effective treatments are available for narcolepsy.

9.3.4 Initial Evaluation and Differential Diagnosis

Although it often goes undiagnosed for years, narcolepsy is not particularly challenging to diagnose. The keys to diagnosis are collecting a careful history and performing a sleep study. The sleep study findings that suggest narcolepsy are average sleep latency (time required to fall asleep) of less than 5 minutes and the onset of REM within the first 15 minutes of sleep. Narcolepsy can therefore usually be diagnosed with an overnight sleep study. When the sleep study results are inconclusive, narcolepsy can also be diagnosed by measuring hypocretin-1 levels in cerebrospinal fluid (CSF) collected during a lumbar puncture. A hypocretin-1 level less than 110 pg/mL in CSF is considered diagnostic of narcolepsy.

Despite the reliability of these diagnostic tests, there are a few alternative conditions that must be considered when entertaining a diagnosis of narcolepsy.

Other Hypersomnias. Narcolepsy is not the only hypersomnia, but it is by far the most common. Primary hypersomnia shares sleep attacks and excessive daytime sleepiness with narcolepsy but does not feature cataplexy or REM-associated abnormalities. Another rare hypersomnia is Kleine–Levin syndrome (KLS), which most often occurs in teenage boys. KLS consists of intermittent bouts of hypersomnia and bizarre behaviors including compulsive eating and sexual inappropriateness. Distinguishing these hypersomnias from narcolepsy may help clarify the patient's prognosis, but the treatment alternatives are very similar.

Insomnia. It may seem odd to include this in the differential diagnosis of a hypersomnia, but insomnia is in fact the most common cause of daytime drowsiness. In addition, it is common for patients with narcolepsy to have some difficulty sleeping at night and for their daytime symptoms to worsen at those times.

Narcolepsy can usually be distinguished from insomnia by the presence of one of the auxiliary symptoms (cataplexy, sleep paralysis, hypnagogic hallucinations). When the diagnosis remains unclear, then a sleep study is necessary.

Seizure Disorders. Narcolepsy is not a form of epilepsy. Although the sleep attacks and cataplexy resemble certain forms of seizures, narcolepsy can easily be distinguished from epilepsy. In particular, those with narcolepsy remain aware of their surroundings during an attack of cataplexy, whereas the epilepsy patient has no recall of events associated with a seizure. Furthermore, the EEG recording during a sleep study typically distinguishes narcolepsy from seizures.

9.3.5 History of Pharmacological Treatment

Stimulants. Treatment for narcolepsy has focused on its most disabling symptoms: namely, sleep attacks and daytime drowsiness. The mainstay of treatment has been stimulants and several have been used including amphetamines, methylphenidate, and pemoline.

Amphetamines. Amphetamine was first synthesized in 1887, and over the years, more than 50 amphetamine-like drugs have been developed. Beginning in the 1930s, narcolepsy was the first psychiatric disorder treated with amphetamine. Amphetamines have since been used to treat a wide variety of problems including Parkinson's disease, obesity, attention deficit–hyperactivity disorder (ADHD), alcoholism and other drug addictions, and treatment-resistant depression. However, we have learned some difficult lessons along the way. Amphetamines themselves are highly addictive. In the late 1960s and early 1970s, amphetamine abuse reached epidemic proportions. In the 1990s, the amphetamine derivative methamphetamine, which can be inexpensively synthesized in small basement laboratories, has emerged as a frequently abused drug. For these reasons and the lack of efficacy in all conditions studied except ADHD, narcolepsy, marked obesity, and perhaps treatment-resistant depression, the clinical use of amphetamines has fallen dramatically. Amphetamine prescriptions are now primarily limited to the treatment of narcolepsy, ADHD, and, occasionally, severe treatment-resistant depression.

Dextroamphetamine (Dexedrine) is commonly initiated at 5 mg taken two to three times daily before meals. Many patients will experience its benefits almost from the first day. The dose can be increased every 5–7 days until the effective dose is found.

Dextroamphetamine does have several side effects that are characteristic of the stimulant class of medications. The most common side effects are insomnia, loss of appetite with associated weight loss, and occasional nausea and diarrhea. Taking the medication just before meals helps to minimize the nausea and diarrhea. To avoid insomnia, dextroamphetamine should rarely, if ever, be taken any later than 6 PM. Some patients will only be able to take the medication with breakfast or lunch, because a dinnertime dose will produce insomnia at bedtime.

Less frequent side effects of stimulants include euphoria, nervousness, irritability, headache, involuntary movements (tics), increased heart rate, and psychosis. If psychosis or tics develop, the patient's doctor should be notified immediately, and the medication should be stopped. Other side effects should also be reported and may necessitate a medication change.

Methylphenidate (Ritalin, Concerta, Focalin). Methylphenidate was introduced in the late 1950s and is now the most widely used prescription stimulant. It was first used to treat ADHD in children but is also effective for narcolepsy. Like dextroamphetamine, methylphenidate should be started at 5 mg per dose given two to three times each day with meals. The average effective dose is 20–30 mg/day, but some patients require as much as 60 mg/day. The benefit of methylphenidate should also be apparent on the first day or so, and the dose can be increased every 5–7 days as needed. Focalin dosing is approximately half that of methylphenidate.

To a lesser extent than the amphetamines, methylphenidate is sometimes abused, though this is a risk to be balanced against the risk of the untreated disease state.

Pemoline (Cylert). Pemoline was introduced as an alternative stimulant in the 1990s. Pemoline has the advantage of being dosed once a day (although longer-acting sustained-release forms of methylphenidate and dextroamphetamine are now available). It is generally believed that pemoline has a gradual onset of action taking several weeks to reach full therapeutic benefit. Some researchers question this assumption and report observing clinical changes in children with ADHD within a few hours of the first dose.

Pemoline is a less potent stimulant than methylphenidate or dextroamphetamine. It should be initiated at 18.75 mg taken each morning with breakfast and can be increased in increments of 18.75 mg every week or so. Typical dosing for pemoline ranges from 60 to 200 mg/day in treating narcolepsy. Because pemoline is less potent than other stimulants, it is more likely to be ineffective, even at its higher doses. When pemoline does not relieve daytime sleepiness or sleep attacks, then the patient should be switched to a different stimulant.

One benefit of pemoline's milder effects is that it appears to have less abuse potential than the other stimulants. Pemoline is a schedule IV drug, in contrast to other stimulants that are schedule II. The side effects of pemoline are similar to other stimulants but in a milder form. The most common side effects are loss of appetite, nausea, and insomnia. Rarer side effects include headache, dizziness, changes in mood, increases in blood pressure or pulse, and psychosis.

On rare occasions, pemoline can cause a chemical hepatitis (liver dysfunction). For this reason, patients with known liver disease should not be prescribed pemoline. A baseline laboratory assessment of liver enzymes before starting therapy with pemoline is advised, and liver function monitoring must be repeated periodically. If liver abnormalities are detected, then pemoline must be discontinued. The recognition of this side effect resulting from therapy with pemoline has markedly restricted its use.

Modafinil (Provigil). Modafinil is a new addition to the wake-promoting agents. At doses between 200 and 400 mg, it appears to treat narcolepsy effectively. In addition, modafinil has milder side effects and little, if any, potential for abuse. The mechanism of action of modafinil is unclear, though it does not appear to affect dopamine or norepinephrine release. Modafinil has the potential to interact with a number of other medications through its effect on the cytochrome P_{450} system. Modafinil induces or increases the activity of the CYP3A4, 1A2, and 2B6 isoenzymes. Additionally, modafinil has the potential to inhibit the 2C9 and 2C19 isoenzymes. The reader is referred to Table 3.10 in Chapter 3 for a listing of medications that could potentially be affected by this activity. Of particular concern is the possibility that oral contraceptives could be rendered less effective when coadministered with modafinil. The most commonly observed side effects of modafinil in clinical trials were headache, nausea, nervousness, anxiety, and insomnia.

Antidepressants. In addition to increasing alertness, the psychostimulants also mildly suppress the REM phase of sleep. Because the auxiliary symptoms of narcolepsy (cataplexy, hypnagogic hallucinations, and sleep paralysis) are basically intrusions of REM brain activity into the waking hours, medications that suppress REM should alleviate these symptoms. Unfortunately, the stimulants are very good at relieving sleepiness but are often not potent enough REM suppressors to relieve the auxiliary symptoms.

Tricyclic Antidepressants (TCAs). TCAs were introduced in the 1950s and over the years have become the mainstay of treatment for cataplexy and the other REM-related symptoms. The doses used are usually less than the doses required in the treatment of depression. Imipramine (Tofranil) is the most widely used TCA for narcolepsy and is usually effective at doses from 10 to 75 mg given once a day. Some doctors prefer the TCA protriptyline (Vivactil) because it has mild stimulant effects, but it has not been as widely used or as thoroughly studied in narcolepsy. The common side effects of TCAs are drowsiness, dry mouth, and constipation, but these are usually not a problem at the lower doses used for narcolepsy. Patients should receive a baseline electrocardiograph (EKG) before starting a TCA and should have blood levels of the medication checked periodically.

TCAs can be lethal in overdose and can cause dangerous heart rhythm abnormalities in susceptible patients. Please refer to Chapter 3 for more complete discussion of the TCAs.

Selective Serotonin Reuptake Inhibitors (SSRIs). Some doctors report that the SSRI antidepressants are also effective treatments for cataplexy. This has not been well studied, but because the SSRIs are generally safer and more tolerable than the TCAs, they may be a welcome alternative.

9.3.6 Current Approach to Treatment

Short-Term Treatment. In the acute phase of treatment, a stepwise approach is often warranted. The medication should be targeted at the most distressing symptom of narcolepsy first. This is almost invariably the sleep attacks and daytime drowsiness.

Currently, treatment choices will focus on a stimulant such as methylphenidate or dextroamphetamine or a wake-promoting agent such as modafinil. Historically, methylphenidate in the regular-release version (in contrast to sustained-release) has been the most popular treatment alternative. Methylphenidate should be started at 5 mg given with breakfast and lunch. A dinnertime dose can be added for symptoms in the evening, though care must be taken to avoid interfering with nighttime sleep. The doses can be increased in 5 mg increments every week or so to a maximum of 20 mg per dose (60 mg/day). Sometimes, the dinner dose is given at about one-half the earlier doses to avoid insomnia at bedtime. A variety of controlled-release methylphenidate formulations are now available and have the advantage of once-daily dosing.

Should the first medication fail to provide satisfactory relief from the drowsiness and sleep attacks of narcolepsy, the patient should be switched to an alternative regimen. The mechanism of action of methylphenidate and dextroamphetamine are not exactly identical, so if one does not work, it is certainly worthwhile to try the other.

It is relatively infrequent that narcolepsy does not respond to treatment with one of these medications. If the patient experiences no improvement with any of the stimulants, a reconsideration of the diagnosis is certainly warranted.

Long-Term Treatment. The key point for long-term management is that narcolepsy is a lifelong condition that almost always requires lifelong treatment. The severity of the symptoms may fluctuate from time to time, but narcolepsy seldom has a sufficiently long remission to allow medication to be discontinued altogether. Long-term maintenance treatment for narcolepsy is generally a continuation of the stimulant therapy that was started during the acute phase of treatment. At times, however, changes in the approach to treatment will need to be made.

One change that is sometimes made during long-term treatment is the addition of a second medication to treat the auxiliary symptoms of narcolepsy. For many patients, these other symptoms do not occur often enough or are not severe enough to require treatment. However, the auxiliary symptoms (especially cataplexy) can be a big problem for some narcolepsy patients. The stimulants used to treat the sleep attacks can also provide some mild relief of cataplexy, but the benefit is often not sufficient.

After checking a baseline EKG to rule out undetected heart rhythm abnormalities, many clinicians use a low dose of imipramine or protriptyline to treat the auxiliary symptoms of narcolepsy. Either of these can be started at 10 mg taken once a day and then slowly increased over several weeks as needed until the symptoms resolve.

ADDITIONAL READING

Banerjee D, Vitiello MV, Grunstein RR. Pharmacotherapy for excessive daytime sleepiness. *Sleep Med Rev* 2004; 8: 339–354.

Benca RM. Diagnosis and treatment of chronic insomnia: a review. *Psychiatr Serv* 2005; 56: 332–343.

Boutrel B, Koob GF. What keeps us awake: the neuropharmacology of stimulants and wakefulness-promoting medications. *Sleep* 2004; 27: 1181–1194.

Brooks S, Black J. Novel therapies for narcolepsy. *Expert Opin Investig Drugs* 2002; 11(12): 1821–1827.

Gatchel RJ, Oordt MS. Insomnia. In *Clinical Health Psychology and Primary Care: Practical Advice and Clinical Guidance for Successful Collaboration*. Washington DC: American Psychological Association, 2003, pp 135–148.

Jindal RD, Buysse DJ, Thase ME. Maintenance treatment of insomnia: What can we learn from the depression literature? *Am J Psychiatry* 2004; 161: 19–24.

Littner M, Johnson SF, McCall WV, et al. Practice parameters for the treatment of narcolepsy: an update for 2000. *Sleep* 2001; 24(4): 451–466.

Mitler MM, Hayduk R. Benefits and risks of pharmacotherapy for narcolepsy. *Drug Safety* 2002; 25(11): 791–809.

Montgomery P. Treatments for sleep problems in elderly people. *BMJ* 2002; 325(7372): 1049.

Reite M, Ruddy J, Nagel K. *Concise Guide to Evaluation and Management of Sleep Disorders, 3rd Edition*. Washington DC: American Psychiatric Publishing, 2002.

Ringdahl EN, Pereira SL, Delzell JE. Treatment of primary insomnia. *J Am Board Fam Pract* 2004; 17: 212–219.

Sanger DJ. The pharmacology and mechanisms of action of new generation, non-benzodiazepine hypnotic agents. *CNS Drugs* 2004; 18(Supplement 1): 9–15, 41–45.

Scammell TE. The neurobiology, diagnosis, and treatment of narcolepsy. *Ann Neurol* 2003; 53(2): 154–166.

Smith MT, Perlis ML, Park A, et al. Comparative meta-analysis of pharmacotherapy and behavior therapy for persistent insomnia. *Am J Psychiatry* 2002; 159(1): 5–10.

Walsh JK. Pharmacologic management of insomnia. *J Clin Psychiatry* 2004; 65(Supplement 16): 41–45.

10

ALZHEIMER'S DISEASE AND OTHER DEMENTIAS

10.1 BRIEF DESCRIPTION AND DIAGNOSTIC CRITERIA

Dementia, a clinical syndrome associated with a variety of distinct pathological causes, is characterized by deterioration in multiple areas of higher intellectual function. As a result, it interferes with the ability to carry out routine daily activities. The symptoms of dementia fall into three categories: intellectual (cognitive) deterioration, functional decline, and behavioral/emotional complications.

Symptoms of Dementia. Loss of memory is the hallmark symptom of dementia. Even in the early stages, individuals with dementia may have problems learning new information (memory registration) or even momentarily retaining that new information (memory recall). Early in the illness, they begin to have trouble remembering conversations and frequently repeat themselves. In addition, they have problems with time-related information about themselves such as what they ate for breakfast or where they left their toothbrush after using it. Later, they may have difficulty learning any new information and eventually may forget old memories.

Although memory is the most conspicuous intellectual problem in dementia, the decline eventually affects other abilities as well. The other losses include:

Principles of Psychopharmacology for Mental Health Professionals
By Jeffrey E. Kelsey, D. Jeffrey Newport, and Charles B. Nemeroff

- Aphasia
- Apraxia
- Agnosia
- Executive functioning

Aphasia is a disturbance in language. This is not a speech problem such as slurred or mumbled words. Instead, it's a mental inability to produce or understand language. Early in the illness, this may mean having difficulty finding words or constructing grammatically correct sentences. Later in the illness, the demented patient may stop speaking altogether.

Apraxia is an inability to carry out coordinated physical activity. This occurs despite no paralysis or weakness. It is believed to result from a decline of visual and spatial abilities. Early in the illness, demented patients may have problems drawing three-dimensional figures. As the illness progresses, they may get lost in familiar neighborhoods or forget how to use a common object like a toothbrush or a hammer. With certain types of dementia they may even forget how to walk (gait apraxia).

Agnosia is an inability to recognize familiar objects or people. This can include not recognizing familiar objects by sight or not recognizing familiar sounds such as the ringing of a telephone.

Finally, *executive functioning*, that is, the ability to plan and carry out complex tasks, is almost always affected. This commonly appears in the early stages of the illness when the patient begins to have trouble paying bills, preparing meals, or cleaning the house, in general, a set of activities that require sequential processing of information.

To fulfill the diagnostic criteria for dementia, memory and at least one other intellectual area must be affected. If only memory is affected, then the disorder is not a dementia, but amnesia. In addition, the intellectual problems must be severe enough to limit the person's function. In particular, the truly demented person will be unable to manage social or occupational functioning and family members will often have begun to take over certain routine tasks. For example, demented patients may no longer drive an automobile because they often become disoriented or have frequent accidents. They may no longer manage the household finances because bills were not being paid or the checking account was repeatedly overdrawn. They may no longer cook because they have burned meals or even started accidental fires. As the illness advances, they may need help dressing themselves and maintaining personal hygiene.

Complications of Dementia. Patients with dementia must have at least two of the following intellectual deficits that are accompanied by a functional decline. They often have other behavioral or emotional complications, but these are not required symptoms. The optional complications listed in the DSM-IV diagnostic criteria are:

- Delirium
- Depressed mood
- Delusions
- Behavioral disturbance

Delirium and depression may exist as separate illnesses that need to be distinguished from dementia or as complications superimposed on dementia. In addition to these four complications that are listed in DSM-IV, demented patients are also frequently troubled by insomnia and anxiety.

Psychosis for demented patients usually takes the form of paranoid delusions. Demented patients may believe family members have turned against them, or they may misidentify their loved ones as intruders in their home. Although hallucinations are not listed in the DSM-IV criteria, they may also occur. When psychosis occurs in a demented patient, it is a serious problem. It is very distressful to the patient, makes it difficult (if not impossible) for family members to provide care, may lead to episodes of violence, and commonly leads patients to be hospitalized or placed in nursing homes. Fortunately, most patients with dementia do not develop delusions or other psychotic symptoms.

Other behavioral disturbances in dementia include personality changes and agitation. The changes in personality traits can be far ranging. Patients with dementia may become more passive, more introverted, more immature, less affectionate, less generous, more unreasonable, more irritable, or more unhappy. Agitation, however, is one of the most troublesome symptoms associated with dementia. This includes disruptive verbal agitation such as incessant screaming or crying, physical aggression, and physical nonaggressive behaviors such as wandering. For family members, these behavioral problems can be the most difficult aspect of caring for their loved ones. It can lead caregivers to feelings of helplessness and anger toward the demented patient.

The behavioral and emotional complications of dementia such as agitation, depression, and psychosis are often the most troublesome aspect of the illness. They can alienate the family members who are trying to provide care and often lead exhausted families to institutionalize these patients whom they would otherwise prefer to keep at home.

10.2 PREVALENCE AND RISK FACTORS

The overall rate of dementia in persons over 65 years of age is 5–10%. As many as 4 million people in the United States suffer from dementia, and these numbers will undoubtedly rise as the population ages. In fact, dementia increases exponentially with age—the rate doubling every 5 years from age 65 to age 90. By the year 2050, we believe that more than 10 million Americans will have Alzheimer's disease, the leading cause of dementia.

10.2.1 Causes of Dementia

There are many causes of dementia. They can be classified into the following groups:

- Degenerative
- Infectious
- Substance-induced
- Nutritional deficiencies
- Other medical conditions
- Head trauma

Degenerative Dementias. Far and away, the most common dementias in the United States are of the degenerative type. These result from gradual deterioration of the brain and include Alzheimer's disease (AD). AD accounts for about 60% of dementias. Vascular dementia, another degenerative dementia, is the second most common form and accounts for another 10%.

The cause of Alzheimer's disease is unknown, but genetic factors clearly play a role. One clue supporting this view is provided by the observation that individuals with Down syndrome, a common cause of mental retardation, frequently develop a dementia similar to Alzheimer's disease during early adulthood. Vascular dementia, which is also called multi-infarct dementia, results from the accumulation of tiny "strokes." Individually, these "strokes" or infarcts are too small to cause any noticeable problem, but as they accumulate, they produce deficits similar to Alzheimer's disease. Other neurological diseases such as Parkinson's disease, Pick's disease, and Huntington's disease cause slow deterioration of the brain that ultimately leads to a degenerative dementia.

Infectious Dementias. One hundred years ago, the most common cause of dementia was an infection: syphilis. Today, syphilis is well treated and seldom left to linger long enough to infect the brain and cause dementia, but a blood test for syphilis remains a routine part of the assessment for patients newly diagnosed with dementia. Today, the most common infectious cause of dementia is HIV/AIDS. Other, rare forms of infection-caused dementia include Creutzfeld–Jakob disease (spongiform encephalopathy) and subacute sclerosing panencephalitis (SSPE), the latter caused by the measles virus in unvaccinated children.

Substance-Induced Dementias. Substances of abuse can also cause dementia. The most common is alcohol-related dementia. Chronic alcoholism leads to dementia in several ways. The poor diet of the alcoholic causes a deficiency of certain essential nutrients such as thiamine. The alcoholic often suffers recurrent head injuries from falls or altercations. Alcohol-induced liver failure can expose the brain to toxic injury. Finally, the direct toxic effects of alcohol itself on the brain can lead to dementia. In addition to alcohol, the abuse of inhalants such as paint thinner and solvents can be especially harmful to the brain and with repeated use cause dementia.

Nutritional Deficiency-Related Dementias. We have already mentioned that chronic alcoholics are subject to thiamine deficiency that can cause dementia. It usually occurs only after heavy, prolonged abuse of alcohol. In developed countries, the other key nutritional concern is vitamin B_{12} deficiency. Vitamin B_{12} deficiency can surprisingly strike even those with a healthy diet. Such people are missing a vital protein, intrinsic factor, which would enable them to absorb it from their digestive tract.

Dementia Due to Other Medical Conditions. Many medical illnesses are associated with symptoms of dementia, and when treated adequately, the dementia is reversible, including endocrine disorders of the thyroid (particularly hypothyroidism) or parathyroid glands and poorly controlled diabetes with repeated episodes of dangerously low blood sugar (hypoglycemia). Brain lesions due to a variety of pathological conditions can also cause dementia, including brain tumors, slow bleeding into the space around the brain (subdural hematoma), or problems with the drainage of the fluid that surrounds the brain (normal pressure hydrocephalus). Other medical conditions associated with dementia include multiple sclerosis, Wilson's disease (toxic accumulation of copper), chronic liver failure, and chronic metabolic disturbances.

Traumatic Dementias. Traumatic brain injury can also result in dementia. This can result from a single massive head injury such as in a motorcycle accident or a gunshot wound. Repeated small head injuries can also cause dementia. The best example is dementia pugilistica, the dementia observed in professional boxers after many years and many prizefights.

10.2.2 Risk Factors for Dementia

Table 10.1 shows the proposed risk factors for Alzheimer's disease, the most common cause of dementia. Heading this list is of course old age. But be careful how you

TABLE 10.1. Risk Factors for Alzheimer's Dementia

Advanced age
Family history of Alzheimer's disease
Down syndrome
Female
Less education
History of significant head injury
Depression
Age of mother at birth (questionable)
Aluminum exposure (questionable)

read this. Although dementia increases exponentially as age increases (doubling every 5 years), most people are not affected even at very advanced ages. Dementia is NOT a normal result of the aging process.

Family history is also important. If you have a parent or sibling who has been diagnosed with AD, you are four times more likely to develop the illness. If two close relatives have AD, you are eight times more likely to have AD. This suggests that there may be a genetic, inherited basis for the disease. In fact, genetic studies have revealed that one-third or more cases of AD may be traceable to a genetic marker known as apolipoprotein E4.

For unknown reasons, women are three times more likely than men to have AD. The rates for African-American women may be even higher that those for Caucasian women.

Those with less education may be at greater risk for developing AD. It is unclear why this may be so. One theory is that extensive education may cause nerve cells to produce a more highly branched interconnected communication network. This in turn may provide duplicate backup circuitry in the brain that prolongs normal brain functioning even as brain cells progressively die.

Other reported risk factors for AD include a history of depression, particularly late onset, exposure to aluminum, and being born when your mother was older than forty. The evidence for the latter two risk factors is not as yet very convincing.

The risk factors for vascular dementia are essentially the same as those for stroke and heart attack. They include high blood pressure, heart disease, diabetes mellitus, sickle cell disease, obesity, smoking, alcohol use, depression, and high cholesterol levels.

10.3 PRESENTATION AND CLINICAL COURSE

With the exception of massive head trauma and certain brain infections, dementias slowly arise in an almost undetectable manner. The first sign of AD is usually short-term memory loss. This is later followed by long-term memory loss. In addition, the patient gradually begins to have difficulty performing daily activities such as personal grooming, shopping, and cooking. The changes are so slow that the patients themselves seldom notice. Family members may not recognize the early changes if they have frequent contact with the patient, but relatives who visit the patient less often may notice the incremental changes that accumulate over the course of several months. When family members do notice changes during the early stage of dementia, they may explain them away as normal aging or forgetfulness. By the time the patient comes for evaluation, other telltale signs of deterioration are usually apparent.

Sometimes, a clinician will notice the impairment before the family does. This is not surprising. For example, if you watch a rose bud, it opens so slowly that you cannot see the change. But if you walk away and return a day later, it is easier to see that the bud has blossomed while you were away. Likewise, by seeing your elderly patients at intervals, you may notice changes that their family members who are around everyday cannot. There are certain signs you should look for as you work with elderly patients. If your patient begins to have problems arriving at the right time for appointments, having difficulty finding words, exhibits some change in their typical dress or behavior, or begins to have problems talking about current events, you should be concerned that the early signs of dementia are becoming apparent.

The course of illness depends on the cause of dementia. As a rule, the degenerative dementias are slowly progressive, taking several years to run their course from initial diagnosis to death. Vascular dementia, like other degenerative dementias, is slowly progressive but in a "stepwise" fashion. A patient with vascular dementia will function at a particular plateau until another small infarct causes a small but noticeable and sudden decline.

Dementias due to trauma usually do not progress in this manner. The injury damages the brain and causes dementia, but further deterioration does not occur. In contrast, a few dementias can be rapidly progressive. This includes most dementias due to infection (although syphilis and AIDS-related dementias are usually slowly progressive) as well as Pick's disease, a dementia associated with a relatively early age of onset, characterized by massive degeneration of frontal and temporal lobe tissue.

As dementia progresses, accompanying behavioral problems often appear. At least 40% of patients with AD develop one or more forms of agitation that interfere with treatment and further worsen intellectual function. Psychosis in the form of paranoid delusions and hallucinations may appear during the early or middle stages of the illness. The delusions of dementia are usually simple and related to the memory loss. They are quite different from the elaborate delusions of patients with schizophrenia or bipolar disorder. Common delusions among demented patients include believing family members are stealing money or personal items, believing the spouse is an impostor, or insisting that a long ago deceased loved one is alive. Depression is another complication that can also occur concurrently in patients with dementia.

During the final stages of dementia, patients are usually bedridden and incontinent and require around-the-clock care. The brain deterioration ultimately leads to a compromise of other body systems and death.

10.4 INITIAL EVALUATION AND DIFFERENTIAL DIAGNOSIS

10.4.1 Initial Evaluation

When evaluating a patient who you think may have dementia, there are two key questions you are trying to answer:

- Is this dementia or something else that resembles dementia?
- If this is dementia, is it a potentially reversible form?

To answer these questions, a complete assessment should include a thorough history from both the patient AND one or more family members, a mental status examination, a physical examination, and diagnostic tests.

Any concerns about a decline in memory or other intellectual skills in an elderly patient should lead you to perform an assessment for dementia. During your interview, you should look for signs of memory-related problems. You should ask the following questions of both the patient and a family member:

- Does (s)he have more trouble remembering conversations, recent events, or appointments?
- Does (s)he frequently repeat him/herself?
- Does (s)he frequently misplace things?
- Does (s)he have trouble performing complex tasks like balancing a checkbook?
- Does (s)he suddenly disregard rules of etiquette or polite social behavior?
- Does (s)he have trouble driving? Has (s)he had recent traffic accidents?
- Has (s)he gotten lost in familiar areas?
- Does (s)he have trouble finding the words to express what (s)he wants to say?
- Has his/her personality changed in any way? More aggressive? More passive? Suspicious?

In addition, you should perform some objective measure of the patient's intellectual functioning. The most commonly used measure is the Folstein Mini-Mental Status Examination (MMSE). The 30 point MMSE assesses many of the intellectual functions that might be impacted by dementia: orientation to surroundings, registration of new information into memory, recall of that same information, concentration, word-finding, following directions, and visuospatial tasks. A score of 25 or lower should raise concern but early dementia is not ruled out even with higher scores.

If your interview or mental status examination suggests the patient has dementia, you should promptly refer the patient to a physician for a medical history, physical examination, and laboratory evaluation. Although there is no available specific diagnostic test to diagnose AD (short of a brain biopsy), a physician, usually a geriatric psychiatrist or neurologist, can reliably diagnose AD in over 90% of the cases. Carefully look for signs or symptoms of potentially treatable causes for dementia. Table 10.2 shows physical findings associated with particular causes of dementia and Table 10.3 shows the laboratory assessments that should be obtained.

10.4.2 Differential Diagnosis

Before diagnosing dementia, you should consider any other condition that might impair intellectual function or that might masquerade as an impairment of intellect. The differential diagnosis of dementia includes:

TABLE 10.2. Findings in Specific Dementias

Cause/Type of Dementia	Symptoms and Physical Findings
AIDS	High risk group
Alcohol	History of alcoholism, frequent falls, liver disease, abnormalities of eye movements, Wernicke–Korsakoff syndrome
Diabetes mellitus	Recurrent episodes of hypoglycemia (low blood sugar)
Huntington's disease	Onset at age 35–45, family history of Huntington's disease, involuntary movements, personality changes
Hypothyroidism	Goiter (enlarged thyroid gland), decreased reflexes, intolerance of cold weather, depression
Normal pressure hydrocephalus	Urinary incontinence, difficulty walking
Parkinson's disease	Tremor, stooped posture, shuffling gait, expressionless face, stiffness
Syphilis	Myoclonus (increased reflexes), abnormality of pupils on eye exam
Thiamine deficiency	History of alcoholism
Tumor (brain)	Headaches, visual disturbances, localized physical weakness
Vascular dementia	High blood pressure, nonsymmetrical reflexes
Vitamin B_{12} deficiency	History of pernicious anemia
Wilson's disease	Onset during childhood or early adulthood, liver disease, involuntary problems, "Kayser–Fleischer" rings during eye examination

TABLE 10.3. Routine Laboratory Evaluation for Dementia

Mandatory studies	Complete blood count
	Blood electrolytes
	Liver enzymes
	Urinalysis
	Vitamin B_{12} level
	Folate level
	Syphilis (RPR/VDRL)
	Thyroid-stimulating hormone (TSH)
	Brain scan (CT or MRI)
	Electrocardiograph (EKG)
Optional studies	HIV antibody screen
	Chest x-ray
	Urine drug screen
	Ceruloplasmin (if Wilson's disease suspected)
	Lumbar puncture (spinal tap)
	Electroencephalograph (EEG)

- Normal aging
- Delirium
- Depression
- Amnesia
- Aphasia
- Hearing loss

Normal Aging. As we previously mentioned, most people experience noticeable changes in intellectual functioning as they age. It may become slightly more difficult to learn new information, but dementia is not part of the normal aging process. A decline that interferes with someone's ability to carry out the routine mental tasks of daily life is not normal. It is not to be expected. It is instead a sign of illness that should be investigated.

Delirium. Delirium, the waxing and waning of consciousness and lucidity, can be difficult to distinguish from dementia. Both affect multiple areas of intellectual functioning. Both tend to affect the same groups of people, namely, the elderly and those with brain injuries. And the two are not mutually exclusive. Patients with dementia can also become delirious; in fact, the brain impairment of dementia increases vulnerability to delirium.

It is extremely important to identify delirium in a timely manner. Delirium is a medical emergency because untreated, it often proves fatal. Delirium generally occurs when some external factor interferes with normal brain functioning. The most common causes of delirium are infection (e.g., pneumonia or bladder infections) and the side effect of prescribed medication or drugs of abuse.

Four factors can help distinguish delirium from dementia. First, delirium usually has a rapid onset whereas dementia invariably has a gradual, often nearly imperceptible, onset and course. Second, delirium is marked by rapid fluctuations from clear, lucid thinking to confusion and agitation. These shifts may occur several times over the course of a single day. The cognitive decline of dementia does not fluctuate in this manner. Third, delirious patients are often stuporous and inattentive whereas those with dementia are alert but confused. Finally, visual and auditory hallucinations are common in delirium but less so in dementia.

Identifying delirium quickly can save your patient's life. Its treatment requires identifying the underlying cause and eliminating it. One important point to remember is that patients with dementia can also become delirious. The most common scenario is a patient with moderate dementia who is incontinent of urine and wears a protective undergarment. If such a patient rapidly deteriorates, it is probably not due to the dementia. Instead, this patient likely has a bladder infection that is superimposing a delirium on the dementia. By treating the bladder infection with antibiotics, the patient can quickly return to their baseline state.

Depression. Like delirium, depression is an illness that is common among the elderly and that can occur either apart from or concurrently with dementia. Elderly depressed patients often have poor concentration and poor motivation and appear to have significant intellectual deficits when formally tested. This syndrome is known as false dementia or pseudodementia. This should be distinguished from patients in the early stages of a true dementia, who often develop depression.

Not surprisingly, it is often difficult to distinguish depression with pseudodementia from dementia with depressed mood. Generally, patients with dementia will try to answer your questions but will make mistakes whereas patients with pseudodementia will more likely say, "I don't know." This distinction is not, however, totally reliable.

Many times the best diagnostic approach is to treat what is most easily treatable. In this case, that is the depression. Once the depression has been treated, the presence of a dementia can be reassessed. The improvement in cognitive function in depressed patients with pseudodementia after successful antidepressant treatment is impressive.

Amnesia. Like dementia, the main feature of amnesia is memory loss. Amnesia, however, does not affect other intellectual abilities in the same manner as dementia. Distinguishing dementia from amnesia is most often a consideration when you evaluate memory problems in a chronic alcoholic. Alcoholics may become demented, but they may also develop an amnestic disorder known as Wernicke–Korsakoff syndrome.

Aphasia. Aphasia is an inability either to produce language (speaking or writing), to understand language, or both. It is in fact one of the most common intellectual impairments in dementia. However, patients without dementia do occasionally develop aphasia. The most common scenario is when a small stroke strikes one of the brain's language centers. Because patients with aphasia have such severe trouble communicating, it may appear that they are demented when they may not be. But two clues usually help distinguish an isolated aphasia from dementia. First, because stroke is the most common cause of an isolated aphasia, the onset is usually abrupt not gradual. Second, when the patient is observed closely, it sometimes becomes apparent that the language impairment is out of proportion to other intellectual deficits. For example, a patient who cannot carry on a simple conversation but who can prepare a full meal likely has an aphasia not a dementia.

Hearing Loss. Like the patient with aphasia, the patient with hearing problems often finds it difficult to communicate. If not mistaken for dementia, hearing problems can certainly complicate the course of mild-to-moderate dementia. Therefore, all elderly patients who appear to be having intellectual problems should have a hearing examination.

10.5 HISTORY OF PHARMACOLOGICAL TREATMENT

10.5.1 Overview and Current Theory

Over the years, there have been many theories to explain the cause of Alzheimer's disease, most specifically, and that of other dementias as well. As a result, many medication strategies based on these theories have been tried. As you will see, most of these treatments have provided little or no benefit.

Before proceeding, it's important to understand the current thinking about Alzheimer's dementia. First, we know that one group of nerve cells in the brain that perform memory processing use the neurotransmitter acetylcholine. We also know that these nerve cells are selectively damaged in Alzheimer's disease and gradually die as the illness progresses. The damaged and dying nerve cells, both cholinergic neurons and other cells, have both neurofibrillary tangles and senile plaques, the pathological hallmarks of Alzheimer's disease. The plaques contain a substance called beta-amyloid, which may be what damages the nerve cells. As the beta-amyloid continues to accumulate and as more and more nerve cells are damaged, the symptoms of dementia worsen. The excess beta-amyloid may not itself be harmful but may merely be a by-product of whatever primary process is harming the cells.

Current research into the treatment of Alzheimer's disease is along two major fronts. First, we are trying to develop medications that boost the availability of acetylcholine, a neurotransmitter known to be involved in cognitive processing. By enhancing cholinergic neurotransmission in the remaining nerve cells, cognitive function should improve or decline more slowly. As you will see, there are now medications available that use this approach and are helpful in the treatment of Alzheimer's disease. Unfortunately, Alzheimer's disease is not a simple acetylcholine-deficiency disorder, and therefore, boosting acetylcholine activity can help only so much. Consequently, we are also trying to develop medications that will slow down or even halt the destruction of the nerve cells. One major research effort seeks to determine if blocking the accumulation of beta-amyloid protects nerve cells from degeneration. There are no treatments currently available to block beta-amyloid accumulation, but this may ultimately prove to be an effective treatment for most cases of dementia. With these considerations in mind, let's now look at the many treatment strategies and theories that have arisen through the years. In the absence of truly understanding the causes of Alzheimer's disease, we largely treat the behavioral sequelae of this disorder by attempting to target specific symptoms (e.g. agitation, psychosis).

10.5.2 Historical Treatment Strategies

Over the years, our attempts to treat dementia have been targeted in four specific areas:

- Dementia reversal
- Brain protection
- Cognitive enhancement
- Behavioral management

Dementia reversal represents attempts to treat the underlying cause of the so-called reversible dementias. Although only a few causes of dementia are to any degree "reversible," these treatments do provide varying degrees of improvement. Brain protection includes a variety of medications or supplements that have been used in the hope of slowing the progression of brain deterioration. Cognitive enhancement includes medications that are used to "replace" what the dementia has taken away. They attempt to treat the illness by replenishing the levels of the brain's chemical messengers (neurotransmitters) that have been lost to the dementing illness. Finally, behavioral management medications are used to treat the symptoms of depression, psychosis, or agitation that sometimes accompany dementia.

10.5.3 History of Dementia Reversal Treatments

The discovery at the turn of the century that untreated syphilis was a common cause of many psychiatric illnesses including dementia revolutionized the field of psychiatry. Although the tools available to investigate brain function were limited at the time, it proved that diseases that attack the brain could cause mental illness. This in turn led to a search for other medical conditions that cause mental illness.

Since that time, we've found that some causes of dementia can be treated. In addition, other treatable conditions as noted earlier cause cognitive impairment that resembles dementia (pseudodementia). Treatment aimed at dementia reversal depends on a careful assessment to identify those patients who have these potentially reversible conditions.

Table 10.4 lists the various medications that can be stopped and medical illnesses that can be treated to reverse dementia. In some cases, such as hypothyroidism or dehydration, the reversal can be complete. More often, the dementia is only partially reversed or its further progression is halted. Examples of these partial improvements include normal pressure hydrocephalus and vitamin B_{12} deficiency.

TABLE 10.4. Potentially Treatable Causes of Dementia or Pseudodementia

Medications	Psychiatric Illnesses	Medical Illnesses
Anticholinergics	Delirium	Adrenal disease
Antihypertensives	Depression	Dehydration
Antipsychotics	Psychosis	Emphysema/COPD
Narcotics (opiates)		Fecal impaction
Sedative-hypnotics (including benzodiazepines)		Hearing loss
Steroids		Liver failure/cirrhosis
Polypharmacy (drug combinations)		Kidney failure
		Normal pressure hydrocephalus
		Parathyroid disease
		Syphilis
		Thiamine deficiency
		Thyroid disease
		Vitamin B_{12} deficiency
		Wilson's disease

The majority of dementias including Alzheimer's disease and vascular dementia are not reversible. However, treatments to protect the brain can theoretically slow the deterioration of these illnesses.

10.5.4 History of Brain Protection Treatments

Increasing Oxygen. It was once believed that the cause of Alzheimer's dementia was poor oxygen supply to the brain. This theory suggested that atherosclerosis, hard plaques of fat and calcium, accumulate in blood vessels and block the arteries that supply the brain, depriving it of oxygen-rich blood. In fact, atherosclerosis does occur in the carotid arteries that supply the brain and is the most common cause of stroke and vascular dementia. There is no evidence that this mechanism is involved in the pathology of Alzheimer's disease.

The treatments used to improve the brain's oxygen supply include vasodilators, anticoagulants, and raising the oxygen content of the blood. Vasodilators work by dilating arteries. When the arteries supplying the brain are opened wide, the plaques of atherosclerosis are less likely to block blood flow. Vasodilators including papaverine, cyclandelate, isoxsuprine, vincamine, and cinnarizine have all been tried.

Anticoagulants, medications that block the formation of clots, have also been used. These work by preventing clots from forming around the atherosclerotic plaques that would further block blood flow. A variety of anticoagulants including warfarin (Coumadin), pentoxifylline (Trental), and aspirin have been used.

Finally, hyperbaric oxygen treatments have also been used to increase the oxygen content of blood. In this way, a smaller amount of blood flowing to the brain might still provide an adequate supply of oxygen.

In controlled trials, all of these treatments provided mixed results at best. A few patients seemed to benefit, but most did not. In retrospect, this is probably because patients with many different types of dementia were lumped together in these older studies. We now believe that these treatments provided no benefit to the Alzheimer's disease patient but may have helped those with vascular dementia.

The greatest benefit for vascular dementia patients may be found with the anticoagulant medications. Unfortunately, elderly demented patients are often at risk of falling. If they fall while taking an anticoagulant, they can have serious and even life-threatening bleeding. A happy medium for many vascular dementia patients may be the mild anticoagulant effects of daily aspirin. However, despite being an over-the-counter medication, daily aspirin should never be started without the full knowledge and consent of your patient's doctor.

Chelation. Chelation (pronounced KEY-lay-shun) medications act by removing trace metals from the body. They are used most often in cases of accidental or intentional overdose of substances containing these elements. Chelators have been used to treat dementia based on evidence that patients with Alzheimer's dementia have abnormally high levels of aluminum in their nerve cells. It's not clear why this may occur. As a result, chelating medications such as desferrioxamine have been used in an attempt to remove aluminum. These treatments have not proved helpful and have been abandoned.

Although chelation is not helpful for Alzheimer's disease patients, it is the key to treating patients with dementia due to Wilson's disease. Wilson's disease is a genetically inherited disorder that usually strikes before age 30. The disease causes toxic levels of copper to accumulate in the liver, brain, eyes, and kidney. Untreated, Wilson's disease leads to tremors, cirrhosis, depression, psychosis, dementia, and ultimately death. Chelation with penicillamine (Cuprimine) can stop and even reverse the accumulation of copper.

Blood Pressure Control. Uncontrolled hypertension (high blood pressure) greatly increases the risk of stroke. Although attaining blood pressure control does not seem to improve Alzheimer's disease, it is extremely important in protecting the brain from the damage of vascular dementia. Excessively high blood pressure increases the rate of damage from vascular dementia. On the other hand, low blood pressures may also worsen dementia due to a reduction of blood flow to the brain.

Blocking Glutamate Activity. An extensive line of research using laboratory animals has shown that nerve cells in the brain can be damaged by excessive stimulation. In particular, uncontrolled release of glutamate, an excitatory amino acid that stimulates neurons by binding the NMDA receptor, can lead to neuronal death by causing toxic accumulations of calcium to collect inside nerve cells in the brain. It should not be surprising, therefore, that medications to block glutamate activity are of keen interest to those studying neurodegenerative disorders like Alzheimer's disease. Memantine (Nemanda) is the most recently approved treatment for Alzheimer's disease, and its mechanism of action is presumably via antagonism of the NMDA receptor. As such, it is the first agent used specifically to protect the brain that has proved successful in the treatment of Alzheimer's disease. Interestingly, memantine has been available in Germany since the early 1980s, where it was used to manage a variety of neurological disorders.

The side effects of memantine are generally mild and include headache, dizziness, and constipation. Memantine is started at an initial dose of 5 mg each morning and is increased to 5 mg twice daily after 1 week. The maximum dose of memantine is 10 mg taken twice daily. A recent study indicates that memantine works synergistically with cholinesterase inhibitors (see Section 10.5.5), and it has quickly become routine clinical practice to coadminister memantine with one of these agents.

10.5.5 History of Cognitive Enhancement Treatments

Using a medication to enhance the cognition of a demented patient is akin to giving insulin to a diabetic patient. In both cases, we are not attempting to cure the disease, but we are trying to replace what has been lost. For the demented patient, this means reawakening activity in the nerve cells. There have been several approaches tried to achieve this goal. They include enhancing metabolism of nerve cells, stimulating nerve cell growth, boosting dopamine transmission, and boosting acetylcholine transmission. Let's look at each of these approaches.

Enhancing Metabolism. Metabolic enhancers theoretically work by promoting activity in relatively inactive areas of the brain. We can infer that these medications enhance brain activity by their ability to increase the brain's use of glucose and oxygen. The metabolic enhancers that have been tried to date include ergot alkaloids, nootropics, and vinca alkaloids.

Ergot Alkaloids. The ergot alkaloid hydergine was introduced in the 1940s and was in fact the first medication approved by the FDA to enhance cognition in dementia patients. It continues to be used occasionally today, but numerous studies have not shown any clear benefit for hydergine or other ergot alkaloids. We therefore do not recommend its routine use.

Nootropics. The nootropic medications (of which piracetam is the best known) are believed to enhance nerve cell activity by improving circulation in the tiniest of blood vessels (capillaries) that provide oxygen-rich blood to the nerve cells. In addition to enhancing nerve cell metabolism, these medications should theoretically protect nerve cells in the same manner as the anticoagulants. Although theoretically sound, the nootropics have not shown any significant benefit for demented patients. Therefore, we cannot recommend their use.

Vinca Alkaloids. Finally, the vinca alkaloid vinpocetine has been shown to enhance learning and memory in laboratory animals. But again, it showed no benefit for patients with dementia.

Why don't any of these medications work? Clearly, they boost nerve cell activity. Some of them do enhance cognition in animals. But they do little for dementia patients. Why is this? The explanation is probably that the small benefit of these medications pales in comparison to the widespread damage to nerve cells caused by dementia. The difference between a dementia's ability to compromise the way the brain works and a medication's ability to enhance brain function is so great that the medication produces no noticeable improvement.

Stimulating Nerve Cell Growth. Although most human brain cells do not reproduce, there are mechanisms in place to maintain and repair damage to nerve cells. One theory is that a defect in these repair mechanisms leads to the progressive deterioration we see in dementia. Along these lines, some researchers have attempted to treat this brain atrophy with nerve growth factor (NGF). It does appear that NGF may slow the rate of deterioration and provide some small benefit to dementia patients. Unfortunately, NGF does not cross the blood–brain barrier and can only be given via a catheter inserted into the brain. This leaves it impractical for routine use at present.

However, estrogen is another substance that has been shown to enhance nerve cell growth. Estrogen therapy has been shown to boost cognition in nondemented postmenopausal women. Any potential cognitive benefit of estrogen therapy, however, must be weighed against the considerable cardiovascular and other medical risks.

Boosting Dopamine Neurotransmission. There is a great deal of evidence that increasing dopamine activity in the brain improves memory, learning, and attention. For example, dopamine-boosting psychostimulants such as methylphenidate (Ritalin) and dextroamphetamine (Dexedrine) enhance intellectual function both in patients with attention deficit disorder (ADD) and in those with no psychiatric or cognitive impairment. It was reasonable to expect that these psychostimulants or other dopamine-promoting medications like bromocriptine might help dementia patients.

Unfortunately, studies have not shown that these dopamine-boosting medications provide any significant cognitive benefit to dementia patients. Nevertheless, there may be some role for these medications in the treatment of dementia. First, the psychostimulants have proved effective in the treatment of apathy experienced by some patients with dementia. Second, when antidepressants are used to treat depressed dementia patients, an argument can be made to use an antidepressant with dopamine-boosting properties. It will do no harm and may provide some modest benefit to cognition while treating the depression. Dopamine-boosting antidepressants include sertraline (Zoloft) and perhaps bupropion (Wellbutrin).

Cholinergic Medications (Boosting Acetylcholine). As we've previously told you, acetylcholine is the primary neurotransmitter that the brain uses for memory and intellectual processing. It was only a matter of time before medications that boost acetylcholine transmission were studied in dementia patients.

There are three ways to increase acetylcholine activity: (1) increase the supply of acetylcholine, (2) directly stimulate acetylcholine receptors (muscarinic agonists), and (3) block the enzyme that inactivates acetylcholine (cholinesterase inhibitors). Let's take a look at each of these approaches.

Acetylcholine Precursors. Your nerve cells produce acetylcholine from certain dietary precursors (choline and lecithin). Many early studies tried dietary supplements of these precursors. A precedent for this approach was established using the dopamine precursor, L-DOPA, a well-established treatment for Parkinson's disease. Unfortunately, this approach is ineffective in dementia. It appears that the daily doses of these fatty acid precursors needed to have any discernible impact on acetylcholine levels far exceed what an individual can reasonably take in a day. This approach has therefore been abandoned.

Muscarinic Agonists. Another approach is to use a medication that directly activates subtypes of the acetylcholine receptors, namely, muscarinic receptor agonists. The muscarinic agonists used in the past have not been effective. This includes bethanecol, pilocarpine, and oxotremorine. This line of treatment, however, has not been entirely abandoned, and several medications are currently in testing.

Cholinesterase Inhibitors

Physostigmine (Antilirium). The first cholinesterase inhibitor available was physostigmine (see Table 10.5). This medication was developed to treat anticholinergic delirium and is still used for that purpose today. However, physostigmine is not a practical medication for treating dementia. It is extremely short acting (1–2 hours) and would therefore need to be taken eight or more times per day. A sustained-release formulation of physostigmine (Synapton) is now available. It is associated with significant cholinergic side effects such as nausea, vomiting, cramping, and diarrhea. It is not FDA approved for the treatment of dementia.

Tacrine (Cognex). Tacrine was first used in the 1940s to reverse the respiratory depressant effects of morphine. In the late 1980s, tacrine was first used to treat dementia. The results were promising. Nearly one-third of dementia patients in the early and middle stages of illness exhibit observable improvement with tacrine.

Tacrine is not without its problems. It produces typical cholinergic side effects (nausea, cramping, loss of appetite, runny nose, and diarrhea). In addition, tacrine can be toxic to the liver in some patients. If liver problems develop while taking tacrine, they reverse when the medication is discontinued. Nevertheless, all patients should routinely undergo blood tests of liver function before starting tacrine and periodically during tacrine therapy.

Although tacrine is longer-lasting than its predecessor physostigmine, it is by today's standards a short-acting medication. It must be taken four times per day with the total daily dose ranging from 80 to 160 mg/day.

Donepezil (Aricept). Donepezil is the second cholinesterase inhibitor approved for the treatment of dementia. Most physicians find it much easier to use than its predecessor. It can be given once a day and carries none of the risk of liver toxicity seen with tacrine. It has been shown in multiple clinical trials to delay the decline in cognitive function in patients with Alzheimer's disease.

Like other cholinesterase inhibitors, donepezil carries the risk of cholinergic side effects. In fact, if the dose of a cholinesterase inhibitor is increased too rapidly, it may even worsen behavior. The principal side effects of donepezil include upset stomach, diarrhea, headache, and dizziness. It is usually started at 5 mg taken once daily in the evening. After 1 month, the dose of donepezil can be increased to 10 mg/day.

TABLE 10.5. FDA Approved Treatments for Alzheimer's Disease

Generic Name	Trade Name	Mechanism	Daily Dosage
Donepezil	Aricept	Cholinesterase inhibitor	5–10 mg
Galantamine	Reminyl	Cholinesterase inhibitor	8–24 mg
Memantine	Nemenda	NMDA receptor antagonist	10–20 mg
Rivastigmine	Exelon	Cholinesterase inhibitor	3–12 mg
Tacrine	Cognex	Cholinesterase inhibitor	80–160 mg

Rivastigmine (Exelon). Rivastigmine has recently been approved for marketing by the FDA. It is also a reversible cholinesterase inhibitor. The common side effects of rivastigmine include nausea, decreased appetite, and weight loss. Rivastigmine is started at 1.5 mg given twice daily and can be increased to 3 mg twice a day after 1 month of treatment. The maximum dose of rivastigmine is 6 mg twice a day.

Galantamine (Reminyl). Galantamine is the newest of the cholinesterase inhibitors approved in the United States. It is started at 4 mg twice a day and can be increased to 8 mg twice daily after 4 weeks of treatment. The maximum dose of galantamine is 12 mg twice a day. The side effects of galantamine include nausea, diarrhea, loss of appetite, and weight loss.

10.5.6 History of Behavioral Management Treatments

We've already described in considerable detail the many complications of dementia including depression, psychosis, delirium, and agitation. In general, the evolution of treatments for these symptoms has been straightforward.

The key has been to avoid using treatments that worsen the disease. In this instance, this means avoiding anticholinergic (acetylcholine-blocking) medications that worsen dementia. As a result, when newer antidepressants such as the SSRIs became available, they quickly replaced the older tricyclic antidepressants because the latter are potent anticholinergics. For the same reason, the low potency antipsychotics like chlorpromazine (Thorazine) were replaced by the higher potency antipsychotics like haloperidol (Haldol) and more recently by the atypical antipsychotics.

However, the evolution of treatment for agitation in dementia deserves further discussion. There have been numerous approaches that have met with varying degrees of success.

Antipsychotics. Antipsychotic medications are also called major tranquilizers. It is for the tranquilizing effect that they have been used to treat agitation. The earliest antipsychotics, especially thioridazine (Mellaril), proved to be effective in reducing agitation; however, this comes at the price of further impairing cognition due to its profound anticholinergic effects.

The high potency antipsychotic haloperidol (Haldol) provides the same calming effects with minimal anticholinergic effects. Although haloperidol is very effective, dementia patients are quite sensitive to its extrapyramidal effects. These include stiffness, shuffling gait, a mask-like facial appearance, and involuntary movements. To minimize these effects, haloperidol is used in very low doses (0.5–1.0 mg) when treating those with dementia.

Atypical antipsychotics may be helpful in managing the delusions and agitated behavior that can accompany dementia. These medications, include risperidone (Risperdal), quetiapine (Seroquel), ziprasidone (Geodon), aripiprazole (Abilify), and olanzapine (Zyprexa). All antipsychotics, typical and atypical, appear to increase the risk of death in patients with dementia and psychosis. This appears as a warning in the package inserts of the newer drugs. A prudent approach is to discuss this risk with the caregiver, use the lowest effective dose, and monitor for effectiveness.

Benzodiazepines. These medications are also known as minor tranquilizers. In general, they have been found less effective than antipsychotics in treating agitation over the long term. However, their relatively quick onset of action makes them effective for acute episodic agitation.

Benzodiazepines should be used with caution in dementia patients. Used improperly, they can disinhibit patients and worsen behavior, or they can accumulate and lead to a state of intoxication. To minimize the risk of accumulation, benzodiazepines that are easily metabolized are preferred for elderly patients. Specifically, lorazepam (Ativan) and oxazepam (Serax) are easier for elderly patients to tolerate than other benzodiazepines.

Mood Stabilizers. First lithium and more recently valproic acid (Depakote, Depakene), carbamazepine (Tegretol), and gabapentin (Neurontin) have been used to treat agitated dementia patients.

Lithium is somewhat effective for the treatment of agitation; however, elderly patients do not tolerate it well. In particular, demented patients are at risk for lithium toxicity, and this toxicity may not be easily detected in these patients. Despite its effectiveness, lithium has been abandoned in the treatment of agitation due to the availability of several effective and better-tolerated treatments, including the atypical antipsychotics described earlier.

Carbamazepine is more widely used for treating chronically agitated dementia patients. Its onset of action is delayed by several days to a couple of weeks; therefore, other tranquilizing medications such as antipsychotics may need to be used when first starting carbamazepine. Carbamazepine doses have problematic side effects that require blood monitoring, and it also interacts with many medications.

In recent years, some physicians have used gabapentin as an alternative treatment for mild but chronic agitation. There are no studies of its effectiveness, but gabapentin is easily tolerated and may be a reasonable alternative for some patients.

Of the mood stabilizers, valproic acid (Depakene, Depakote) is the most widely used. Like the other mood stabilizers, its onset of action can be delayed by several days. Valproic acid is a reasonably well tolerated mood stabilizer. It does occasionally cause tremor, and it can on rare occasion lower platelet counts or cause liver problems. For this reason, blood monitoring is required when starting this medication. In addition, valproic acid can irritate the stomach lining, but this problem is largely overcome by using the buffered form sodium divalproex (Depakote or Depakote ER). Finally, valproic acid can also cause hair loss or drowsiness.

Unlike carbamazepine, valproic acid has few drug interactions, an added benefit for elderly patients. One interaction worthy of mention, however, is that aspirin can increase levels of valproic acid. For this reason, vascular dementia patients taking an aspirin a day may need a lower dose of valproic acid or at least more careful monitoring of blood levels when starting valproic acid.

Antidepressants. Antidepressants are used to treat not only depression but also chronic mild-to-moderate agitation in demented patients. In particular, serotonin-boosting antidepressants appear to be effective at reducing agitation. The best studied in this regard are trazodone (Desyrel), sertraline (Zoloft), and paroxetine (Paxil).

Trazodone is quite effective at treating agitation and given at bedtime can also alleviate insomnia and nighttime wandering. Many physicians consider it the treatment of choice for sundowning (severe nighttime agitation). It is reasonably well tolerated at low doses of 50–100 mg/day given at bedtime. Unfortunately, elderly patients can seldom tolerate the higher doses needed to treat depression. At these higher doses, excessive drowsiness and dizziness (which increases the risk of falls) become too problematic. Therefore, trazodone is not used to treat depression in demented patients.

Sertraline, on the other hand, can be used to treat both mild-to-moderate agitation and also depression. Its primary side effects are indigestion, diarrhea, and sexual dysfunction. Paroxetine works in a fashion similar to sertraline and therefore also appears to treat both depression and mild-to-moderate agitation. However, paroxetine does have a mild anticholinergic action (acetylcholine-blocking) that can theoretically worsen the cognitive impairment of dementia. Finally, fluoxetine (Prozac) likely has the same benefits in demented patients as sertraline and paroxetine, but some physicians shy away from using fluoxetine in these patients because its long duration of action may make it difficult to discontinue it quickly if side effects develop.

Before the arrival of the new antidepressants, the older tricyclic antidepressants were widely used to treat depression and agitation in demented patients. They have now largely been abandoned in these patients as their prominent anticholinergic effects tend to worsen dementia and the increased risk for cardiac toxicity can be especially dangerous in geriatric patients.

Buspirone (Buspar). Buspirone is a nonbenzodiazepine anxiety-reducing medication. It can be an effective treatment for demented patients with chronic anxiety. Buspirone is not sedating like the benzodiazepines and in fact probably has the fewest side effects of any available psychiatric medication. Buspirone does have a delayed onset of action; therefore, it is not useful for acute treatment of anxiety or agitation.

Other Medications. A variety of other medications have been tried. These include hormone treatments and certain blood pressure medications (e.g., clonidine and the beta blockers). For the most part, these have met with minimal success and should not be considered a part of routine treatment.

In recent years, however, physicians have used medroxyprogesterone to treat sexual aggression in men with dementia. Although this has not been well studied, anecdotal reports suggest it may be effective.

10.6 CURRENT APPROACH TO TREATMENT

The overall goal of treatment in dementia is to maximize the patient's ability to function independently as long as possible and to shorten the period of severe disability as much as possible. This requires distinct approaches at different stages of the illness.

10.6.1 Current Treatment Options at Different Stages of Dementia

The stages of dementia (early, moderate, and late) are somewhat arbitrarily defined. There is no clear demarcation between the stages of illness. There is also no specific timeline that will place an individual within a specific stage. Different types of dementia progress at widely different rates, and there is considerable variation from person-to-person. Nevertheless, some grouping of patients into stages of illness can help the patient's family know what to expect and how best to help.

During the early stage of dementia, the impairment first becomes noticeable and interferes with complicated tasks such as driving a car, paying the bills, or preparing a full meal. These patients should not live alone but do not require 24 hour supervision. In the moderate stage of dementia, the disability begins to affect simpler tasks. Moderately demented patients often need help dressing, maintaining personal hygiene, and carrying on a conversation. These patients should probably not be left at home alone; it is at this stage of illness that wandering from home and getting lost may become a problem. Finally, during the late stage of dementia, patients need total care. They often need to be fed, they usually have lost control of both bladder and bowel function, and they may not talk at all. Family members often cannot provide the round-the-clock care needed at this stage of illness, and many patients at this stage are placed in nursing homes.

As the dementia progresses through these stages, different care strategies (including medication strategies) are needed. But one rule of treatment prevails at all stages. Before starting or changing medications aimed at enhancing cognitive abilities or protecting brain function, any coexisting behavioral or emotional problems should be treated first. This is essential for two reasons. First, it is difficult to determine the severity of the dementia and whether your patient is being helped by the dementia treatment when other problems are present. Second, starting too many medications at once should always be avoided, and this is especially so in patients with dementia. If the behavior worsens or side effects develop after simultaneously starting several medications, which medication should be stopped? It would be impossible to know with certainty.

When first encountering a patient who appears to be in the early stages of dementia, this is the time to search for any treatable causes. The first step in treatment is therefore to refer your patient for a medical evaluation. If any treatable conditions are identified (see Table 10.4), they should be the immediate focus of treatment. Thereafter, during the early-to-moderate stages of dementia, medications that enhance cognition should be a mainstay of therapy. In addition, medications or nutritional supplements that protect the brain and delay the progression to the severely disabling end stage of the illness may be useful.

In the final stages of illness, cognitive enhancers do not provide any noticeable improvement in the patient's day-to-day functioning and therefore are usually not used. But some physicians believe that cognitive enhancers may be helpful in managing the behavioral problems of dementia. This has not been well studied, but if it proves true, then cognitive enhancers may be useful even in the late stages of illness. Brain protecting medications are usually not used during the final stages of dementia.

Medications to manage behavioral problems may be needed at any or all stages of dementia. The key issue is the same at all three stages. The behavioral problem should be eliminated (or at least minimized) without worsening the patient's intellectual difficulties further. This is sometimes no small task because dementia patients may be quite sensitive to the sedative or anticholinergic effects of many psychiatric medications.

10.6.2 Current Options for Cognitive Enhancement

As noted earlier, cognition-enhancing medications are most helpful during the early and moderate stages of dementia. These medications proved effective for both Alzheimer's disease and vascular dementia; it's unknown whether they are helpful for other dementias.

We recommend that all patients in the early and moderate stages of Alzheimer's disease or vascular dementia be given a trial of a cognitive enhancer. Families should be counseled when starting these medications. They must understand that these medications will not stop the progression of the illness and will not return their loved one to a predementia level of functioning. The family should also be told to be patient because any improvement will be gradual, unfolding over many weeks. These medicines can be tried in patients with other forms of dementia, but it's not certain whether their acetylcholine-boosting effects will be helpful in other dementias.

The oldest of the cholinesterase inhibitors, physostigmine and tacrine, have been supplanted by the newer agents that are simpler to use and easier to tolerate. These newer agents, donepezil, rivastigmine, and galantamine, need only be administered once daily and do not require periodic liver testing. They are now routinely coadministered with memantine (cf. Section 10.6.3) that is used to protect the brain and thereby slow the progression of the dementing illness.

10.6.3 Current Options for Brain Protection

The key to successful brain protection for Alzheimer's disease is the newly introduced NMDA receptor antagonist, memantine. Family members should be advised that the protection provided by memantine will slow the progression of Alzheimer's disease, but it does not halt or reverse the course of the illness. Memantine is now commonly coadministered with a cholinesterase inhibitor.

Most of the other medications studied to slow the course of Alzheimer's dementia presumably work as an antioxidant to protect nerve cells from damaging free radicals. Of the antioxidants, vitamin E is the safest and has the best evidence of efficacy. Thus, we recommend that all patients receive 2000 IU of vitamin E each day during the early and moderate stages of Alzheimer's disease. It will do no harm, is reasonably inexpensive, and may prove helpful.

Some families and physicians may choose to use several brain protecting medications. We advise caution here. Medications, even over-the-counter herbs like ginkgo biloba, have side effects, and combining multiple medications (although sometimes necessary) increases the risk of delirium and other medical complications in these often-fragile patients.

We do not recommend the routine use of selegiline, nonsteroidal anti-inflammatory drugs like ibuprofen, or herbs such as ginkgo biloba for patients with dementia. These all have the potential for problematic side effects that may outweigh their benefit. If they are used, please be sure that a physician closely monitors your patient.

During the early-to-moderate stages of vascular dementia, an aspirin a day can provide some protection from additional infarcts. However, daily aspirin does carry risks of bleeding and stomach irritation and should only be used under the supervision of a physician.

10.6.4 Current Options for Treatment of Behavioral and Emotional Problems

Many behavioral problems can complicate dementia, and these problems can strike at any phase of the illness. It is often this aspect of the illness that is most distressing to both the patients and their caregivers. Behavioral disturbance is the most frequent cause of hospitalization and long-term institutionalization for patients who would otherwise be at home with their families. Therefore, treating these behavioral problems not only provides emotional relief for dementia patients and their families but can also lower the tremendous economic burden of dementia. The key, as we have said before, is to control the behavioral disturbance without worsening the dementia. (See Table 10.6)

Delirium. Anytime you notice a sudden decline in a dementia patient, you should suspect delirium. Any time you notice a drowsy, stuporous patient, you should suspect delirium. If you suspect delirium, immediately send the patient for a medical examination.

The medical treatment of delirium includes finding and removing the cause of the delirium and controlling the behavioral consequences of delirium. When searching for the cause of delirium, your patient's physician will perform a thorough physical exam, will review the recent medical history, will review the current medications, and will order a battery of laboratory tests. Because medications can cause or contribute to delirium, any medications that are not absolutely necessary and can safely be discontinued (at least temporarily) should be stopped.

While the medical evaluation is being performed, treatment may be needed to control the patient. A frightened, combative, confused patient is dangerous both to him/herself and those trying to help. Therefore, medication may be needed to calm

TABLE 10.6. Treating Behavioral Complications of Dementia

Behavioral Complication	Preferred Medications	Alternative Medications	
Anxiety (acute)	Lorazepam	Oxazepam	
Anxiety (chronic)	Buspirone	Lorazepam Oxazepam	
Agitation (acute, mild)	Trazodone Lorazepam	Buspirone Sodium divalproex SSRI	
Agitation (acute, severe)	Lorazepam Ziprasidone Risperidone	Trazodone Olanzapine Quetiapine	Haloperidol
Agitation (chronic)	Sodium divalproex	Risperidone Olanzapine SSRI	Trazodone Ziprasidone Haloperidol
Delirium	Risperidone Ziprasidone	Haloperidol Lorazepam	
Depression	SSRIs SNRIs	Mirtazapine Bupropion Nortriptyline Desipramine	
Insomnia	Trazodone Quetiapine	Zolpidem Temazepam Chloral hydrate	
Psychosis (acute)	Risperidone Ziprasidone	Olanzapine Quetiapine	Aripiprazole Haloperidol
Psychosis (chronic)	Risperidone Ziprasidone	Olanzapine Quetiapine	Aripiprazole Haloperidol

the patient. But remember, medications that calm or tranquilize a patient may also worsen the delirium. Careful medication selection is warranted.

The medication of choice was for many years haloperidol (Haldol), a high potency antipsychotic, that can be given orally or by injection. When used, haloperidol should be administered in low doses (0.5–1.0 mg) and only on an as-needed basis. Due to concerns regarding the tolerability of haloperidol in patients with dementia, its role in the management of agitation associated with delirium has largely been supplanted by atypical antipsychotics. A number of atypical antipsychotics are available by either an oral or intramuscular (injection) route of administiation.

Although many physicians routinely use benzodiazepines to treat combative, delirious patients, this is not recommended. First, benzodiazepines can cloud consciousness and actually worsen the confusion of delirium. Second, benzodiazepines can worsen the breathing problems of patients with pneumonia or emphysema, two common causes of delirium. The lone exception is a delirium that is caused by alcohol or benzodiazepine withdrawal. A benzodiazepine MUST be used for alcohol or benzodiazepine withdrawal. When a benzodiazepine is used, a low dose of a short-acting medication that is less likely to accumulate in elderly patients is preferred. We recommend lorazepam (Ativan), which meets all these requirements and can be given orally or by injection.

Depressed Mood. The preferred treatment for depression in a demented patient is an antidepressant of the SSRI or SNRI class. They are usually effective and reasonably well tolerated. When choosing an antidepressant, potential interactions with the many other medications that older patients are often taking must be considered. Please refer to Chapter 3 (Mood Disorders) for more information on potential drug interactions.

When prescribing antidepressants to the geriatric patient with both depression and dementia, the initial dose should be reduced compared to that given a younger adult. Examples include sertaline (Zoloft) 12.5–25 mg/day or paroxetine (Paxil) 10 mg/day. If paroxetine (Paxil) is used, its dose should not be too high because it has anticholinergic effects that can worsen dementia at high doses.

The so-called atypical antidepressants such as venlafaxine and bupropion can be tried, but their safety and efficacy in treating patients with dementia have not been well studied. The older tricyclic antidepressants and monoamine oxidase inhibitors are not tolerated well by demented patients and should be avoided. Two possible exceptions are nortriptyline (Pamelor) and desipramine (Norpramin), but even these should be tried only after the newer antidepressants have proved ineffective.

For very severe cases of depression, electroconvulsive therapy (ECT) can be tried. However, you must remember that demented patients are especially sensitive to the adverse memory effects of ECT.

The antidepressant trazodone (Desyrel) is commonly used in low doses to treat agitation or insomnia in dementia patients. However, older patients often do not tolerate the higher doses of trazodone needed to treat depression.

Delusions/Psychosis. Demented patients who are acutely psychotic and agitated should be treated in much the same manner as demented patients with delirium. Low doses of a high potency conventional antipsychotic like haloperidol were once preferred. This was mainly because it can be given both orally and by injection. In recent years, the atypical antipsychotic ziprasidone, which is now also available in oral and injectable forms, has superseded haloperidol as the preferred agent when treating the acutely psychotic and agitated patient with dementia. As previously noted, ziprasidone affords the same tranquilizing benefit as haloperidol, it can now be administered via injection when necessary, and it avoids the problematic extrapyramidal symptoms of haloperidol to which patients with dementia are often keenly sensitive.

The side effects of conventional antipsychotics are of even greater concern when treating chronic psychosis in a patient with dementia. With sustained administration of a typical antipsychotic, these patients will be highly vulnerable to the extrapyramidal effects of the medication, which can increase the risk for falls. Thus, atypical antipsychotics have also been rapidly accepted as first-line agents when treating chronic psychosis in a patient with dementia. Like the typical antipsychotics, the atypical agents should be administered at doses that are considerably lower than those used to treat schizophrenia. Any of the atypical antipsychotics could benefit patients experiencing the psychosis that accompanies dementia, though this has been difficult to demonstrate consistently in controlled clinical trials and no antipsychotics currently have the indication for this use.

Anxiety. Like psychosis, choosing a medication to treat anxiety in demented patients depends in large part on whether the anxiety is acute or longstanding. Acute severe anxiety requires rapid relief. For this, we recommend a benzodiazepine. Our first choice is lorazepam (Ativan) that is given as needed at 0.25–0.5 mg per dose. We prefer lorazepam because elderly patients tolerate it well (i.e., they metabolize it easily), and it is available in both oral and injectable forms. Oxazepam (Serax) is another benzodiazepine that older patients metabolize easily, but it is only available in oral form. When using benzodiazepines, be careful that your patients do not become overly sedated or delirious.

We do not recommend benzodiazepines for the long-term treatment of anxiety. The risk of sedation, falls, and worsening memory is usually not warranted. Our first choice for the long-term treatment of anxiety in demented patients is buspirone. It should be started at 5 mg given twice daily and raised as tolerated to 30 mg/day. Doses may be raised as high as 50–60 mg/day. Buspirone may take several weeks to begin relieving anxiety, but it has few side effects and is very unlikely to interact with other medications. The primary alternatives to buspirone are a variety of antidepressants including trazodone, the SSRIs, nefazodone, and venlafaxine.

Insomnia. The medicines used to treat insomnia are the same as those used to treat insomnia in other patients. As with other complications of dementia, the crucial task is to relieve the insomnia without worsening the dementia.

We recommend trazodone (Desyrel) as a first-line treatment for insomnia in dementia patients. It has the added advantage of reducing nighttime agitation due to sundowning. Trazodone should be started at 25–50 mg given at bedtime. It should not be increased above 100 mg as higher doses increase the risk of dizziness and falls.

Other medications that can be considered are zolpidem (Ambien), the benzodiazepine temazepam (Restoril), quetiapine (Seroquel), and chloral hydrate.

Other sleep-inducing benzodiazepines should be avoided. They are more difficult to metabolize and can accumulate in elderly, demented patients. Sedating, low potency antipsychotics should also be avoided. Their strong anticholinergic (acetylcholine-blocking) effects can worsen dementia or cause delirium.

Agitation. Of all the behavioral and emotional problems that accompany dementia, agitation is the most troublesome. As a result, a multitude of book chapters and articles have appeared in recent years discussing precisely this problem.

As with delirium the first step is to identify any treatable causes of agitation. The most common causes are interactions from medications, bladder or respiratory infection, pain, constipation, recent stroke, or undetected head injury from a recent fall. Your patient's physician can usually rule out these possibilities with a thorough physical examination and a few laboratory studies.

Environmental changes can also help alleviate agitation. Often the agitation results from confusion or overstimulation. It can be helpful to simplify the surroundings by reducing noise levels or ensuring adequate lighting. Once these problems have been eliminated or treated, the treatment of any remaining agitation can be chosen. Several factors should guide medication selection: the duration of the agitation, the severity of the agitation, the usual time of day of the agitation, and whether any psychotic symptoms are also present.

Brief Mild Agitation. For the acute treatment of mild agitation without physical aggression, low doses of trazodone are preferred. If this mild agitation persists, several options are available. Your patient's physician may continue to use trazodone or may prefer sodium divalproex (Depakote), buspirone (Buspar), or any of the SSRI antidepressants. These are all well tolerated but should be started at low doses and slowly raised upward as needed.

Among these choices, buspirone is preferred if the patient is also experiencing anxiety. If the patient is depressed and agitated, a SSRI should be tried first. Second line choices include carbamazepine (Tegretol) or one of the atypical antipsychotics—ziprasidone (Geodon), risperidone (Risperdal), olanzapine (Zyprexa), quetiapine (Seroquel), or aripiprazole (Abilify) can be tried. If psychotic symptoms are present, one of the atypical antipsychotics should be tried first.

Brief Severe Agitation. Acute management of severe agitation with physical aggression requires more definitive treatment. The first choice is haloperidol given in low doses (0.25–1 mg) as needed. Lorazepam can also be helpful if used briefly. Risperidone, olanzapine, quetiapine, or trazodone can also be used but are not available in injectable forms.

Chronic Agitation. For chronic agitation with physical aggression, sodium divalproex is the preferred treatment. If divalproex is ineffective, haloperidol or an atypical antipsychotic can be added or substituted. Other options include trazodone, carbamazepine, and SSRI antidepressants.

For milder forms of chronic agitation, antidepressants are the preferred treatment. When sexually aggressive behavior occurs in demented male patients, we have found that 20–40 mg daily doses of oral medroxyprogesterone (Provera) can be helpful. Weekly injections of medroxyprogesterone have also been used but are more likely to cause weight gain, elevated blood pressure, muscle cramps, or gynecomastia (breast enlargement) than the oral form.

ADDITIONAL READING

Bonelli RM, Wenning GK, Kapfhammer HP. Huntington's disease: present treatments and future therapeutic modalities. *Int Clin Psychopharmacol* 2004; 19: 51–62.

Bullock R. Treatment of behavioural and psychiatric symptoms in dementia: implications of recent safety warnings. *Curr Med Res Opin* 2005; 21: 1–10.

Cummings JL. Use of cholinesterase inhibitors in clinical practice: evidence based recommendations. *Am J Geriatr Psychiatry* 2003; 11: 131–145.

Doody RS. Current treatments for Alzheimer's disease: cholinesterase inhibitors. *J Clin Psychiatry* 2003; 64(Supplement 9): 11–17.

Finkel S. Pharmacology of antipsychotics in the elderly: a focus on atypicals. *J Am Geriatr Soc* 2004; 52: S258–S265.

Hardy J, Selkoe DJ. The amyloid hypothesis of Alzheimer's disease: progress and problems in the road to therapeutics. *Science* 2002; 297: 353–356.

Hay DP, Klein DT (eds). *Agitation in Patients with Dementia: A Practical Guide to Diagnosis and Management. Clinical Practice Series.* Washington DC: American Psychiatric Publishing, 2003.

Herrman N. Cognitive pharmacotherapy of Alzheimer's disease and other dementias. *Can J Psychiatry* 2002; 47: 715–722.

Lee PE, Gill SS, Freedman M, et al. Atypical antipsychotic drugs in the treatment of behavioural and psychological symptoms of dementia: systematic review. *Br Med J* 2004; doi:10.1136/bmj.38125.465579.55.

Lichtenberg PA, Murman DL (eds). *Handbook of Dementia: Psychological, Neurological, and Psychiatric Perspectives.* Hoboken, NJ: John Wiley & Sons, 2003.

Madhusoodanan S. Introduction: antipsychotic treatment of behavioral and psychological symptoms of dementia in geropsychiatric patients. *Am J Geriatr Psychiatry* 2001; 9(3): 283–288.

Michaelis ML. Drugs targeting Alzheimer's disease: some things old and some things new. *J Pharmacol Exp Ther* 2003; 304: 897–904.

Rabheru K. Special issues in the management of depression in older patients. *Can J Psychiatry* 2004; 49(3 Supplement 1): 41S–50S.

Rubey RN. The cholinesterase inhibitors. *J Psychiatr Pract* 2003; 9(6): 422–430.

Ryan JM. Newer generation antipsychotics for the management of psychosis in older patients with dementia. *J Clin Psychiatry* 2003; 64(11): 1388–1390.

Sink KM, Holden KF, Yaffe K. Pharmacological treatment of neuropsychiatric symptoms of dementia. *JAMA* 2005; 293: 596–608.

Sun MK, Alkon DL. Depressed or demented: common CNS drug targets? *Curr Drug Targets CNS Neurol Disord* 2002; 1(6): 575–592.

Tariot PN, Federoff HJ. Current treatment for Alzheimer disease and future prospects. *Alzheimers Dis Assoc Disord* 2003; 17: S105–S113.

11

PERSONALITY DISORDERS

11.1 INTRODUCTION

11.1.1 How Little We Know

The area of pharmacotherapy for the personality disorders represents what may be the largest gap between practice and research in the field of psychiatry. What this statement is intended to communicate is the remarkable lack of data regarding the use of psychotropic medications to treat personality disorders, yet many patients with personality disorders are, and probably should be, prescribed various medications. Certainly, some of these prescriptions are for comorbid conditions such as major depressive disorder or anxiety disorders, but many drugs are utilized to target specific symptoms of the personality disorder. Thus, medication regimens being used to treat patients with personality disorders are often more complicated than those used to treat patients with Axis I disorders alone. This is in part due to the inherent challenge in treating personality disorders, but the relative lack of evidence-based medicine that can be used to formulate treatment strategies in this population is likely the major factor underlying this phenomenon.

Principles of Psychopharmacology for Mental Health Professionals
By Jeffrey E. Kelsey, D. Jeffrey Newport, and Charles B. Nemeroff

How then has our routine clinical practice come to be so divergent from any research-generated database? There are three major reasons that help explain this inconsistency. First, the DSM-IV personality disorders were largely conceived from a psychodynamic framework. Psychotherapy has therefore traditionally been seen as the cornerstone of treatment for personality disorders, and perhaps rightfully so, though it is also clearly effective in the treatment of major depression and certain anxiety disorders. However, psychotherapy should not necessarily be the sole treatment. Unfortunately, an understanding of the biology of personality disorders has only recently begun to emerge. Likewise, our knowledge of how medications fit into the management of personality disorders has lagged as well.

Second, our patterns of clinical practice have often led us to overlook the role of medications in the treatment of personality disorders. Either out of habit, due to genuine comorbidity, or in order to satisfy insurance and managed-care demands, some practitioners might tend to diagnose an Axis I disorder as the target of treatment when initiating a course of psychiatric medication in patients with a personality disorder. At some level, after recognizing that the target symptoms arise primarily from the personality disorder, the focus of treatment might change, but the initial diagnosis persists. For example, even when a patient with severe borderline personality disorder (BPD) has been admitted to a psychiatric hospital for the fifth or sixth time when decompensating under stress, the patient invariably leaves the hospital with a diagnosis of major depressive disorder, adjustment disorder, brief psychotic disorder, impulse control disorder, or some other seemingly appropriate Axis I diagnosis. In reality, the impulsivity, paranoia, mood disturbance, and/or suicidality can often be directly attributable to the personality disorder. This tendency to think of medications solely as treatments for Axis I disorders has led to little reflection as to how these medications might be useful in the treatment of a personality disorder.

Finally, personality disorders are seldom given serious consideration in clinical research except as an exclusion criterion. Researchers, particularly when conducting a clinical trial to study the efficacy of a medication, typically recruit homogeneous patient groups. For example, in studying a novel antidepressant, excluding patients who have other disorders comorbid with depression leads to a more easily interpretable outcome. By contrast, studying the treatment of personality disorders is notoriously difficult. It is difficult to arrive at a homogeneous sample of personality disorder patients simply because they so commonly have secondary complicating illnesses such as substance abuse, mood, anxiety, or eating disorders. Because of these inherent difficulties, researchers have largely neglected the study of personality disorder treatment, at least in medication trials. They have either excluded patients with personality disorders or simply failed to assess whether a personality disorder may be present. Perhaps the growing awareness of the need for "real world" or effectiveness research—that is, studies that include homogeneous patient samples *and* also patients representative of those we see in our offices, will hopefully lead to more research into the treatment of personality disorders.

11.1.2 Defining a Personality Disorder

One's personality is a panoply of qualities, attitudes, and behaviors that make one person distinct from another. It is composed of the various traits that determine an understanding and way of relating to the surrounding world. There is often a certain fluidity or flexibility in the way particular traits are emphasized in different social situations. For instance, one is more likely to tease friends, be deferential with a boss, and be nervous when speaking in front of an audience. One may be shy and awkward when meeting new people but gregarious and at ease among old acquaintances. This flexibility helps an individual adapt to different situations. Despite this adaptability, the set of behavioral traits from which an individual draws defines a cohesive personality that others know and recognize.

For some, a particular personality trait can become inflexible and exaggerated, so much so that it dominates and overrides other aspects of their persona. In moderation, there may be no problem with the particular trait in and of itself, but its unyielding presentation causes problems. For example, a measure of obsessionality can be a helpful trait for the college student who needs to organize his/her studies, but taken to extremes, an obsessive preoccupation with detail can make it impossible to complete assignments in a timely manner. Similarly, a degree of suspiciousness can be a good trait for a police officer, but in excess, this same suspiciousness drives away friends and family. When a particular trait becomes fixed in this exaggerated form, it is by definition maladaptive. In other words, it is more trouble than it is worth. At this point, personality traits are transformed into a personality disorder.

There are ten personality disorders defined in DSM-IV. In each of the disorders, one or more personality traits have become entrenched in a maladaptive pattern. This aberrant personality trait alters the way the person thinks, responds emotionally, relates to others, and/or manages impulses. In addition, it must be fixed both across time and throughout varying social situations (see Table 11.1 for the diag-

TABLE 11.1. General Diagnostic Criteria for Personality Disorders

A. Thinking and acting in a way that does not fit with the surrounding culture. It is seen in at least two of the following ways:
   1. Has an unusual way of understanding him/herself and the world
   2. Has unusually intense, rapidly shifting, or inappropriate emotional responses to others
   3. Has difficulty relating to others
   4. Has difficulty controlling his/her impulses
   5. Has unusual behavior that does not change despite different situations
   6. Has unusual behavior that causes problems in relationships and at work

B. Begins no later than early adulthood.

C. Not due to another psychiatric disorder.

D. Not due to a medication, a drug of abuse, or a medical illness.

Source: Adapted from DSM-IV.

nostic criteria for a personality disorder) and invariably markedly interferes in social and occupational functioning.

11.1.3 Prerequisites to Beginning Treatment

Completing a thorough evaluation before choosing a patient's treatment is just as important with personality disorders as it is with other psychiatric disorders, but typically requires a longer period of evaluation. This assessment includes a psychiatric history of both the current problems and longstanding difficulties. While it is difficult, if not poor practice, to diagnose a personality disorder during an initial evaluation, the seasoned clinician can often obtain some sense of maladaptive personality traits. Therefore, during an initial evaluation it is appropriate to focus on all five axes of the diagnosis, including the personality disorders (Axis II) not just Axis I disorders. In addition, collecting a history of childhood development, medical illnesses, and substance abuse are important as well as collecting collateral information from family members, because patients with personality disorders often find it difficult to recognize the degree of impairment associated with their illness. Direct observation of the patient (i.e., the mental status examination) can also provide telltale clues regarding the likelihood of a personality disorder. Finally, laboratory evaluation and in some cases a brain imaging study should complete the evaluation process.

In general, Axis I disorders will be the initial focus of treatment, particularly as it pertains to choosing psychotropic medication as a component of treatment. However, once the symptoms of the Axis I disorder yield to treatment, then addressing the personality disorder becomes an important focus. It is critical to have a sound philosophy of what can and cannot be accomplished with medication when treating personality disorders. Obviously, medication alone rarely "cures" a personality disorder. Even long-term psychotherapy seldom results in anything resembling a cure. Optimal treatment for personality disorders is undoubtedly a combination of psychotherapy and pharmacotherapy. A realistic goal of treatment is improvement in the severity of the signs and symptoms of the disorder.

There are two major ways to conceptualize the use of psychiatric medications to treat personality-disordered patients. First, one can use medication to treat Axis I illnesses that commonly plague patients with personality disorders such as episodes of major depression. Very often, antidepressants are used to treat depression in patients with personality disorders. In this sense, one is not so much treating the personality disorder as treating the comorbid condition. In a similar fashion, patients with diabetes are prone to foot infections. When a diabetic takes an antibiotic for an infected foot, the antibiotic is not treating the diabetes per se but is treating a comorbid condition or complication of the diabetes. However, treating the infection often makes the diabetes easier to manage. We see this as analogous to treating depression and other Axis I illnesses in patients with personality disorders.

Second, medications can be used to manage symptoms of the personality disorder itself. Among the list of personality disorders, troubling symptoms include impulsivity, paranoia, anxiety, and affective instability. These are all symptoms that can to some degree be addressed with medication as well as with psychotherapy. It is important to realize that the personality disorder itself is not necessarily being treated; instead, medications are used to attenuate certain target symptoms. Thus, an individual with narcissistic personality disorder who is taking medication still has the personality disorder, but with successful treatment may experience less distress and dysfunction.

DSM-IV divides the personality disorders into three clusters, and within each of the three clusters, the respective disorders have a number of overlapping characteristics. To some extent, the medications that are suitable for one personality disorder are likely to be helpful treatments for the other disorders within the same cluster. This is an important consideration, because several of the personality disorders have been overlooked altogether in the treatment literature that has accumulated to date. For this reason, we will discuss treatment recommendations not for each individual personality disorder but for each of the three clusters.

11.2 CLUSTER A: ODD AND ECCENTRIC PERSONALITY DISORDERS

11.2.1 Brief Description and Diagnostic Criteria

The Cluster A personality disorders, described as the odd and eccentric disorders, include paranoid personality disorder (PPD), schizotypal personality disorder (STPD), and schizoid personality disorder (SPD). Each of these three disorders bears certain similarities to schizophrenia, yet none of the three meets the full criteria for an Axis I psychotic disorder. Some have described the Cluster A disorders as attenuated or mild forms of schizophrenia. In Chapter 4, we noted that the symptoms of schizophrenia have commonly been divided into positive and negative symptoms. The positive symptoms include delusions and hallucinations; the negative symptoms include social withdrawal, affective flattening, and lack of volition. In one sense, these personality disorders represent milder presentations of these positive or negative symptoms. PPD, for example, is chiefly comprised of a softer version of the paranoid delusions that often contribute to the positive symptoms of schizophrenia. On the other hand, the social isolation of SPD bears striking resemblance to the negative symptoms of schizophrenia. Meanwhile, STPD exhibits lesser variations of both the positive (e.g., illusions, paranoia, and magical thinking) and negative (e.g., social withdrawal) symptoms of schizophrenia. Recognizing this debatable relationship to schizophrenia may help to understand the direction that research has taken into the causes and possible treatments of Cluster A personality disorders.

In distinguishing the Cluster A disorders one from another, the unique feature of a paranoid personality is a constant distrust of others. Paranoid people may be interested in having friends; however, they repeatedly drive them away. They become convinced that others are plotting against them, jealously guard their privacy, and bear grudges against those who presumably have slighted them. In this way, there is a repeated rejection of the people whom they want to befriend them and they often end up hostile and alone.

The patient with a SPD is also alone and socially isolated. However, it does not result from a fearful and hostile pushing away of others so much as it does from having no or minimal interest in pursuing relationships with others. The schizoid person simply does not want to be around other people; however, the schizoid person is not troubled by the paranoia of the person with a PPD.

Those with STPD also have few friends, and they are likewise seen as aloof and eccentric. While the schizotypal patient may be paranoid, similar to the patient with PPD, there are other features that set him/her apart. Namely, the schizotypal patient is prone to preoccupations with magical or superstitious thinking and reports unusual sensations including bodily illusions. (S)he may find special personal meaning in the way things are arranged about him/her or in events reported in the news.

11.2.2 Prevalence and Risk Factors

The rates of the Cluster A personality disorders range from 1% to 3% of the general population. STPD appears to be somewhat more common than its counterparts. Of the three, the rate for SPD is probably the hardest to determine. Schizoid patients are least likely to seek treatment on their own, and their unobtrusive (although eccentric) life style seldom leads others to insist they seek treatment. So it is difficult to be entirely certain just how many people have schizoid personalities.

Research into the risk factors for Cluster A personality disorders has focused on genetic factors. In particular, many researchers have looked for a shared genetic linkage between these disorders and schizophrenia. Only schizotypal personality appears to be genetically linked to schizophrenia. It may be that STPD exists on a biological continuum with schizophrenia. In other words, STPD could theoretically be a far milder variant of Axis I schizophrenia. There is less evidence linking PPD or SPD to schizophrenia; nevertheless, certain characteristic symptoms of these other disorders also overlap with schizophrenia.

Other research has studied how childhood experiences may contribute to the development of a Cluster A personality disorder. Psychosocial explanations revolve around the observation that there is a degree to which distrust is a rational response to certain experiences. Some have theorized that cold and indifferent parenting can contribute to the disinterest in relationships that characterizes Cluster A disorders. It is in fact likely that a genetic predisposition to subclinical personality traits that mirror the positive and/or negative symptoms of schizophrenia may combine with certain developmental experiences that conspire to the development of a Cluster A personality disorder.

11.2.3 Initial Evaluation and Differential Diagnosis

The evaluation should include a careful history and a thorough mental status examination. At the time of the initial visit, the patient will likely be in crisis. It will be this crisis that has brought him/her into treatment, and its resolution will be the first order of business. However, as longer-term care is anticipated, one will do well to screen for potential maladaptive personality traits and personality disorders even at this juncture. This of course means collecting not only a cross-sectional history of the acute events but a longitudinal history as well. This history is ideally obtained not only from the patient but also from close friends or family members as well. Friends or family can usually give a clearer picture of how the patient was doing both before the crisis that led to evaluation and in its aftermath. The mental status examination is an essential part of the evaluation. Even a casual conversation will often uncover some of the odd and eccentric beliefs in behavior of these patients. But some skill is needed to distinguish between these oddities and the more severe disturbances of thought and perception that characterize Axis I psychotic disorders.

Schizophrenia and Schizophreniform Disorder. As mentioned earlier, the Cluster A personality disorders share many features with schizophrenia but are generally less severe and do not produce the same degree of social and occupational impairment that is seen with schizophrenia. Cluster A patients may have vague suspicious thoughts, but they will not suffer from the systematized delusions of schizophrenia. They may also have unusual sensory experiences but not the frank hallucinations seen in schizophrenia. Finally, these patients may have trouble organizing their thoughts when under stress, but the gross disorganization of thought and behavior that characterizes schizophrenia will not be seen in patients with Cluster A personality disorders. In essence, the difference between the Cluster A personality disorders (especially STPD) and schizophrenia is quantitative not qualitative. The symptoms of schizophrenia generally have less severe parallels in these personality disorders.

Delusional Disorder. It can be particularly difficult to distinguish patients with delusional disorder from those with a PPD. Again, the key difference is one of degree. The patient with a paranoid personality has vague suspicious thoughts, but these do not reach delusional intensity. In addition, the delusions of someone with a delusional disorder are often very focused and circumscribed, whereas the paranoia of the patient with PPD is more generalized.

Major Depressive Disorder with Psychotic Features. One severe subtype of depression is characterized by both depressive and psychotic symptoms. Unless a longitudinal history is available, it can be difficult to distinguish a patient with a psychotic depression from a depressed patient who has a comorbid Cluster A personality disorder. Some qualitative features may be helpful, but these are not wholly reliable. The most prominent psychotic symptoms of a psychotic depression tend to be delusions and auditory hallucinations, but these sometimes present in an attenuated form more reminiscent of Cluster A symptoms.

The key to distinguishing a Cluster A personality disorder from a psychotic depression is to obtain a history of the patient prior to the acute episode of depression. This includes both the past history from medical and psychiatric records and collateral history provided by friends and family. In the case of a psychotic depression, the odd, eccentric behavior will be a recent development only in the context of the depression. The patient with the Cluster A personality disorder will be said to have always been a bit odd. But exercise caution here; for patients with a Cluster A personality disorder can become depressed and that depression can occasionally have psychotic features. Whether the patient has always been known to be odd and eccentric or not, if (s)he is now having frank hallucinations or delusions then this cannot be explained by a personality disorder.

Obsessive-Compulsive Disorder (OCD). The obsessions and compulsive rituals of OCD can sometimes resemble the odd behavior of a Cluster A personality disorder. The most helpful difference may be that the rituals of OCD are ego-dystonic while the eccentricity of Cluster A personality disorder tends to be ego-syntonic. Usually, the OCD patient is aware of the excessive nature of the obsessions and wishes to be rid of them. The Cluster A patient tends to embrace the odd behavior and draw comfort from it.

Avoidant Personality Disorder (APD) and Social Anxiety Disorder. These illnesses share the tendency toward social withdrawal and isolation with the Cluster A disorders. There is, however, a critical difference that can help make the distinction. The patient with social anxiety disorder is greatly troubled by the fact that (s)he may have so few friends or feel uncomfortable around them. (S)he would, in general, much prefer to feel more at ease in a social setting. This differs from the Cluster A personality disorders. The patient with SPD is indifferent to the fact that (s)he has few friends; in fact, (s)he prefers to not have any. The patient with STPD is in a somewhat more intermediate position, feeling very anxious around others and perhaps preferring to have more friends, but also finds it easy to withdraw into a life of isolated fantasy.

11.2.4 History of Pharmacological Treatment

Antipsychotics. Of the three Cluster A disorders, only STPD has received any attention in medication research. A handful of studies have evaluated the effectiveness of low doses of high potency typical antipsychotics in treating STPD. These preliminary studies suggest that typical antipsychotics can produce modest benefit for the odd behavior, paranoia, and social isolation of STPD. But it also appears that these patients may be more sensitive to the side effects of these medications than patients with schizophrenia. These limited studies all used low doses of antipsychotics. To our knowledge, there have been no long-term studies to evaluate the risk of tardive dyskinesia in patients with STPD as compared to those with schizophrenia.

Formal study of the newer, atypical antipsychotics in the treatment of STPD is limited to a pilot study of risperidone (Risperdal). This study suggested that risperidone, given in low doses (0.5–1.0 mg/day), is well tolerated by patients with STPD and helps reduce the paranoia and social isolation of the disorder. Despite this limited formal study, atypical antipsychotics are increasingly used on an empirical basis by clinicians treating patients with STPD and other Cluster A personality disorders.

Antidepressants. A few studies of the treatment of depression in patients with personality disorders have included subjects with STPD. This limited data also suggests that antidepressants may be helpful additions for these patients.

11.2.5 Current Approach to Treatment

Paranoid Personality Disorder (PPD). There is a relative lack of data to support the usefulness of medications in the treatment of PPD. Nevertheless, clinical observation suggests that psychiatric medications may be helpful for some patients. The biggest problem is typically in getting the paranoid patient to agree to pharmacotherapy.

Most patients with PPD have difficulty acknowledging that their paranoia is a problem. In the perceived absence of a problem, it can be difficult to make the case for treatment to the patient.

In the event that one is able to convince the paranoid patient to take a medication, a trial of a low dose atypical antipsychotic may be warranted.

We prefer low doses of atypical antipsychotics as a first-line treatment. In this way, the threat of extrapyramidal symptoms is largely avoided without having to use a second anticholinergic medication to offset antipsychotic side effects. Risperidone 0.25–0.5 mg/day, olanzapine 2.5 mg/day, quetiapine 25 mg/day, ziprasidone 20 mg/day, or aripiprazole 2.5–5 mg/day are reasonable starting doses. The typically higher doses used to treat schizophrenia are usually not necessary.

Schizoid Personality Disorder (SPD). Again, there is very little research to guide in the selection of medications to treat the schizoid patient. If we conceptualize the symptoms of SPD as most resembling the negative symptoms of schizophrenia, the choice of agents would tend to favor the atypical antipsychotic drugs as opposed to the older typical antipsychotics. Consequently, we also recommend low doses of an atypical antipsychotic as a first-line treatment for SPD.

Schizotypal Personality Disorder (STPD). Patients with STPD most closely resemble those with schizophrenia. They have parallels to both the positive and negative symptoms of schizophrenia. Of the three Cluster A personality disorders, most medication research has been conducted in STPD though it is also quite limited.

Antipsychotics in a few small studies have been shown to be helpful. To date this research is limited to typical antipsychotics. Nevertheless, the excellent track record of atypical antipsychotics in treating schizophrenia and the lower burden of side effects lead us to recommend atypical antipsychotics as a first-line treatment for STPD as well. Low doses of risperidone, olanzapine, quetiapine, ziprasidone, or aripiprazole are all reasonable options. If no therapeutic effect is observed, doses should be increased.

The limited research data available also suggests a role for antidepressants in the treatment of patients with STPD. We recommend using a SSRI/SNRI antidepressant that could theoretically address both depressive symptoms and those of the personality disorder. In our experience, schizotypal patients can usually tolerate a more conventional dose increase schedule than can patients with PPD.

11.3 CLUSTER B: DRAMATIC AND EMOTIONAL PERSONALITY DISORDERS

11.3.1 Brief Description and Diagnostic Criteria

Cluster B includes the so-called dramatic and emotional disorders. This group is comprised of antisocial personality disorder (ASPD), borderline personality disorder (BPD), narcissistic personality disorder (NPD), and histrionic personality disorder (HPD). In each of these disorders, the person is attention seeking, is emotionally unstable, and finds it difficult to conform to social norms. Unlike the odd and eccentric Cluster A patients and the anxious and withdrawn Cluster C patients, those with Cluster B personality disorders seldom escape clinical attention for very long. The disruptive nature of these personality disorders often leads them to psychiatric or legal intervention no later than their early adult life.

From a clinical perspective, there are two dimensions of Cluster B symptoms that are targeted with medication treatment: impulsivity and affective instability. By impulsivity, we mean poor self-control, which can take several forms ranging from childish acting out to dangerous fits of rage. When upset by some stressful life event, Cluster B patients can be dangerously aggressive toward themselves or others. These patients may get into fights or arguments, and they are prone to suicidal threats and gestures. The second component, affective instability, describes severe disturbances in mood that can fluctuate very rapidly. With minimal provocation, these patients can plunge into a severe depression or an agitated state that resembles the manic phase of bipolar disorder.

Despite overlapping symptoms in the Cluster B personality disorders, there are key distinguishing characteristics of each. Antisocial personality disorder (ASPD) is characterized by a patient's lack of concern for and repeated victimization of others. For this reason, the popular terms sociopath and psychopath have been applied to those with an antisocial personality. This indifference toward the feelings of others can also be seen in those with a narcissistic personality, but in that case it serves to feed the narcissist's need for admiration. The antisocial patient instead uses others as a means to gain some material or financial benefit. Of course, there are patients who fulfill the diagnostic criteria for both narcissistic and antisocial personality disorders.

Borderline personality disorder (BPD) is the most common and best described of all the personality disorders. These patients lack stability in their relationships, have a clouded concept of their own identity, and have trouble modulating their mood. Their lives are often characterized by chaos as they frantically seek intensely close relationships to fill the emptiness of their lives but then destroy those relationships for fear of losing their own identity. They are prone to repeated and abrupt emotional decompensation that can be manifested by paranoia, hallucinations, depression, and a variety of dissociative symptoms.

The patient with histrionic personality disorder (HPD) craves attention from others and resorts to excessive displays of emotion to obtain it. Like the narcissistic patient, the histrionic demands to be the center of attention but typically without the haughty arrogance of the narcissist. They are also manipulative and easily frustrated like the antisocial patient but able to experience remorse and are generally more law abiding. Finally, the histrionic patient experiences mood instability much like the borderline patient but is typically not as severely impaired. Whereas the borderline patient is frequently self-destructive and feels chronically empty, the histrionic patient is usually not prone to these more severe disturbances.

The last of the four Cluster B disorders, narcissistic personality disorder (NPD), is chiefly characterized by an arrogant demand for admiration from others who are seen as tools to achieve those ends. The narcissistic patient's haughty persona is a thin veneer; (s)he is extremely vulnerable to criticism and may react in rage when perceiving that (s)he is being attacked. The narcissistic patient exhibits a superficial charm reminiscent of those with histrionic and antisocial personalities. The narcissist, however, uses this charm to gain social recognition and status, whereas the antisocial patient uses it for material gain.

11.3.2 Prevalence and Risk Factors

The prevalence of the Cluster B disorders parallels that of the other personality disorders. Rates range from 1% to 2% of the general population for each of the Cluster B disorders. Despite these rates that parallel the other personality disorder clusters, Cluster B patients command a considerable bulk of our clinical resources. In particular, BPD is the most common of the personality disorders receiving care in most psychiatric settings. The dramatic nature of the Cluster B disorders leads to severely disruptive and erratic behavior that commands clinical attention as opposed to the quiet and unobtrusive psychopathology seen in the Cluster A and Cluster C disorders.

Of particular interest is the gender distribution of the Cluster B personality disorders. Three out of four patients diagnosed with BPD are women. Likewise, most patients diagnosed with HPD are females as well. In contrast, ASPD is much more common among men. There has been considerable discussion as to whether these are true differences or whether they result from diagnostic biases.

Similarly, there has also been considerable research into genetic contributions to the Cluster B disorders. There does appear to be a genetic contribution to the vulnerability for developing ASPD, which parallels similar findings in HPD. By contrast, there is less evidence of genetic inheritance of NPD and BPD, though this cannot be ruled out at present.

Even more emphasis has been placed on psychological and sociological theories of Cluster B personality disorders. Much of this centers on the frequent observation that children who are victims of physical or sexual abuse are at increased risk for developing BPD as adults. These early traumatic experiences may lead to insecure attachments that ultimately contribute to the adulthood fears of abandonment and disturbances in self-image. Although the ties to child abuse are not as clear with ASPD, parents who are critical or who mete out harsh or erratic discipline appear to increase the risk that their children will develop ASPD. In contrast, NPD is often though not always associated with neglectful and unfeeling parents. It is postulated that adults with NPD may have, as a child, missed out on the parental warmth and encouragement that fosters a personal sense of intrinsic self-worth. Instead, the child develops a sense that his/her value is contingent on success and accomplishment. The result of course is a fragile individual who desperately seeks adulation from others as a reaffirmation of self-worth.

11.3.3 Initial Evaluation and Differential Diagnosis

Patients with Cluster A disorders may go unnoticed for years until some crisis leads to the need for acute psychiatric treatment. By contrast, Cluster B patients more often come with an extensive history dating back to childhood of encounters with mental health professionals, school counselors, and legal authorities. However, like other personality-disordered patients, Cluster B patients typically present for treatment when in crisis.

The symptoms of Cluster B disorders resemble a spectrum of Axis I disorders including mood disorders, anxiety disorders, impulse control disorders, and even certain medical illnesses. For this reason, a careful assessment including the collection of a longitudinal history is essential to achieving an accurate diagnosis. If a haphazard evaluation leads one to overlook the potential presence of a Cluster B diagnosis, then even short-term crisis management can be compromised. There are a number of diagnoses that need to be entertained as part of the differential diagnosis of the Cluster B disorders.

Bipolar Disorder. Each of the Cluster B disorders, but in particular BPD, can be difficult to distinguish from a bipolar spectrum illness. The attention seeking of HPD and NPD, the grandiosity of NPD, the pleasure seeking of HPD and ASPD, and the legal encounters of ASPD are all reminiscent of the symptoms of mania or hypomania. But these pale in comparison to the patient with BPD who at times may be indistinguishable from a bipolar patient during the manic and hypomanic phases of bipolar disorder.

The diagnosis can be clarified by collecting a retrospective history both from the patient and from a collateral source, such as a friend or family member. A history of bipolar disorder will include episodes of illness that typically arise spontaneously, last for days or weeks, and often result in a decreased need for sleep during times of hypomania or mania. The periods of affective lability in the patient with a Cluster B personality generally do not arise in this spontaneous fashion but are instead triggered by a stressful life event. In addition, they seldom last as long as the typical hypomanic/manic phase of bipolar illness and are generally not associated with a decreased need for sleep.

Delusional Disorder and Schizotypal Personality Disorder. In our experience, patients with BPD at times resemble those with Cluster A personality disorders or those with an Axis I psychotic disorder. Psychotic symptoms in the BPD patient, although intense, tend to arise in the context of some stressor and to be relatively short-lived. This usually takes the form of a brief psychotic disorder. Placing the BPD patient in a structured and supportive environment usually hastens the resolution of these psychotic symptoms. By contrast, the psychotic symptoms of a patient with a delusional disorder or a Cluster A personality disorder are long-term and potentially intractable even with antipsychotic treatment.

Substance Use Disorder. Patients abusing alcohol or other substances may be prone to erratic behavior reminiscent of the Cluster B personality disorders. If these behaviors occur exclusively in a context of intoxication or during periods of heavy substance use, then the diagnosis of a Cluster B personality disorder is not warranted. Instead, treatment should be focused on the substance use disorder. This is not to say, however, that substance use disorders and Cluster B personality disorders cannot occur together. In fact, the difficulty that these patients have in self-soothing leaves them especially vulnerable to substance abuse.

Dependent Personality Disorder (DPD). Like the borderline patient, those with DPD have an intense fear of abandonment. The two disorders, however, can be distinguished by the way that the patient responds to this fear. The DPD patient makes attempts at appeasement in an effort to sustain the relationship that (s)he fears losing. The borderline patient, however, may react with rage or resort to extortion to keep from losing the relationship.

Dissociative Identity Disorder (DID). There are numerous similarities between this dissociative illness, which includes multiple personality disorder, and BPD. Patients with both disorders are commonly victims of physical or sexual abuse as children and experience intense shifts in affect and periods of dissociation. Some clinicians in fact discount the validity of DID as a psychiatric diagnosis, contending that the phenomena of DID can be explained by BPD. In fact, severely ill BPD patients very much resemble the prototypical patient with DID.

The observation that certain regressive forms of psychotherapy may contribute to the emergence of personalities lends some credence to this argument. Some argue that DID is an iatrogenic ally created when the shifting mood states of a borderline patient are assigned personalities. This issue obviously needs further research, and its resolution is beyond the scope of our discussion. However, it reminds us that those with severe dissociative disorders should carefully be screened for BPD.

11.3.4 History of Pharmacological Treatment

Of the Cluster B personality disorders, only BPD has received any significant degree of attention in terms of psychopharmacology research. However, the implications of that research as well as other studies into the treatment of nonspecific aggression may be applicable to antisocial, narcissistic, and histrionic personalities as well.

Tricyclic Antidepressants (TCAs). The tricyclic antidepressants are believed to act mainly by increasing norepinephrine and/or serotonin reuptake inhibition. The few studies that have evaluated their use in the treatment of BPD were not promising. Given those disappointing results in conjunction with the prominent side effects and danger in overdose, TCAs are not generally recommended for the treatment of BPD.

Monoamine Oxidase Inhibitors (MAOIs). The MAOIs work in a unique fashion by blocking the activity of an enzyme that degrades each of three key brain transmitters: norepinephrine, dopamine, and serotonin. These widespread effects on several brain transmitter systems make the MAOIs a potentially very effective class of medications for a variety of disorders. A few small studies have evaluated the usefulness of the MAOIs in the treatment of BPD and found them moderately helpful for the impulsivity associated with this illness. Unfortunately, the requirements for strict dietary restrictions due to a risk of hypertensive crisis severely limit the usefulness of MAOIs in the treatment of BPD. These restrictions are a particular concern when treating patients who have problems with impulsivity and are therefore likely to have difficulty maintaining the dietary regimen. For this reason, although they may theoretically be helpful, MAOIs should only be used to treat BPD after other more easily tolerated medications have been tried and have failed. In the near future, so-called reversible MAOIs that appear to avoid the need for diet restrictions may become available. If so, this will allow us to reconsider their use in the treatment of BPD. For more information regarding the use of MAOIs, please refer to Chapter 3.

Serotonin-Boosting Antidepressants. Many of the new generation of antidepressants including the SSRIs and several of the so-called atypical antidepressants act primarily by increasing serotonin neurotransmission. There is good evidence that increasing serotonin activity provides a calming effect that may counteract both the impulsivity and the affective lability characteristic of the Cluster B personality disorders. Of these medications, fluoxetine has received the most study. It appears to reduce aggression, lability, and impulsivity in BPD patients.

The serotonin-boosting antidepressants are a reasonable first choice in the treatment of impulsivity and mood lability in patients with BPD. They have proved effective in the limited studies conducted thus far and are also easy to tolerate and safe in overdose. This last factor is an important consideration when treating BPD patients prone to impulsivity and at times suicidal behavior with little advance warning. When these antidepressants are used, they should be started and titrated in a similar fashion to that used in the treatment of major depression and other mood disorders, though in our experience patients with BPD may at times require doses far in excess of what is typically prescribed. For more information on the use of fluoxetine and the other serotonin-enhancing antidepressants refer to Chapter 3.

Lithium. Lithium is a mood stabilizer that clearly treats both the manic and the depressive phases of bipolar disorder. Because the affective instability of the Cluster B disorders resembles the mood fluctuations of bipolar disorder, it is easy to understand why lithium has been studied in the treatment of BPD. Lithium appears to be effective in decreasing impulsivity and reducing mood lability in patients with BPD, though again the available data is limited. For this reason, lithium may have a role in the treatment of Cluster B personality disorders. However, like the MAOIs, this usefulness is limited by its side effects and danger in overdose. Lithium should be prescribed at doses similar to those used to treat bipolar disorder with target therapeutic lithium blood levels from 0.8 to 1.2 mEq/L. Common side effects of lithium include frequent urination, drowsiness, and tremor. Lithium can also cause birth defects if ingested during the first trimester of pregnancy. Appropriate laboratory testing must be performed before starting lithium and repeated during ongoing treatment. For more information on the safe use of lithium please refer to the discussion of bipolar disorders in Chapter 3.

Norepinephrine-Blocking Medications. There is some evidence that exaggerated norepinephrine activity plays a part in the affective instability, aggression, and impulsivity seen in a variety of psychiatric illnesses including the personality disorders. This may in fact explain why the TCAs, which tend to increase norepinephrine activity, have not proved helpful for BPD. Based on this theory, beta blockers, which interfere with norepinephrine activity at the beta-adrenergic receptor, may help in the treatment of impulsivity and aggression in those with BPD.

The beta blocker propranolol (Inderal) has been studied in the treatment of impulsivity and appears to provide a slight benefit to some patients. It can be started at a dose of 10 mg taken three times per day and increased gradually to a maximum of 200 mg/day. Side effects of propranolol include depression, fatigue, lowered blood pressure, impotence, and a worsening of symptoms in patients with asthma.

Anticonvulsants. The similarity of BPD not only to bipolar disorder but also to the mood lability seen in temporal lobe epilepsy (TLE) has led to trials of the anticonvulsants (some of which are also mood stabilizers) carbamazepine (Tegretol) and valproic acid (Depakote, Depakene) in treating BPD. Both of these antiseizure medications appear to provide some benefit in reducing the aggression, impulsivity, and mood lability seen in patients with BPD. One recent controlled study of valproic acid in the treatment of BPD found it helpful for the core symptoms of depressed mood, suicidality, irritability, and aggression; however, the study was plagued by a high dropout rate, highlighting the difficulty in sustaining treatment adherence in these patients.

Of the two, valproic acid is somewhat easier to tolerate, is less likely to cause interactions with other medications, and has more data supporting its effectiveness in BPD. Therefore, when anticonvulsants are to be used, we typically recommend valproic acid as the first-line agent. Valproic acid can be started at 500 mg/day and increased as needed up to 2000 mg/day in a stepwise fashion. The common side effects of valproic acid include indigestion, hair loss, and tremor. Valproic acid rarely causes an irritation of the liver as well as a reduction in platelet count. In addition, valproic acid, like lithium, is known to cause birth defects and should be avoided during pregnancy. There is some evidence that, in women of reproductive age, valproic acid may cause polycystic ovary syndrome (PCOS), a cause of diminished fertility. Like lithium, certain laboratory tests must be conducted before starting valproic acid. For more information on the safe use of valproic acid, please refer to the discussion of bipolar disorders in Chapter 3.

Carbamazepine is believed to be effective in BPD, though the data is far less robust than with valproic acid. It is prescribed at doses up to 1200 mg/day. Like valproic acid, it can also cause birth defects and requires laboratory monitoring including serum levels. For more information on the use of carbamazepine, please refer to the discussion of bipolar disorder treatment in Chapter 3.

Other anticonvulsants such as oxcarbazepine, gabapentin, and lamotrigine may also be helpful in treating the affective lability and impulsivity seen in BPD, though little data is available. Each of these medications is discussed in Chapter 3.

Benzodiazepines. Benzodiazepines have not been well studied in patients with Cluster B personality disorders; however, they do appear to be used on a relatively common basis. There are two scenarios in which benzodiazepines have been used to treat BPD. First, they have been used on an as-needed basis in the inpatient setting to manage severe agitation and aggression. Lorazepam (Ativan) is often preferred because it can be administered either orally or by injection. Usually, 0.5–2 mg of lorazepam can help to calm an agitated patient with BPD. This can then be repeated as needed every 2–4 hours, though care should be taken not to overly sedate the patient.

Some clinicians also use oral benzodiazepines on an outpatient basis for the long-term management of impulsivity and aggression. Two benzodiazepines have been most commonly used in this setting. These are the short-acting alprazolam (Xanax) and longer-acting clonazepam (Klonopin). In the limited research on benzodiazepines in the treatment of BPD, it appears that benzodiazepines can at times worsen the impulsivity of these patients. To our understanding, this is similar to the disinhibiting effects of alcohol. For this reason, we cannot recommend benzodiazepines for routine outpatient use in the treatment of BPD, though the relative risks and benefits should be weighed for each patient and some patients do benefit from the anxiolytic effects of the benzodiazepines. See Chapter 4 for a comprehensive discussion of the benzodiazepines.

Antipsychotics. Paranoia has long been a recognized symptom of BPD. In addition, these patients are at risk for psychotic decompensation in the face of acute stress. This typically takes the form of an Axis I brief psychotic disorder and often quickly resolves with increased social support and the alleviation of the stressors.

Nevertheless, patients with severe BPD may be especially vulnerable to repeated psychotic decompensation and therefore arguably need prophylactic treatment with an antipsychotic. In addition to their proven ability to treat psychotic symptoms, antipsychotics also have tranquilizing effects that can counteract impulsivity and mood lability. They do so while avoiding the potential disinhibition that can be caused by benzodiazepines.

Several studies have evaluated the use of low doses of the typical antipsychotics. These include studies of high potency antipsychotics such as haloperidol, medium potency antipsychotics such as loxapine, and low potency antipsychotics such as chlorpromazine and thioridazine. In general, the studies have shown that antipsychotics reduce impulsivity and protect from psychotic decompensation.

There are, of course, risks with long-term use of conventional antipsychotics. The most concerning is an irreversible movement disorder known as tardive dyskinesia. Nevertheless, some particularly fragile patients with BPD may require long-term antipsychotic treatment. If so, atypical antipsychotics are recommended.

Recently, atypical antipsychotics have been used, not surprisingly, in the treatment of Cluster B personality disorders. The atypical antipsychotics include risperidone, olanzapine, quetiapine, ziprasidone, and aripiprazole. In addition to the published data on atypical antipsychotics in the treatment of Cluster B personality disorders, their proven track record in treating schizophrenia and other psychotic disorders, their growing popularity in treating the lability of the bipolar disorders, and their superior side effect profile when compared to the typical antipsychotics have led many clinicians to prefer them when treating fragile BPD patients. Preliminary studies with risperidone and olanzapine in the treatment of BPD indicate that atypical antipsychotics can, for some patients, effectively manage both the depressive symptoms and aggressive behaviors associated with the disorder.

Despite the limited formal study, atypical antipsychotics are increasingly used in the management of BPD and other Cluster B syndromes. We have found the atypical antipsychotics to be remarkably helpful in low doses (e.g., ziprasidone 20–40 mg/day, risperidone 0.25–1.0 mg/day, quetiapine 25–100 mg/day, aripiprazole 2.5–5 mg/day) when treating more severe forms of BPD, though additional research is needed. Because of the common side effects of weight gain, and possibly diabetes, we would discourage the long-term use of either clozapine or olanzapine in this group. See Chapter 5 for a comprehensive discussion of the antipsychotic drugs.

Omega-3 Fatty Acids. There has been at least one report that the omega-3 fatty acid ethyl-eicosapentaenoic acid, administered at 1 gram daily under study as an antidepressant, may be helpful in the treatment of moderately severe BPD. It is tempting to speculate that the omega-3 fatty acids might possess mood-stabilizing properties, but this needs to be studied in controlled trials.

11.3.5 Current Approach to Treatment

Borderline Personality Disorder (BPD). In selecting a treatment for BPD, there are two key considerations. First, one should choose the treatment that will address each of the primary symptoms of the disorder: impulsivity, associated aggression, and mood instability. Second, the medication should be safe, both in terms of side effects at therapeutic levels and in the event of a deliberate overdose attempt. As mentioned previously, the safety and tolerability of the medication are especially important when considering that patients with BPD are prone to impulsive acts such as intentional overdose as well as repeated periods of medication noncompliance.

Of the various medications available, we believe that the serotonin-boosting antidepressants best fit these dual goals as a first-line treatment. They are easy to take, possess a favorable side effect profile, and require a once daily dosing regimen that improves adherence. They are also comparatively safe in overdose. They provide a moderate degree of improvement in impulsivity, as well as in mood lability. Fluoxetine is the best studied in this patient population and therefore is a reasonable first choice; however, in our experience any of the SSRIs and the serotonin-boosting atypical antidepressants venlafaxine, duloxetine, nefazodone, and mirtazapine all appear to be effective in some patients.

Often, BPD may not respond adequately to antidepressant therapy alone. In such cases, atypical antipsychotics or anticonvulsants are reasonable choices for augmentation. One can use the prevailing target symptoms to guide treatment selection. When vague paranoia or periods of frank psychotic decompensation are most prevalent, we suggest using an atypical antipsychotic to augment the antidepressant, though we have also found them exceptionally helpful in patients with severe impulsivity and mood lability.

Alternatively, severe impulsivity or aggression can also be treated by anticonvulsant augmentation, particularly with valproic acid. When these initial steps have failed, other therapies can be tried including augmentation with lithium or propranolol or initiation of a monoamine oxidase inhibitor.

It is important to recognize the fact that the cornerstone of treatment for BPD is psychotherapy. All patients should ideally be treated with a combination of psychotherapy and pharmacotherapy.

Antisocial Personality Disorder (ASPD). As mentioned earlier, there have been no studies that have specifically investigated the use of medications to treat ASPD. Nevertheless, medications may provide some benefit. The target symptoms of ASPD for medications are impulsivity and aggression. Thus, we can apply what we have learned from BPD and other nonspecific studies of aggression. In our experience, serotonin-boosting antidepressants and anticonvulsants may provide a modest degree of benefit for patients with ASPD.

When using these medications, just as when conducting psychotherapy with an antisocial patient, it is important that the treatment be designed in a manner that the patient will remain motivated and adherent. The focus of treatment should not be directed toward developing a superego, but instead on helping the patient see the adverse consequences of antisocial behaviors. If the ASPD patient can recognize how his/her impulsivity and aggression are harmful to him/herself, it may increase the motivation for treatment.

Histrionic Personality Disorder (HPD). HPD has also received remarkably little study, but we can perhaps extrapolate from our experiences with BPD. HPD shares with BPD the target symptom of mood instability. Although medications seldom play a significant role in the treatment of HPD, SSRIs/SNRIs may provide some benefit in alleviating depression as well as in reducing affective lability.

Narcissistic Personality Disorder (NPD). Medications have not been studied to any extent in the treatment of NPD. In our experience, antidepressants are often used to treat these patients, but more so for the common comorbid depression than for the personality disorder itself. It is not clear to what extent, if any, medications may be helpful in treating the target symptoms of NPD itself.

11.4 CLUSTER C: ANXIOUS AND FEARFUL PERSONALITY DISORDERS

11.4.1 Brief Description and Diagnostic Criteria

The so-called anxious disorders of Cluster C include avoidant personality disorder (APD), dependent personality disorder (DPD), and obsessive–compulsive personality disorder (OCPD). Like the Cluster A disorders, these personality disorders are typically unobtrusive and may escape clinical detection for many years. Over time, patients adapt their life styles to these illnesses by decreasing their social contacts in an effort to minimize anxiety. In so doing, they further decrease the likelihood of encountering mental health professionals.

APD is distinguished by its pervasive pattern of social introversion. Avoidant patients feel inadequate and are particularly sensitive to criticism from others. As a result, they structure their lives to minimize contacts with others, thereby decreasing the potential for finding themselves in an embarrassing situation. They are loath to try new activities and avoid meeting people for fear of stumbling into an embarrassing situation. They are restrained in their relationships and have difficulty expressing emotions for fear of embarrassment and ridicule.

Like those with an avoidant personality, patients with OCPD also have difficulty expressing emotions. They complain that they have difficulty experiencing any emotion and consequently feel that life is passing them by. The key characteristic of obsessive–compulsive personality is control. These patients are driven to maintain strict control of themselves and of the surrounding environment. As a result, they become inflexible and inefficient. They often are incapable of completing assignments at work or school due to an exaggerated insistence on perfection but cannot delegate work to others for fear they will not do it correctly. They have difficulty expressing their feelings in relationships for fear of being emotionally vulnerable. They so dread making any wrong decision that they may seek advice from an inexhaustible supply of confidants for even the most trivial of decisions. Ultimately, they have difficulty making any decision and find themselves stuck in a life without change or progress as they watch others move on and leave them behind.

DPD patients also have extreme difficulty making decisions. They do not trust themselves to make the right decision, but unlike the OCPD patient who does not trust anyone else's judgment, the dependent patient will gladly hand over decision-making to others. The defining characteristic of the dependent personality is an exaggerated need to be cared for such that patients develop an intense fear of abandonment. They allow others to make decisions for them and take responsibility for their lives.

11.4.2 Prevalence and Risk Factors

Like the other personality disorders, Cluster C disorders occur at a rate of about 1–2% in the general population. APD appears to be evenly distributed between men and women. DPD is somewhat more common in women, but OCPD is slightly more common in men.

Genetic studies of these disorders have focused on the likelihood that introversion is an inherited character trait. There does appear to be a considerable genetic component to introversion that in turn increases the risk of developing a Cluster C personality disorder. In addition to introversion, the obsessionality seen in OCPD also appears to have an inherited basis that may contribute to the risk of developing that disorder.

Psychological theories of the Cluster C disorders have focused on parent–child interaction. It is believed that APD may arise when parents who are overly cautious and overprotective raise a child with an introverted temperament. Similar parent–child interactions may contribute to the risk of DPD. By contrast, most theorists believe that OCPD emerges from the combination of an introverted and obsessional temperament in a child raised by authoritarian yet detached and unemotional parents.

11.4.3 Initial Evaluation and Differential Diagnosis

These patients will often present with complaints of depressed mood or anxiety. The depression frequently takes the form of dysthymic disorder although these patients are at increased risk for major depressive disorder as well. Anxiety is often a symptom of the personality disorder itself, though comorbid Axis I anxiety disorders are occasionally present. Similar to the other personality disorders, there is a differential diagnosis that should be considered in patients who have a Cluster C personality disorder.

Schizoid Personality Disorder, Schizotypal Personality Disorder. Like the patient with APD and to a lesser extent DPD, those with Cluster A disorders also have limited social interaction. The key difference is that the patient with a Cluster A disorder is not interested in pursuing social contact, preferring isolation and with a general lack of concern about his/her degree of social contact. Cluster C patients, on the other hand, are quite distressed by their solitude, and it often becomes a primary motive for treatment.

Social Anxiety Disorder. The generalized subtype of social anxiety disorder can be quite difficult to distinguish from APD. In fact, they appear to occur on a continuum of severity. In both social anxiety disorder and APD, patients are afraid of potentially embarrassing social situations and are generally shy in interpersonal interactions. APD is typically diagnosed when the social inhibition pervades almost all social interaction and has been present since childhood. Thus, differentiating between APD and social anxiety disorder can be diagnostically challenging.

Borderline Personality Disorder, Histrionic Personality Disorders. The patient with DPD shares with these Cluster B patients a fear of abandonment. The two Cluster B disorders can be distinguished from DPD largely on the basis of how the patient attempts to manage this fear. Dependent patients will go to great lengths to preserve a relationship they are fearful of losing. The histrionic patient instead tends to become more flamboyant in order to attract attention in an effort to sustain the relationship. The borderline patient often reacts with anger and may resort to blackmail and manipulation to try to preserve the relationship.

Obsessive-Compulsive Disorder (OCD). Certainly the name suggests that OCD and OCPD are closely related. This is actually somewhat misleading. With OCD, the obsessions are intrusive and distressful (i.e., ego dystonic) thoughts that lead the patient to develop rituals (i.e., compulsions) to alleviate the resultant anxiety. With OCPD, we use the term obsession in a somewhat different way. The OCPD patient is not necessarily prone to obsessions in the form of intrusive thoughts; instead, they display a perfectionistic preoccupation with detail that characterizes their obsessionality. Furthermore, this obsessionality is ego-syntonic. Patients with OCPD purposefully harbor these obsessions in an effort to exert control over themselves and their environment.

Agoraphobia. Agoraphobia also resembles the Cluster C disorders (in particular APD). In both APD and agoraphobia, patients avoid social interaction. The difference lies in the underlying motivation. The patient with APD avoids social contact for fear of criticism and potential humiliation. The agoraphobic patient instead fears being trapped in a situation in which escape would be difficult or embarrassing, especially in the event of a panic attack.

11.4.4 History of Pharmacological Treatment

Of the three disorders that make up Cluster C, only APD has received much attention in medication treatment studies. In addition, much of this has been an extraction of the results of social anxiety disorder treatment studies.

Monoamine Oxidase Inhibitors (MAOIs). As mentioned earlier, the MAOIs are excellent treatments for both depression and anxiety. They act by increasing neurotransmission of three neurotransmitter systems: serotonin, norepinephrine, and dopamine. The MAOIs have been shown to be excellent treatments for generalized social anxiety disorder and therefore may be helpful for APD as well. They appear to help patients feel more at ease and self-confident in social situations.

When treating APD, MAOIs are used in doses similar to those used to treat depression. The primary limitation of the MAOIs is their potential to interact dangerously with certain foods and other medications. This limits their usage in many illnesses, but they remain a viable option for patients who have failed other treatments and can tolerate the life-style changes mandated by taking a MAOI. Please refer to Chapter 3 for more information regarding the MAOIs.

Serotonin-Boosting Antidepressants. The SSRIs have also been studied in the treatment of generalized social anxiety disorder, and paroxetine, sertraline, and venlafaxine are effective. Preliminary data suggests that the serotonin-boosting atypical antidepressants (mirtazapine and nefazodone) may also be helpful. Like the MAOIs, they appear to be effective at doses comparable to those used to treat depression. They may help avoidant patients to gradually increase their social interaction and become more assertive.

These medications are generally well tolerated. Patients with APD should be warned, however, that the treatment effects will not be immediate. In addition, one would be wise to warn them that anxiety can actually be transiently worse for a few days when they begin treatment with one of these medications.

Benzodiazepines. Longer-acting clonazepam and shorter-acting alprazolam have also been used in the treatment of social anxiety disorder, and controlled trials have shown them to be quite effective. In our experience, alprazolam is best suited for discrete periods of intermittent anxiety, though both clonazepam and the new long-acting alprazolam (Xanax XR) are likely effective for long-term treatment.

Norepinephrine-Blocking Medications. As noted in Chapter 5, exaggerated norepinephrine activity has been posited to play a key role not only in impulsivity but in anxiety as well. Therefore, norepinephrine-blocking medications, such as the beta blocker propranolol, have been studied in social anxiety disorder but have been found to be ineffective in the treatment of generalized anxiety disorder. Propranolol and other beta blockers do not reduce anxiety per se, but they can alleviate the physical symptoms that accompany anxiety, namely, profuse sweating, racing heart, dry mouth, and tremor. This can be helpful in patients with APD who are very self-conscious regarding the physical symptoms of their anxiety. They worry that others "see them sweating" and this can set up a vicious cycle in which the anxiety continues to escalate. By blocking these physical symptoms, a beta blocker can help to circumvent this escalation. Propranolol is prescribed at a dose of 10 mg three times per day and can be increased slowly to as much as 200 mg/day. Atenolol is dosed at 50–150 mg/day. The most common side effects of propranolol and other beta blockers are low blood pressure and worsening of asthma symptoms.

11.4.5 Current Approach to Treatment

Avoidant Personality Disorder (APD). We generally recommend following the same pharmacological treatments for APD that are used for the generalized subtype of social anxiety disorder. Because APD is so pervasive, medications should be used on a daily basis as opposed to "as-needed" dosing.

Serotonin-boosting antidepressants or longer-acting benzodiazepines are also both suitable first-line treatments for APD. For APD patients who are also troubled by depression, an antidepressant is obviously preferable. We also prefer to use antidepressants rather than benzodiazepines to treat APD patients who have a history of substance abuse. The current data suggests that any of the SSRIs as well as nefazodone, mirtazapine, and venlafaxine may be helpful. When these do not work, a MAOI is a reasonable alternative provided the patient is willing to commit to the dietary regimen.

Of the benzodiazepines, we prefer using clonazepam or long-acting alprazolam. These can be prescribed once or twice per day.

Dependent Personality Disorder (DPD). Apart from psychotherapy, which is essential, there is simply no data at this time to guide us in making psychopharmacological treatment recommendations for DPD. However, these patients often suffer from comorbid depression or anxiety disorders that invariably require medication treatment.

Obsessive-Compulsive Personality Disorder (OCPD). Despite the similarity in name, OCD and OCPD are not closely related. Therefore, the medications used to treat OCD are not necessarily helpful for OCPD. As a result, we also cannot offer any specific medication recommendations for the treatment of OCPD. The overall anxious nature of the illness and the likelihood that such patients have comorbid depression or anxiety disorders may, however, guide medication selection.

ADDITIONAL READING

Bohus M, Schmahl C, Lieb K. New developments in the neurobiology of borderline personality disorder. *Curr Psychiatry Rep* 2004; 6(1): 43–50.

Koenigsberg HW, Woo-Ming AM, Siever LJ. Pharmacological treatments for personality disorders. In Nathan PE, Gorman JM (eds), *A Guide to Treatments that Work, 2nd Edition*. London, Oxford University Press, 2002, pp 625–641.

Markovitz PJ. Recent trends in the pharmacotherapy of personality disorders. *J Pers Disord* 2004; 18(1): 90–101.

Newton-Howes G, Tyrer P. Pharmacotherapy for personality disorders. *Expert Opin Pharmacother* 2003; 4(10): 1643–1649.

Rivas-Vazquez RA, Blais MA. Pharmacologic treatment of personality disorders. *Prof Psychol Res Pract* 2002; 33(1): 104–107.

Trestman RL, Woo-Ming AM, de Vegvar M, et al. Treatment of personality disorders. In Schatzberg AF, Nemeroff CB (eds), *Essentials of Clinical Psychopharmacology*. Washington DC: American Psychiatric Press, 2001, pp 271–287.

Zanarini MC. Update on the pharmacotherapy of borderline personality disorder. *Curr Psychiatry Rep* 2004; 6(1): 66–70.

12

TRAUMATIC BRAIN INJURY

12.1 INTRODUCTION

12.1.1 Brief Description and Diagnostic Criteria

Although traumatic brain injury (TBI) is not, in and of itself, a psychiatric illness, it nonetheless warrants attention in our discussion of psychiatric medicines for two important reasons. First, it is not unusual for TBI to produce psychiatric symptoms severe enough to require pharmacological treatment. Second, treatment with psychiatric medicines after TBI often raises clinical concerns that are unique to these patients. More specifically, an injured brain is often especially vulnerable to medication side effects. Thus, the medical axiom "first, do no harm" is particularly important when treating TBI patients and must be considered when deciding whether to use psychiatric medicines, and if so, what medicines to use, and at what doses.

12.1.2 Prevalence and Risk Factors

Approximately 2 million people suffer head injuries each year in the United States alone. Of these, nearly 500,000 will be hospitalized and nearly 100,000 will suffer

Principles of Psychopharmacology for Mental Health Professionals
By Jeffrey E. Kelsey, D. Jeffrey Newport, and Charles B. Nemeroff

long-term disability as a result. The most common cause for head trauma, accounting for over one-half of all cases, is motor vehicle accidents. Other frequent causes include accidental falls, assaults, and sports-related injuries. Not surprisingly, men are twice as likely to suffer head trauma. Further, head injuries are most likely to occur in young adults, most often due to motor vehicle accidents. Another increase in the vulnerability to head injuries occurs late in life with falls being the most common cause in this group.

12.1.3 Presentation and Clinical Course

By definition, most patients who suffer a serious TBI present to an emergency room in the immediate aftermath of the traumatic event. However, patients may also be brought to medical attention days or even weeks after an apparently mild head injury when the symptoms are delayed or so subtle that they initially escaped detection. In some instances, patients may even visit a clinic unaware that their psychiatric symptoms are attributable to a remote head injury. One extreme example is so-called dementia pugilistica that occurs after years of repeated minor TBIs over the course of a boxer's career.

Well-defined emergency medical protocols guide the initial treatment of a patient immediately after TBI in an effort to limit the scope of the injury. Those treatment steps are beyond our discussion and won't be recounted here. Instead, we'll focus on the reasons that patients who have suffered a TBI come to the attention of mental health care providers. Four factors influence the presentation and course of psychiatric symptoms in brain-injured patients. First is the location of the injury. As we discussed at length in Chapter 2, the brain is a highly organized organ that carries out distinct and highly specific functions within each brain region. Thus, an injury to one area may be likely to cause a mood disturbance, to another area psychotic symptoms, and to yet other areas no psychiatric symptoms at all.

The second factor is the extent of the injury. Obviously, a more extensive injury is likely to cause a wider range and more severe set of psychiatric symptoms. In addition, because the brain heals slowly and sometimes incompletely, the extent of TBI also affects the patient's clinical course. Patients with greater injury experience a more prolonged period of recovery and are more likely to be left with residual deficits once the healing is complete. The extent of a brain injury depends both on the mechanical force of the trauma and the body's attempts to respond to the trauma. Blunt trauma is associated with brain swelling, a dangerous situation because the brain is confined to the space available within the skull. Consequently, brain swelling can lead to brain tissue compression. Moreover, the natural inflammatory response to injury sometimes releases substances that are toxic to nerve cells and can actually damage more brain matter in the hours after a traumatic injury. This is why well-conceived emergency and critical medical care is important. Immediate care can limit the secondary damage done after the initial injury.

The third factor to influence the likelihood of psychiatric complications after TBI is the patient's health prior to the injury. Elderly patients, those with preexisting medical disease or psychiatric illness, and those who have abused alcohol and other substances are more likely to experience psychiatric complications after TBI.

Finally, disruptions in the patient's social support network contribute to the risk of psychiatric complications after TBI. This can be a problem both during the patient's initial grief shortly after the TBI, or later, during the long and often arduous process of rehabilitation. For example, a family's initial optimism for full recovery may turn to disappointment and even disillusionment when their loved one develops behavioral problems such as impulsivity or lability that interfere with their efforts to be helpful and supportive. The patient may even become a target of the family's unconscious (or conscious) anger for being injured, which in turn can engender guilt and even suicidal thoughts on the part of the patient.

Clinical Vignette

Mr. Thomas was a 54-year-old male veteran who had served in Vietnam where he received a gunshot wound to the front of his skull. Over the previous 5 years he had been admitted to the psychiatric unit of the local Veterans Administration hospital and received a variety of diagnoses including bipolar disorder, major depressive disorder, alcohol abuse, borderline personality disorder, and schizoaffective disorder. On a Friday afternoon, he was admitted with alcohol intoxication and suicidal ideation. Late that evening a call came from the ward for a request to involuntarily commit him and transfer him to a locked unit. The nursing staff explained that he became belligerent and would not follow directions. Upon asking Mr. Thomas his understanding of what they wanted him to do he was not able to answer with any degree of detail. Informal mental status testing revealed evidence of frontal lobe dysfunction with perseveration, he was stimulus bound and with a significant degree of confabulation. The next day on rounds these deficits were still present. Formal neuropsychological testing revealed significant impairment of his frontal lobe functioning and led to placement in a brain injury rehabilitation program with moderate results.

This is an example of a patient with TBI who had not previously been diagnosed. The nature of his injury was such that it was difficult, if not impossible, for him to follow more than a two-step command. After each hospitalization he would quickly progress to a situation where he was not cognitively equipped to respond appropriately. Only after looking for evidence of a TBI was an appropriate treatment setting procured for him.

In our experience, victims of TBI most often come to the attention of mental health care providers when referred by other clinicians. Their first psychiatric encounter may be a consultation during the initial postinjury hospitalization or later during active rehabilitation. Patients may also be referred for mental health treatment during the postconvalescent phase when faced with the realization that some of their physical deficits may be permanent. As we mentioned earlier, TBI patients infrequently seek psychiatric care on their own, because they are often unaware that their psychiatric symptoms are a consequence of a past brain injury.

12.1.4 Initial Evaluation and Differential Diagnosis

During the initial interview with a patient who has suffered a head injury, a complete description of the occasion when the injury occurred should be obtained. Where was your head struck and by what? Did you lose consciousness? How long were you out? Did you go to the hospital? How long did you stay there? Did you have headaches, dizziness, nausea, or visual problems after the injury? Were you confused or especially sensitive to light after the injury? How severe were these problems and how long did they last? These are all important questions that can provide clues as to how severely the "brain" was injured during a "head" injury. It's also important during the first evaluation to gather certain collateral information such as: (1) the patient's psychiatric and medical history prior to the injury; (2) the patient's history of substance use prior to the injury; (3) a list of the patient's current medications including over-the-counter remedies and "as-needed" doses of sedatives and pain relievers; and (4) the character and time course of both physical and psychiatric symptoms since the injury, taking care to identify any temporal association between the two. Collecting this information at the beginning of the evaluation can not only aid in determining the severity of the brain injury but also in identifying the often overlooked contributing factors to your patient's psychiatric problems.

Unless the TBI has caused severe cognitive impairment (i.e., dementia), most patients after TBI can provide an accurate and insightful description of their physical and cognitive impairment. However, they often have less insight into the nature and severity of many of the common psychiatric symptoms that follow TBI. For this reason, the initial assessment should also include an interview with the patient's family members and friends, if they are available. Interviews with other health care providers (e.g., doctors, nurses, physical and occupation therapists) can also be extremely helpful.

In many, if not most, instances the TBI victim has had an extensive medical evaluation prior to referral for mental health care. If this is not the case, or if there has been a marked change in the patient's mental status since the most recent medical workup, then a thorough medical assessment is again mandatory. A comprehensive evaluation will also include a battery of neuropsychological tests. Neuropsychological testing is helpful in assessing attention, memory, concentration, and several aspects of the brain's executive function such as abstraction and problem solving. Performed by a neuropsychologist, these tests can not only help identify the regions of the brain that have been most severely injured but can also detect subtle cognitive and behavioral changes that may dictate certain modifications in the approach to treating the patient.

Brain imaging (preferably MRI) to look for evidence of structural damage is essential after TBI. MRI, while more expensive and time-consuming, can sometimes detect small brain lesions that are missed by CT, especially in the frontal and temporal lobes that are common sources of psychiatric complications after TBI. In addition, an electroencephalogram (EEG) can detect seizure activity or other signs of abnormal brain function. Although they are not yet part of the routine post-TBI evaluation, the so-called functional brain imaging techniques such as positron emission tomography (PET) or functional MRI (fMRI) may be able to identify areas of abnormal brain function when CT, MRI, and EEG have detected no problems.

Because TBI is not itself a psychiatric syndrome, there is no differential diagnosis to review. However, there are two dimensions to consider in understanding the psychiatric complications of TBI. The first is whether the brain trauma is a direct or indirect cause of the psychiatric syndrome. Using post-TBI depression as an example, we may ask if the mood disturbance is an immediate consequence of dysfunction in the injured part of the brain. If so, then the depression is a "neuropsychiatric" illness. On the other hand, the depression may be triggered by the stress arising from the other disabilities imposed by the injury and/or the imposing demands of prolonged rehabilitation. This is a "psychiatric" illness. At an earlier time, this distinction was called functional versus organic, but as we discussed in Chapter 2, such labels can be misleading. Although it may be reasonable to argue that the direct "neuropsychiatric" consequences of TBI can (at least theoretically) be distinguished from its indirect "psychiatric" consequences, this distinction is often hard to draw in clinical practice. We believe, in fact, that most psychiatric problems after TBI are likely a consequence of interacting neurobiological, psychological, and social factors: that is, they are biopsychosocial in origin and require a biopsychosocial orientation to treatment.

12.2 APPROACHES TO TREATMENT

12.2.1 Post-TBI Depression

The full spectrum of depressive symptoms including depressed mood, anhedonia, lack of energy, and even suicidal thoughts may strike as many as 25% of patients who experience a TBI. Depression in these patients not only exacts a tremendous psychosocial toll but also interferes with their participation in physical and occupational rehabilitation. As a result, long-term functional recovery from TBI can be sorely compromised by depression. Potential treatments for post-TBI depression include conventional antidepressants and stimulants (see Table 12.1).

Antidepressants. Depression after TBI is routinely treated with antidepressant medicines. Although all antidepressants are potentially helpful, antidepressants prone to burdensome side effects, particularly sedative and anticholinergic side effects, should generally be avoided, as they are likely to be tolerated poorly by these patients. In addition, antidepressants that may increase the risk for seizure, such as many of the older tricyclic antidepressants (TCAs) and bupropion (Wellbutrin), should be avoided because post-TBI patients as a rule are already more vulnerable to seizures.

The TCAs were once widely used to treat depression in brain-injured patients, but they have been replaced as first-line treatments by the so-called selective serotonin reuptake inhibitors (SSRIs) including citalopram (Celexa), fluoxetine (Prozac), fluvoxamine (Luvox), paroxetine (Paxil), sertraline (Zoloft), and, most recently, escitalopram (Lexapro). In addition to relieving depression, these serotonin-enhancing antidepressants have the advantage of treating anxiety and behavioral disturbances that can also follow TBI. The newer atypical antidepressants have not been used extensively in these patients, but they may be considered in those patients who fail to respond to an adequate SSRI trial.

Although the ultimate therapeutic dose of an antidepressant when treating a depressed patient after TBI often parallels those used when treating other depressed patients, the starting dose and the frequency of dose increases should generally be cut in half to help ensure that the brain-injured patient isn't saddled with problematic side effects. One exception to this conservative approach occurs when the depression has become immediately life threatening. In other words, your patient may need to be treated more aggressively if (s)he is actively suicidal or the neurovegetative symptoms of the depression are leading to medical compromise. Please refer to Chapter 3 for more detailed information regarding the use of antidepressants.

Stimulants. Stimulant medicines, particularly methylphenidate (Ritalin) and dextroamphetamine (Dexedrine), may also be helpful for treating depressed patients after TBI. The stimulants especially deserve consideration when (1) the patient is not responding to treatment with an antidepressant alone, (2) the patient's depression is so disabling that his/her health is being compromised and rapid clinical improvement is necessary, or (3) the patient's depression is marked not by anxiety and agitation but by lethargy and disinterest that is interfering with rehabilitation. In addition to depression, stimulants have also been used to treat apathy and chronically diminished arousal in patients who have suffered TBI. Interestingly, some evidence suggests that stimulants paradoxically increase the appetite of many patients after TBI.

Stimulants must, of course, be used with caution after TBI. They may rarely cause psychotic symptoms such as paranoia but are more likely to cause uncomfortable nervousness, insomnia, or agitation. In addition, sudden discontinuation of stimulants may even worsen depression. Like the antidepressants, stimulants should be started at half the usual dose and titrated more slowly. Please refer to Chapter 8 for more detailed information about stimulant medicines.

12.2.2 Post-TBI Apathy

Injury to certain areas within the brain's frontal lobes may produce a syndrome that resembles depression but without depressed mood or a sad affect. Instead, this apathetic syndrome is marked by a lack of motivation, little emotional response, profound psychomotor slowing, and disengagement from social interaction. Antidepressants, stimulants, and medicines that specifically boost dopamine activity have been tried when treating apathy after TBI (see Table 12.1).

Antidepressants. As a rule, medicines that increase dopaminergic activity in the brain seem to work best when treating post-TBI apathy. Most antidepressants, however, work primarily by increasing serotonergic and/or noradrenergic activity.

TABLE 12.1. Medication Strategies for Traumatic Brain Injury Syndromes

Medicine	Post-TBI Syndrome								
								Behavioral Disturbances	
	Depression	Apathy	Mania	Psychosis	Anxiety	Delirium	Dementia	Mild	Severe
Anticonvulsant carbamazepine			2					3	2
Anticonvulsant valproic acid			1					3	1
Antidepressant SSRI	1	3			1			1	2
Antidepressant, atypical	2	3						2	3
Antipsychotic, typical			3	2		2			3
Antipsychotic, atypical			2	1		1			2
Benzodiazepine			3		3			3	3
Beta blocker								3	2
Buspirone					2			2	2
Cholinergic enhancers							1		
Dopamine enhancers	3	2							
Lithium			2						3
Stimulant	3	1				3			3

Key: 1—first-line treatment; 2—second-line treatment; 3—may also be considered.

Consequently, most conventional antidepressant medicines have not proved especially helpful for treating patients who have become apathetic after TBI.

A handful of antidepressants do activate the dopaminergic system and at least theoretically may be helpful for apathy. For example, the older monoamine oxidase inhibitors (MAOIs) increase dopamine activity in addition to serotonin and norepinephrine, but MAOIs are not a wise choice for most patients who have suffered TBI. The MAOIs require adherence to a strict diet, have problematic and even dangerous interactions with a wide range of other commonly used medicines, and can complicate blood pressure control. MAOIs should only be used to treat apathy or depression in brain-injured patients when other alternatives have been exhausted. Bupropion (Wellbutrin) has been reported to increase dopaminergic activity, though its effect in this regard is quite small. However, immediate-release bupropion, as we mentioned earlier, increases the risk for seizure and is generally avoided in these patients. Among the antidepressants that are more tolerable and more widely used after TBI, sertraline has the greatest impact on the dopaminergic system, but no data is available on the effectiveness of sertraline especially at higher doses for treating apathy after TBI.

Stimulants. Methylphenidate (Ritalin) and dextroamphetamine (Dexedrine) are the most widely used and perhaps the most effective medications when treating post-TBI apathy. They act by enhancing the activity of dopaminergic, noradrenergic and, to a certain extent, serotonergic brain systems. Stimulants act quickly to relieve the core symptoms of apathy, and they may also improve the impairments in attention and short-term memory that often follow TBI. Please refer to Chapter 8 for more information about the stimulants.

Dopamine-Boosting Medications. Amantidine and bromocriptine, which work almost exclusively by enhancing dopaminergic activity, also appear to be beneficial for apathy in patients who have suffered TBI. These medicines are most commonly used to treat Parkinson's disease and as such are widely prescribed by neurologists. Although they have not found widespread use in the psychiatric community, they are perfectly reasonable alternatives for treating post-TBI apathy, especially when the patient is having trouble tolerating stimulants. Bromocriptine is started at 2.5 mg given twice daily. The dose can be increased every 5–7 days until reaching a maximum of about 60 mg/day. Amantidine is also taken twice daily and is started at 50 mg per dose. The maximum daily dose of amantidine is 400 mg/day. The newer anti-Parkinsonian dopamine agonists, pramipexole and ropidirole, are also theoretically useful when treating post-TBI apathy but have not been studied.

12.2.3 Post-TBI Mania

As many as 1 in 10 patients experience episodes of mania akin to those seen in bipolar disorder after TBI. Right-sided brain injury, particularly in the frontal lobe or so-called limbic structures, has the greatest potential to produce a "secondary mania." The manic symptoms include euphoric or irritable mood, decreased need for sleep, mood lability, rapid speech, impulsivity, and disinhibited and sometimes aggressive behavior. Potential treatments for post-TBI mania include lithium, anticonvulsants, and the so-called atypical antipsychotics (see Table 12.1).

Lithium. Despite arguably remaining the single most effective medication for bipolar disorder, lithium is less often used when treating patients who experience manic episodes due to TBI. For one thing, lithium is often less effective for these patients than the anticonvulsants. Perhaps more importantly, lithium is more likely to produce a neurotoxic syndrome that can worsen any cognitive impairment that may already accompany TBI. Nevertheless, lithium remains a viable alternative when other treatments have failed. If lithium is used in these patients, it should be started at a single 300 mg/day dose and slowly increased to ensure that the patient tolerates it well. The target blood lithium level is just above the lower end of lithium's therapeutic range (i.e., slightly above 0.5 mEq/L). This may improve its tolerability in these sensitive patients. If an adequate response is not witnessed at these lower levels, then the dose can be escalated in a stepwise fashion with frequent monitoring of medication concentrations. Please refer to Chapter 3 for a more comprehensive discussion of the risks, benefits, and guidelines for lithium therapy.

Anticonvulsants. Although there has been little systematic study in TBI patients, the anticonvulsant medications valproate (Depakote, Depakene) and carbamazepine (Tegretol, Equetro) have gained widespread acceptance as the preferred treatments for post-TBI mania. In addition to treating mania, the anticonvulsants, unlike lithium, offer the added advantage of protecting the post-TBI patient from seizures. Of the two, valproate is less prone to problematic drug–drug interactions and perhaps easier to tolerate, and consequently, it is generally used as a first-line treatment. The dosing and laboratory monitoring guidelines when treating brain-injured patients with valproate or carbamazepine follow those used when treating patients with bipolar disorder, though the post-TBI patient may have more difficulty tolerating medication levels in the higher end of the accepted therapeutic range. Please see Chapter 3 for a more extensive discussion of valproate and carbamazepine.

The newer anticonvulsants, lamotrigine (Lamictal), gabapentin (Neurontin), oxcarbazepine (Trileptal), topiramate (Topamax), and zonisamide (Zonegran), among others, have not often been used to treat secondary mania after TBI. Furthermore, they may not be as effective as the primary mood stabilizers when treating bipolar disorder. Thus, we cannot vouch for their effectiveness or tolerability when treating post-TBI patients and cannot recommend them for routine use. However, they may find use as second- or third-line treatments for post-TBI patients who experience manic episodes that are not responding to valproate, carbamazepine, or lithium.

Antipsychotics. Because the primary mood stabilizers typically have a delayed onset of action by several days to as long as a week or two, other medications are commonly used to manage the acute symptoms of mania during the interim period between beginning treatment and achieving a therapeutic response. Antipsychotics have been widely used in this regard in treating both bipolar patients and patients who experience manic episodes after TBI. For years, the most common medications used in this regard were the high potency typical antipsychotics such as haloperidol (Haldol) and fluphenazine (Prolixin). The typical antipsychotics are now seldom used when treating brain-injured patients except in low doses and for very brief periods of time. This change is in part due to evidence that the typical antipsychotics may interfere with the brain's healing capacity after injury. As a result, we reserve our use of typical antipsychotics, particularly during the first few months after TBI when the brain is actively healing, until other treatment alternatives have failed.

With the arrival of the newer atypical antipsychotics including olanzapine (Zyprexa), quetiapine (Seroquel), risperidone (Risperdal), ziprasidone (Geodon), and aripiprazole (Abilify), we now have alternatives that avoid the problematic side effects of the older antipsychotics. As a group, the newer atypical antipsychotics are clearly efficacious in managing the symptoms of acute mania, but there is little data with these drugs in TBI. In contrast to lithium and the anticonvulsants, the atypical antipsychotics offer the added advantage of treating not only manic but psychotic symptoms. Furthermore, both olanzapine (Zyprexa) and aripiprazole (Abilify) are indicated for maintenance therapy in bipolar disorder, though not in the context of traumatic brain injury. These are some of the issues that surround the use of atypical antipsychotics when treating mania secondary to TBI. We certainly cannot at this time recommend atypical antipsychotics as the primary treatment for mania after TBI, but they can certainly be useful. Specifically, atypical antipsychotics can be used for treating post-TBI mania (1) when beginning the acute phase of treatment while waiting for a primary mood stabilizer to take effect, (2) when the manic post-TBI patient also has psychotic symptoms, and (3) as part of a long-term augmentation strategy when the response to the primary mood stabilizers has been unsatisfactory. Please refer to Chapters 3 and 5 for more information regarding the use of atypical antipsychotics.

Benzodiazepines. Like the atypical antipsychotics, benzodiazepines, most commonly lorazepam (Ativan) and clonazepam (Klonopin), can be used to manage the symptoms of acute mania while awaiting the response to a newly started primary mood stabilizer. Long-acting clonazepam offers the convenience of infrequent dosing (one to three times daily), while lorazepam offers the versatility of an intermediate duration of action coupled with several modes of administration (oral, intramuscular, intravenous). We must recommend, however, that special care be taken when giving benzodiazepines to brain-injured patients. These patients are especially vulnerable to certain problematic side effects of benzodiazepines such as confusion, excessive sedation, and disinhibited behavior. As a result, we discourage the use of benzodiazepines on any long-term basis when treating the brain-injured patient, but they may be helpful on a short-term as-needed basis.

12.2.4 Post-TBI Psychosis

Psychotic symptoms such as delusions, hallucinations, or disorganized thinking may be both a transient and a chronic complication after TBI. Furthermore, psychotic symptoms after TBI can occur both independently or in conjunction with depression, mania, dementia, or delirium. The potential treatments for psychosis after TBI include the typical and atypical antipsychotics (see Table 12.1).

Typical Antipsychotics. Low doses of high potency typical antipsychotics such as haloperidol or fluphenazine (0.5–2 mg given once or twice daily) are generally quite effective for psychotic symptoms after TBI. Unfortunately, as noted earlier, many post-TBI patients are susceptible to the extrapyramidal side effects of these medicines, especially if there was any injury to brain regions such as the basal ganglia. Low potency antipsychotics are not a viable alternative, because their anticholinergic and sedative effects are equally, if not more, problematic for patients who have suffered TBI. We recommend using typical antipsychotics, even for psychotic symptoms, as briefly as possible and in the lowest effective dose, if at all. Fortunately, there are now alternatives.

Atypical Antipsychotics. Although they have never been thoroughly studied in the treatment of brain-injured patients, the problems associated with the older typical antipsychotics have by default led to an increasing preference for the newer atypical antipsychotics. These medicines are generally better tolerated by patients who have suffered TBI, though drowsiness can be a problem. The atypical antipsychotics are now generally regarded as first-line treatments for the brain-injured patient with psychotic symptoms. Doses should be started low (e.g., aripiprazole 5–10 mg, olanzapine 2.5 mg, quetiapine 12.5–25 mg, risperidone 0.25–0.5 mg, ziprasidone 10 mg) and increased slowly over several days to weeks. Please refer to Chapter 4 for a more thorough discussion of atypical antipsychotics.

12.2.5 Post-TBI Anxiety

The full complement of anxiety syndromes including panic, generalized anxiety, obsessive–compulsiveness, and post-traumatic stress disorder can arise in the aftermath of TBI. In fact, anxiety may be the most common neuropsychiatric complication of TBI. Anxiety appears to be most likely to arise when the injury occurs to the right side of the brain. The treatment alternatives for post-TBI anxiety parallel those used when treating anxiety disorders and include serotonin-boosting antidepressants, buspirone (Buspar), and the benzodiazepines (see Table 12.1).

Antidepressants. The most widely used psychiatric medicines with the broadest range of application in TBI patients are undoubtedly the SSRI antidepressants. They are well tolerated, unlikely to worsen any of the preexisting deficits associated with TBI, and offer relief from not only depression but also impulsivity and virtually all variants of anxiety in these patients. As such, SSRIs are the preferred first-line treatment for all anxiety disorders after TBI. Other newer antidepressants that also work (at least in part) by boosting serotonin activity, namely, mirtazapine (Remeron), nefazodone (Serzone), venlafaxine (Effexor XR), and duloxetine (Cymbalta) can also be considered, but they have not been well studied in patients with TBI. In general, apply the "start low and go slow" philosophy even with the well-tolerated SSRIs, to treat a brain-injured patient. Please refer to Section 12.2.1 in this chapter for more information about the use of antidepressants after TBI. You may also refer to Chapter 5 for a comprehensive discussion of the treatment of anxiety disorders.

Buspirone (Buspar). Buspirone also warrants consideration for post-TBI anxiety. Its usefulness is limited to the generalized form of anxiety, though it may also be helpful for TBI patients who are struggling with agitation and impulsivity. Although buspirone has not been well studied in patients after TBI, they have little trouble tolerating it. In fact, buspirone's most noteworthy feature is perhaps that it causes such minimal side effects. Buspirone should be started at 10 mg/day given in two divided doses. The daily dose can be increased by 5 mg every 4 or 5 days. Please refer to Chapter 5 for more information regarding buspirone.

Benzodiazepines. We've already discussed the potential problems of using benzodiazepines when treating brain-injured patients, namely, confusion, sedation, and disinhibition. These problems largely preclude their use when treating anxiety disorders after TBI. In our experience, the problems of benzodiazepines generally outweigh their potential benefits in this group of patients. As a rule, we recommend avoiding the use of benzodiazepines when treating anxious TBI patients except those experiencing severe and frequent panic attacks that require more rapid relief than can be provided by an antidepressant.

12.2.6 Post-TBI Dementia and Delirium

It goes without saying that TBI can impair cognition. In the first few days to a month after an injury to the brain, some patients suffer from a delirium characterized by disorientation, periodic agitation, and a fluctuating level of consciousness. Once this delirium resolves, the brain-injured patient with cognitive impairment may gradually regain intellectual function over the next several months. Unfortunately, some patients will not fully recover and will permanently suffer from the cognitive and functional impairments of dementia.

The treatment of post-TBI delirium generally consists of minimizing medication use to avoid further compromise of the patient's level of arousal. The introduction of medications to manage the agitation of delirium is, however, occasionally warranted. Interestingly, the options that have been suggested employ two diametrically opposed theoretical approaches. The only current treatment options for dementia due to TBI are the acetylcholine-enhancing medicines used to improve cognition in patients with Alzheimer's disease (see Table 12.1).

Antipsychotics. Dopamine-blocking antipsychotics can be used to manage the agitation and psychotic symptoms that accompany delirium. Generally, low doses of high potency antipsychotics such as haloperidol have been most often used, though risperidone, ziprasidone, and other atypical antipsychotics are gaining increased acceptance. Because, as we mentioned earlier, some evidence indicates that typical antipsychotics may slow the brain's recuperative processes after injury, these medicines should be used sparingly. Please refer to Section 12.2.4 of this chapter and Chapter 10 for recommendations regarding the use of antipsychotics when treating cognitively impaired patients.

Stimulants. An alternative approach that has been suggested for post-TBI delirium is to use a dopamine-enhancing psychostimulant such as methylphenidate (Ritalin) or dextroamphetamine (Dexedrine). In using these medicines, the theory is to treat not the agitation of delirium, but the impaired arousal that underlies it. Stimulants have the added advantage of improving memory and attention, which may prove helpful during rehabilitation, but they have the potential to worsen the agitation that often accompanies delirium. For this reason, we do not recommend the routine use of stimulants for post-TBI delirium. If a stimulant is going to be used, start at low doses that are increased only with careful ongoing observation. Please see Section 12.2.2 of this chapter and Chapter 8 for a more comprehensive discussion of stimulant therapy.

Acetylcholine-Boosting Medications. Medicines used to treat Alzheimer's disease and other forms of dementia, which act by slowing the elimination of acetylcholine, have shown some benefit in limited studies of patients with dementia due to TBI. These medicines, including tacrine (Cognex), donepezil (Aricept), galantamine (Reminyl), and rivastigmine (Exelon), need to be studied further in TBI patients. Until then, they represent a reasonable treatment alternative for patients with mild-to-moderate dementia after TBI. In other words, what do you have to lose? These medicines may be helpful with only a small chance of problematic side effects. The dosing guidelines for treating Alzheimer's disease should be applied when using these medicines to treat TBI patients with dementia. Please see Chapter 10 for a more extensive discussion of these medicines.

12.2.7 Post-TBI Behavioral Disturbances

Yet another neuropsychiatric complication of TBI is a set of behavioral disturbances including impulsivity, irritability, disinhibition, and/or aggression. These symptoms appear to be more likely to arise when the brain injury involves the temporal or orbitofrontal brain regions. Treatment options for these disruptive behavioral syndromes include antidepressants, buspirone, anticonvulsants, antipsychotics, beta blockers, and stimulants (see Table 12.1).

Antidepressants. In our experience, clinicians who are trying to manage the behavior of impulsive or aggressive patients too often overlook antidepressants. Antidepressants are often just as effective as anticonvulsants, antipsychotics, or benzodiazepines, especially when managing mild-to-moderate behavioral disturbances. Furthermore, antidepressants are generally easier to use and easier to tolerate than these alternatives. Once again, the SSRIs are best studied and so represent the favored first-line treatment for managing mild-to-moderate behavioral lability in TBI patients. The new so-called atypical antidepressants may also be considered though they have yet to be studied.

One particular variant of the post-TBI behavioral disturbances, nighttime agitation, can be managed successfully with low bedtime doses of sedating antidepressants such as trazodone (25–50 mg) or nortriptyline (10 mg). These antidepressants may calm the patient and help him/her to sleep while avoiding the potential for confusion or disinhibition posed by other commonly used sleep medicines.

Buspirone. In addition to its primary indication for generalized anxiety, buspirone may also be helpful for mild agitation and impulsivity in brain-injured patients. As we discussed in Section 12.2.5, the potential for significant side effects when taking buspirone is quite small. Starting at low doses (5 mg given twice daily) and increased in 5 mg/day increments every 3–5 days, most patients require a total daily dose of 45–60 mg/day before significant benefit is observed.

Anticonvulsants. Given their effectiveness in treating patients with bipolar illness, valproate and carbamazepine have gained considerable favor for treating behavioral lability in other patients as well. They are often quite effective and may, in fact, be the most effective medicines for the long-term treatment of patients prone to especially severe behavioral disturbances. However, these medicines do require regular laboratory monitoring and are more likely to cause problematic side effects than antidepressants or buspirone. For this reason, we reserve our use of valproate or carbamazepine for those patients with severe behavioral disturbances or those who have not responded well to more conservative measures. To our knowledge, the newer anticonvulsants have not been widely used to treat patients who experience behavioral lability after TBI; therefore, we cannot recommend their use. Please refer to Section 12.2.3 and Chapter 3 for more information regarding the anticonvulsants.

Lithium. With a long history of effectively managing the agitation that accompanies manic episodes of bipolar disorder, lithium has also been used to treat aggression and lability in other groups of patients. Although lithium is sometimes helpful for patients with impulse control disorders, it has not proved especially beneficial for TBI patients with behavioral disturbances (other than mania) and is prone to inducing neurotoxicity in these vulnerable patients. Thus, we discourage the use of lithium for TBI patients with behavioral lability that is not due to mania.

Benzodiazepines. The benzodiazepines have long been used when treating behavioral lability, yet with mixed results. Some studies indicate that benzodiazepines are helpful for TBI patients who experience behavioral disturbances, while others suggest that they may actually worsen aggression and other behavioral problems. Given these inconsistent results and recognizing that benzodiazepines can cause confusion and increase the risk of accidental falls, they should seldom be used on a long-term basis for TBI patients. Nevertheless, they remain valuable for short-term use to provide rapid control of severely agitated behavior. For this indication, we prefer using from 0.5 to 2 mg lorazepam, which can be given either orally or as an intramuscular injection.

Antipsychotics. There is also a long history of using the typical antipsychotics to manage severe agitation. In fact, antipsychotics and benzodiazepines are often coadministered when attempting to gain control of an acutely agitated patient in the emergency room or hospital setting. Although low doses of haloperidol or fluphenazine (0.5 mg of either medicine given twice daily) may be beneficial for TBI patients who repeatedly experience episodes of behavioral lability, we generally resort to using typical antipsychotics for these patients only after several alternatives (e.g., antidepressants, anticonvulsants, beta blockers) have failed. We believe that, especially in the absence of psychosis, it is difficult to justify exposing a TBI patient to the side effects and possibility of diminished nerve cell recovery posed by a typical antipsychotic.

The so-called atypical antipsychotics represent one of the newest options for managing disruptive behavioral syndromes. Because they have yet to be studied in patients who have suffered a TBI, we certainly cannot recommend the atypical antipsychotics for routine first-line use. Nevertheless, an atypical antipsychotic might prove helpful when other medicines aren't providing satisfactory results in the management of severe behavioral disturbances. Ziprasidone (Geodon) is available in an injectable form that we have found to be particularly helpful in TBI patients.

Beta Blockers. The beta blockers, which act by interfering with noradrenergic transmission, have been used to manage aggression and other behavioral disturbances in patients who have suffered brain injury due to trauma and stroke for over 25 years. Several beta blockers have been tested including propranolol (Inderal), pindolol (Visken), nadolol (Corgard), and metoprolol (Lopressor). Fat-soluble beta blockers such as propranolol and pindolol more readily cross the blood–brain barrier and are thus better suited to managing psychiatric symptoms such as behavioral lability.

The beta blockers can cause a wide array of side effects including low blood pressure, slowed heart rate, dizziness, fatigue, and impotence. They may exacerbate asthma and depression, though this remains controversial, in vulnerable patients. Symptomatic bradycardia (slow pulse) and depression are probably less problematic when using pindolol, which in addition to blocking noradrenergic activity also increases serotonergic activity.

Propranolol and pindolol have been the most used beta blockers for psychiatric indications. Propranolol can be started at 10–20 mg given two or three times each day, and the dose can be increased every week until a therapeutic benefit is achieved. The total daily dose of propranolol can reach as high as 800 mg when attempting to manage disruptive or aggressive behavior. For ease of use, propranolol can then be switched to the long-acting formulation (Inderal LA) permitting once daily dosing. Pindolol is started at 10 mg given twice daily, and the dose can be increased by 10 mg/day every week until reaching 60–80 mg/day. Pindolol is not available in a controlled-release formulation. If symptoms of dizziness, unsteady gait, or wheezing occur while your patient is taking a beta blocker, the dose should be decreased, or the medicine should be discontinued.

Stimulants. A handful of case reports hint that treatment with stimulants (methylphenidate or dextroamphetamine) can help manage behavioral agitation in patients who have suffered a TBI. Certainly, stimulant therapy helps control the impulsivity and hyperactivity of children with attention deficit–hyperactivity disorder. Despite these encouraging signs, we have to discourage any routine use of stimulants when attempting to manage behavioral lability in TBI patients. Because stimulants have the potential to exacerbate behavioral lability, we recommend that they only be considered when other medication alternatives have been exhausted.

ADDITIONAL READING

Flanagan SR. Psychostimulant treatment of stroke and brain injury. *CNS Spectrums* 2000; 5(3): 59–69.

Glenn MB. A differential diagnostic approach to the pharmacological treatment of cognitive, behavioral, and affective disorders after traumatic brain injury. *J Head Trauma Rehabil* 2002; 17(4): 273–283.

Glenn MB, Wroblewski B. Twenty years of pharmacology. *J Head Trauma Rehabil* 2005; 20: 51–61.

Kennedy R, Burnett DM, Greenwald BD. Use of antiepileptics in traumatic brain injury: a review for psychiatrists. *Ann Clin Psychiatry* 2001; 13(3): 163–171.

Kraus MF, Levin HS. The frontal Lobes and traumatic brain injury. In Salloway SP, Malloy PF (eds), *The Frontal Lobes and Neuropsychiatric Illness.* Washington DC: American Psychiatric Publishing, 2001, pp 199–213.

Perino C, Rago R, Cicolin A, et al. Mood and behavioural disorders following traumatic brain injury: clinical evaluation and pharmacological management. *Brain Injury* 2001; 15(2): 139–148.

Perna RB, Bordini EJ, Newman SA. Pharmacological treatment considerations in brain injury. *J Cogn Rehabil* 2001; 19(1): 4–7.

Rao V, Lyketsos C. Neuropsychiatric sequelae of traumatic brain injury. *Psychosomatics* 2000; 41(2): 95–103.

Whyte J, Vaccaro M, Grieb-Neff P, et al. Psychostimulant use in the rehabilitation of individuals with traumatic brain injury. *J Head Trauma Rehabil* 2002; 17(4): 284–299.

13

MANAGING SIDE EFFECTS

13.1 INTRODUCTION

13.1.1 Organizing This Discussion

What Is a Side Effect? This chapter picks up where Chapters 1 and 2 left off. As we discussed in the earlier chapters, all medications, psychiatric and otherwise, have multiple effects. One takes a medication to achieve a therapeutic effect. Occasionally, a single medication may have more than one therapeutic effect. All other effects are side effects. Different medications may have differing therapeutic and side effects depending on the intended use. For example, trazodone and quetiapine are often prescribed to aid in sleep, and in this instance sedation is the desired effect, yet when used as an antidepressant and antipsychotic, respectively, the sedation is often an unwanted effect. Psychotropic medications typically have multiple effects. First, they usually interact with more than one nerve cell protein, be it a transporter or a receptor. Quite often, one of the medication's receptor or transporter interactions produces the therapeutic effect. The other interactions tend to not be involved in the therapeutic effect and only serve to produce side effects. Sometimes a neurotransmitter will have multiple different receptor types, but the medication interacts with

Principles of Psychopharmacology for Mental Health Professionals
By Jeffrey E. Kelsey, D. Jeffrey Newport, and Charles B. Nemeroff

many of them. Serotonin selective reuptake inhibitors (SSRIs) block the reuptake of serotonin into the cell that released it, and thus increase the action of serotonin, albeit indirectly, at a number of different serotonin receptors. Of these, some help to exert the antidepressant or antianxiety effects of these drugs whereas others mediate the transient nausea or persistent sexual dysfunction. The body has the advantage of what could be called "anatomical specificity"; serotonin is released at a specific cluster of synapses in a particular part of the brain or body. When we prescribe a psychotropic medication, it must pass through the blood–brain barrier to work, and this means that it travels to all parts of the body and interacts not only with the targets that produce the therapeutic effect, but also those targets that produce side effects.

Don't, however, jump to the conclusion that it's always a bad thing when a medication interacts with more than one type of receptor. Sometimes, the combination of interacting with two different receptor types can produce even greater therapeutic benefit or can circumvent certain side effects.

Organizing This Chapter. We debated how to organize this chapter so that it would be user friendly. There are basically three ways to organize this information. First, we could discuss the side effects of each particular medication or class of medications and how they might be managed. This would make the chapter a handy reference for looking up the side effects of a single medication. The problem is that it would be outdated by the time the book is published. New medications are arriving all the time, and an encyclopedic listing of side effects without a context to evaluate them in is not especially useful.

Second, we could organize our discussion by particular types of side effects, such as sedation, sexual problems, or appetite changes. At first glance, this seems rational, but there are shortcomings with this approach as well. The main problem is that a single side effect can occur in several very different ways. For example, benzodiazepines and antidepressants produce a qualitatively and quantitatively different drowsiness. Likewise, antidepressants and antipsychotics cause sexual side effects in different ways. This is an important distinction, because the remedy to a side effect depends in large part on what is causing it. Organizing this chapter in this way could very quickly become quite confusing.

Finally, we could organize our discussion according to the effects that we anticipate when a medication interacts with a particular neurotransmitter system. For example, we could discuss the effects of blocking dopamine, enhancing serotonin, or blocking histamine. We've chosen to organize the chapter in this way. We believe that in so doing, you will not only learn something about managing the side effects of medications, but also be better prepared to anticipate what side effects may arise before the patient even takes a particular medication. This will better position you not only to anticipate a given medication's side effects but also to predict what may happen when two medications are taken together. Furthermore, you'll be better able to take what you learn from this chapter and apply it to new medications in the coming years as they are approved for use.

As we move forward with our discussion, we'll devote a section of this chapter to each of the key neurotransmitter systems that psychotropic medications interact with. We will discuss the following systems: norepinephrine, dopamine, serotonin, GABA, acetylcholine, and histamine. Within each of the sections is a description of the effects that can be anticipated when a medication enhances the activity of that transmitter (reuptake inhibitors or agonists), and the effects to expect when a medication interferes (receptor antagonists) with the activity of that same transmitter. We will then describe strategies that can be implemented to help minimize and/or manage these side effects.

Know that some side effects will not fall neatly within this scheme, because they do not arise from their activity at the nerve cell. Side effects can also occur through direct effects on end organs such as the liver, kidneys, and bone marrow. Such side effects can range in severity from inconvenient to life threatening. Examples of the latter include agranulocytosis (essentially stopping the production of white blood cells), which can be caused by clozapine and carbamazepine, diabetic ketoacidosis, which can be caused by olanzapine or clozapine, Stevens–Johnson syndrome, which can be caused by lamotrigine, changes in kidney or thyroid function, which can be caused by lithium, chemical hepatitis, which can be caused by valproic acid and carbamazepine, and heart beat irregularities, which can be a side effect of tricyclic antidepressants. Clinical management of these side effects includes patient education about their signs and symptoms as well as periodic laboratory testing as a means to detect them sooner rather than later. If and when such a symptom develops, the medication generally is stopped. Because we have discussed these issues in previous chapters, we will not devote any discussion in this chapter to side effects that are not due to effects on nerve cell function.

13.1.2 Recognizing Side Effects

Before a side effect can be treated, one first has to recognize that there is a side effect present. We know this sounds somewhat silly; however, distinguishing a medication side effect from a symptom of the illness that is being treated can be a daunting task. This is no small matter. When the observed symptoms represent a medication side effect, the appropriate response is different than if they are due to the illness. In one case, the dose would likely be reduced, whereas in the other, it might be increased (see Table 13.1). Choosing the wrong direction could either worsen the side effect burden or lead to premature discontinuation of an otherwise successful treatment course. There are several circumstances in which a medication side effect resembles the illness that is being treated. Let's review a few examples.

Loss of Interest in Sex. One of the prominent symptoms of depression is anhedonia, a lack of interest or pleasure in life. Anhedonia is commonly manifested by a decreased libido or a lack of interest in sex. This is different from the sexual dysfunction of delayed ejaculation, delayed orgasm, or anorgasmia seen with all antidepressants that block serotonin reuptake. The problem, however, is that loss of

TABLE 13.1. Side Effects Associated with Neurotransmitter Changes

Transmitter	Side Effects from Increasing	Side Effects from Decreasing
Acetylcholine	Nausea Diarrhea Slow heart rate	Confusion Poor memory Delirium Dry mouth Blurred vision Constipation Difficulty urinating Increased heart rate
Dopamine	Psychosis Loss of appetite Nausea Tics	Sexual dysfunction Parkinsonism Dystonic reactions Tardive dyskinesia Akathisia Menstrual irregularities Breast enlargement Depression (?)
GABA	Drowsiness Lack or coordination Amnesia	
Histamine		Drowsiness Weight gain
Norepinephrine	Anxiety Loss of appetite Insomnia	Depression Dizziness
Serotonin	Anxiety (short-term) Nausea Diarrhea Sexual dysfunction	Depression

sexual desire is also a potential side effect of many of the newer antidepressants, particularly the SSRIs. When beginning treatment for depression, it is often helpful to ask about sexual interest in order to establish a baseline for later comparison. Once treatment has commenced, a periodic review of side effects/symptoms is indicated, such as asking about sexual desire. At times it is often difficult to tell whether the loss of sexual desire is due to a medication side effect or residual depression. In one case, the side effect should be addressed, in the other, a more vigorous treatment of the depression is indicated. One clue to this conundrum is whether the other symptoms of depression have abated in response to antidepressant therapy in the face of worsening sexual function. In that event, the sexual dysfunction is likely a medication side effect.

Akathisia. This is a restless inability to sit still. It is an extremely unpleasant sensation that can arise when a patient is treated with an antipsychotic drug (this is seen much more frequently with older style antipsychotics than with the newer atypical medications) or on rare occasions a serotonin-boosting antidepressant. Unfortunately, worsening psychosis, worsening anxiety, agitated forms of depression, and even mania all resemble akathisia. Again, if this is not recognized as a medication side effect, then raising the patient's dose of medication typically worsens the akathisia. In addition, patients may be treated with anxiety-reducing medications such as benzodiazepines that would otherwise be unnecessary.

There is no definitive way to differentiate akathisia from a worsening of the underlying psychiatric disorder. However, patients with akathisia will often endorse a feeling of needing "to get up and move around," though this does not tend to bring relief. Once there is awareness that this may be a side effect, then judicious use of a medication trial may help to clarify the problem. This is an important point: sometimes, a trial of medication is used to clarify the diagnosis. In this case, if there is a suspicion that the patient is having akathisia, it should be treated. If the symptoms resolve, then the problem is solved. Should the psychotic symptoms worsen, however, the illness itself should be treated more aggressively.

Parkinsonism. As will be discussed later, dopamine-blocking antipsychotics and rarely other psychotropic medications can produce symptoms that resemble Parkinson's disease. This includes an expressionless face, slowed movement, and a stooped posture. In many respects, medication-induced parkinsonism resembles both depression and the negative symptoms of schizophrenia. Again, one must decide if it is the illness or the medication. Do you decrease the medication to remedy the side effect? Or do you increase the medication to treat the illness, anticipating that a higher dose may prove more beneficial (though this is not always what is found)?

In this case, a more careful psychiatric and physical examination can be of help. Although there are admitted similarities to depression and the negative symptoms of schizophrenia, Parkinson's disease is also associated with a resting tremor, called "cogwheel rigidity," and at times drooling. These other symptoms are not typically due to psychiatric illness. If these symptoms are present, one should investigate the possibility of a medication side effect or the presence of Parkinson's disease.

Medication-Induced Delirium. Delirium is an acute confusional state that has a wide range of potential etiologies including infection, metabolic and vascular changes, and as a side effect of medication, the latter perhaps the most common reason. Among psychotropic medications, sedatives, anticholinergics, and toxic levels of lithium, tricyclic antidepressants, or anticonvulsants can all produce delirium. However, a medication-induced delirium may also resemble the agitation of a psychotic illness or the disorganization of an acute manic episode.

Fortunately, there are differences between delirium and psychotic illnesses. Delirious patients will more often experience visual or tactile as opposed to auditory hallucinations. In addition, they will often be disoriented; that is, they cannot tell you where they are, what time it is, or who you are. By contrast, psychotic patients more commonly experience auditory hallucinations (i.e., they hear voices), and although they may make misinterpretations, they are usually well oriented to their surroundings. Physical symptoms can also provide an indication of medication toxicity. Blood pressure or pulse may be abnormal; pupils may be widely dilated or pinpoint and sluggish. The patient may be drowsy, uncoordinated, and staggering about or be incontinent. All of these can help distinguish delirium from psychosis.

13.1.3 General Approach to Managing Side Effects

There are several general approaches to managing the side effects of psychiatric medications. These vary somewhat depending on the severity of the side effect, the anticipated duration of the side effect (transient or longstanding), the availability of countermeasures to control the side effect, and the availability of alternative medications to use thereby avoiding the side effect altogether. Although specific recommendations will be reserved for the discussion of individual classes of medication, there are nevertheless a few general recommendations that apply across the board. Let's take a look at these broader concepts.

Be Patient. Probably the simplest way to manage a side effect is just to wait it out. Granted, this is easier said than done, but sometimes, a side effect that occurs upon starting a new medication resolves within a few days. For example, this is typically the case with the gastrointestinal side effects often experienced by patients prescribed serotonin reuptake inhibitors. Within a few days, a patient beginning a SSRI will become adjusted to the increased levels of serotonin and the stomach queasiness resolves. We find that when advising patients of potential side effects, it helps to reassure them that certain side effects will likely be short-lived.

Change the Medication Schedule. Sometimes simply taking the medication at a different time can relieve a side effect. For example, if drowsiness is a problem, then taking the medication at bedtime may resolve the issue. By contrast, when insomnia is a problem, changing the dose from the evening to the morning may eliminate or at least reduce the problem. If a medication causes nausea or queasiness when taken on an empty stomach, then you should recommend taking the medication after meals. Knowing in advance what potential side effects a medication might have allows us to guide the patient and recommend a schedule before (s)he takes the first dose.

Take a Medication Holiday. Some side effects are not a problem on a daily basis; nonetheless, they can be quite disturbing. The best examples are sexual side effects of some antidepressants or the possible effects of stimulants upon the growth of children with ADHD. One approach has been to skip taking the medication for a brief period of time. For example, those with antidepressant-induced sexual dysfunction have sometimes circumvented this problem by skipping a single day's dose when they plan to have sex. In a similar fashion, parents concerned with the effects of stimulants on their child's growth may have their child skip doses on the weekends or stop taking the medication altogether during the summer break from school. The medication holiday approach can be successful, but it is not without risk. The key dilemma is that skipping doses can undermine the treatment. If too many doses are skipped, the illness may reemerge or in the case of some short half-life antidepressants a discontinuation syndrome may emerge. Defining how many doses are "too many" is a question that can be very difficult to answer.

Split the Dose. Some side effects emerge only when a medication is at its highest (peak) levels. The level of a medication is continually fluctuating in your patient's system between doses. Peak levels usually occur within the first hour or so after each dose though with the advent of a number of sustained-, controlled-, or extended-release preparations, the peak level often occurs 2–4 hours after ingesting the pill. The lowest level, known as the trough level, occurs just before taking the next dose. These swings from peak to trough generally hover around a fairly consistent midpoint known as the steady state.

Even though the steady state remains consistent, the degree to which the peaks and troughs vary from steady state depends on how often the medication is taken. Taking a large dose once a day produces a larger swing from the midpoint to the peak level as compared to twice a day dosing. Taking half the dose twice a day (e.g., taking 50 mg twice a day as opposed to 100 mg once a day) can lower this peak level. The average medication level stays the same, but the peak levels are not as high and the trough levels are not as low. Lowering the peak levels can bypass side effects that emerge only when the medication is at high levels; it is not clear if raising the trough level provides any better treatment outcome.

Splitting the dose is not without drawbacks. Clearly, it is harder to remain adherent with multiple doses per day than it is with a single daily dose. Remembering to take one dose per day is hard enough; remembering a second dose becomes even harder. So by recommending that a patient split the dose, we increase the chance that the patient will forget to take the medication. Fortunately, the various slower release agents on the market remove the need for this strategy, and indeed, in controlled clinical trials the advantage of the extended-release forms appears to be in the realm of fewer side effects, especially early in treatment.

Take a Second Medication as a Countermeasure. Sometimes despite problematic side effects, it may be necessary that a patient remain on a particular medication. This is a good time to address the risk–benefit approach to side effects. The best comparison is not the side effects associated with a particular medication compared to the lack of side effects without taking the pill; it is the side effects of treatment versus the consequences of the untreated disease state. So what if a patient is on a medication that works for them when previous trials have proved unsuccessful, but there is the presence of one or more uncomfortable side effects? This does not necessarily leave you powerless to deal with the side effects. One approach is to use a second medication to counteract the side effect of the first medication. One common example of this approach is using anticholinergic medications such as diphenhydramine (Benadryl) or benztropine (Cogentin) to counteract certain side effects of antipsychotic drugs. Another is the addition of any of a wide range of medications in an attempt to treat the sexual dysfunction associated with serotonin reuptake inhibitors. There are, however, shortcomings to this approach as well. Adding a second medication increases the expense and the potential for drug interactions, as well as adding the side effect burden of the additional medicine.

Change Medications. This, of course, is the most drastic measure, but one that may need to be taken. If, for example, a patient does not tolerate a particular antidepressant, especially early on in the course of treatment, there are so many alternatives that work in different ways that it is often best to switch to a different antidepressant. By so doing, one can avoid a problematic side effect but still offer potentially effective treatment for depression.

As newer medications are continually being introduced, the need to tolerate a particular side effect may change. For example, the introduction of new classes of antidepressants in the 1980s and antipsychotics in the 1990s has revolutionized treatment. In the 1980s, most chronically psychotic patients in the United States received a high potency typical antipsychotic such as haloperidol. They were almost always also prescribed an anticholinergic medication to help manage its side effects. Currently, high potency typical antipsychotics are no longer the first line of treatment for psychotic disorders. The so-called atypical antipsychotics either greatly minimize or eliminate many of these side effects altogether. On occasion, one will come across a patient who has been on a typical antipsychotic for years and has never tried one of the newer atypical medications. Although that patient may be stable on the older medication, it may make sense to change to one of the newer medications. In so doing, you'll often find that the patient does just as well (or even better) clinically, yet avoids the problematic side effects or the need for a second medication to treat those side effects.

13.2 NOREPINEPHRINE-RELATED SIDE EFFECTS

13.2.1 Side Effects of Norepinephrine-Boosting Medications

Medications that enhance norepinephrine activity can do so in one of several ways. First, they can block the reuptake of norepinephrine back into the nerve cell once it has been released. This keeps the norepinephrine in the synapse longer and therefore makes it more active. The tricyclic antidepressants (TCAs), duloxetine (Cymbalta), and venlafaxine (Effexor) act in this manner, as does paroxetine (Paxil) at higher doses. Atomoxetine (Strattera), a treatment for ADHD, also works in this way.

Blocking the norepinephrine alpha-2 receptor can also increase norepinephrine activity. The alpha-2 receptor provides feedback to the neurons to stop releasing norepinephrine and, for that matter, serotonin. By blocking the alpha-2 receptor, norepinephrine and serotonin are more readily released. The atypical antidepressant mirtazapine (Remeron) acts in part in this manner (see Table 13.2).

TABLE 13.2. Medications that Enhance Norepinephrine Activity

Medication	Means of Increasing Norepinephrine (NE) Activity	Prominent Effects on Other Transmitters	Clinical Uses
Tricyclic antidepressants	Blocks NE reuptake	⇑Serotonin ⇓Acetylcholine ⇓Histamine	Depression Anxiety disorders ADHD Pain Insomnia
Monoamine oxidase inhibitors	Blocks enzyme that destroys NE	⇑Serotonin ⇑ Dopamine	Depression Anxiety disorders Parkinson's disease ADHD
Venlafaxine	Blocks NE reuptake	⇑ Serotonin	Depression Anxiety disorders
Mirtazapine	Blocks NE alpha-2 receptor	⇑ Serotonin ⇓Histamine	Depression Anxiety disorders
Reboxetine	Blocks NE reuptake	None	Depression
Duloxetine	Blocks NE reuptake	⇑ Serotonin	Depression Anxiety disorders (?)
Psychostimulants	Trigger release, block reuptake of NE	⇑ Dopamine	ADHD Augmentation for depression (?)
Atomoxetine	Blocks NE reuptake	None	ADHD

A third way of promoting norepinephrine activity is to interfere with the enzyme that inactivates norepinephrine, monoamine oxidase (MAO). The monoamine oxidase inhibitors (MAOIs) work in this way. Incidentally, inhibiting monoamine oxidase also increases serotonin and dopamine activity.

Finally, you can increase norepinephrine activity by directly stimulating norepinephrine alpha-1 and beta receptors. Some medicines that are used to treat asthma and cardiogenic shock work in this manner, but no psychiatric medications do so.

Medications that enhance norepinephrine activity are used to treat depression and ADHD. Boosting norepinephrine can also produce numerous side effects including nervousness and anxiety, insomnia, and loss of appetite. With mirtazapine and the TCAs, these side effects are usually not a problem because these antidepressants also block histamine receptors. Their antihistamine effects promote increased appetite and drowsiness that tend to offset the side effects that might be experienced from increased norepinephrine activity.

However, these side effects can be experienced with reboxetine or atomoxetine. Although they are seldom severe, one may need to take steps to remedy the side effects. The first step is to use the smallest effective dose. When this fails, using a second medication such as a benzodiazepine to counteract sleep difficulties or anxiety can be tried. However, without compelling reasons to stay with one of these medications, the best remedy is often to change to a different antidepressant.

13.2.2 Side Effects of Norepinephrine-Blocking Medications

Blocking the Beta Receptor. Blocking norepinephrine activity can be accomplished in one of three ways. One way is to block the so-called beta receptor. Beta blockers don't interfere with norepinephrine release; instead, they prevent norepinephrine that has already been released from binding to its receptors on neighboring nerve cells. If the norepinephrine can't reach the adjacent nerve cell, the signal is not passed along. Examples of beta blockers used by psychiatrists are propranolol (Inderal), atenolol (Tenormin), and pindolol (Visken). Propranolol and atenolol are used to treat the physical symptoms of anxiety in social anxiety disorder. They can also help counteract akathisia or a lithium-induced tremor. Psychiatrists most often use pindolol as a method to augment the effects of antidepressants, though this effect is far from established. It does so not through its norepinephrine-blocking activity but because it modestly enhances serotonergic activity (see Table 13.3).

Blocking the beta receptor can lower blood pressure, slow heart rate, trigger erectile dysfunction (impotence), or worsen breathing difficulties in patients with asthma or emphysema. The best way to manage these side effects is to use the lowest effective dose. If the side effects remain intolerable at the least effective dose, then it's probably necessary to switch to an alternative medication.

Blocking the Alpha-1 Receptor. Blocking the alpha-1 receptor can also reduce norepinephrine activity. There is no apparent psychiatric benefit to blocking alpha-1 receptors, and unfortunately, many psychiatric medications do just that, resulting in side effects.

Blockade of alpha-1 receptors is associated with orthostatic hypotension. Have you ever gotten dizzy when you got out of bed or stood up from a chair too quickly? This happens because your blood pressure falls briefly when you abruptly change

TABLE 13.3. Medications that Reduce Norepinephrine Activity

Medication	Means of Reducing Norepinephrine (NE) Activity	Prominent Effects on Other Transmitters	Psychiatric Uses
Clonidine	Stimulates NE alpha-2 receptor	None	ADHD Agitation Opiate detoxification
Guanfacine	Stimulates NE alpha-2 receptor	None	ADHD
Propranolol	Blocks NE beta receptors	None	Specific social anxiety disorder Agitation Lithium tremor Akathisia
Pindolol	Blocks NE beta receptors	⇑ Serotonin	Depression (with SSRIs)

positions like this. Medications that block alpha-1 receptors exaggerate this effect. This, of course, causes dizziness and increases the risk for falls. This is a significant problem in elderly patients who are already prone to falls and can easily break a hip, an arm, or a leg. The only reasonable way to control this side effect is to minimize the dose of medications that block alpha-1 receptors. In addition, patients who are taking medications that block alpha-1 receptors need to be aware of the importance of getting out of bed slowly to avoid falling. When waking, they should sit up on the side of the bed for a minute or so before standing. Finally, it is important to review the list of medications that a patient is taking. Although a single medication may have mild effects on the alpha-1 receptor, the combined effect of several medications that block this receptor can be additive and result in problematic side effects.

Stimulating the Alpha-2 Receptor. Some medications reduce norepinephrine activity by stimulating the alpha-2 receptor. This causes nerve cells to slow down their release of norepinephrine (and serotonin as well). Clonidine and guanfacine, two medications most often used to treat high blood pressure, work in this way. These medications are sometimes used by psychiatrists to treat aggression that occurs in association with several psychiatric disorders including dementia, ADHD, and certain personality disorders. They are also used to manage physical symptoms of withdrawal during detoxification from opiates, alcohol, and occasionally benzodiazepines.

The alpha-2 stimulating medications essentially reduce the concentration of norepinephrine that would otherwise be available to stimulate both the alpha-1 and beta receptors. Therefore, these medications can produce all of the side effects of both beta blocking and alpha-1 blocking medications. The best approach to managing such side effects is to use the lowest effective dose. If the patient cannot tolerate clonidine or guanfacine, do not stop these medications abruptly, because dangerous rebound high blood pressure may ensue. When discontinuing these medications, they must be tapered gradually over several days.

13.3 DOPAMINE-RELATED SIDE EFFECTS

13.3.1 Side Effects of Dopamine-Boosting Medications

Dopamine activity can be enhanced in one of four main ways. Medications can stimulate dopaminergic nerve cells to release dopamine into the synapse. This is the way that stimulants such as methylphenidate (Ritalin), dextroamphetamine (Dexedrine), and dextroamphetamine/amphetamine (Adderall) work. In addition, certain drugs of abuse, notably cocaine and methamphetamine, act in part in this way. Providing more of the raw material that nerve cells use to manufacture dopamine can also increase dopamine activity. This is the approach that neurologists use when they prescribe L-DOPA (Sinemet) to patients with Parkinson's disease. Nerve cells convert L-DOPA into dopamine. L-DOPA otherwise has little place in the treatment of psychiatric disorders. Dopamine activity can also be increased by medications that directly stimulate dopamine receptors. Bromocriptine, another medication used to treat Parkinson's disease, works in this way as does pramipexole (Mirapex) and ropinirole (Requip). Bromocriptine is seldom used by psychiatrists except to treat neuroleptic malignant syndrome, whereas there is evidence that pramipexole and ropinirole are effective as augmenting agents in refractory depression. A fourth means of increasing dopamine activity is to block its reuptake into the nerve cell after it has been released. There is some evidence that sertraline (Zoloft) works in this manner, in addition to its SSRI effect. Finally, medications can increase dopamine activity by blocking the enzyme that inactivates dopamine. This is the way that the monoamine oxidase inhibitors (MAOIs) work. MAOIs include both selegiline (Eldepryl), used to treat Parkinson's disease, and certain antidepressants, phenelzine (Nardil), and tranylcypromine (Parnate) (see Table 13.4).

Increasing dopaminergic neurotransmission can cause several side effects including insomnia, irritability, decreased appetite, and nausea. On rare occasions, increasing dopamine tone can trigger paranoia, hallucinations, or involuntary movements known as tics. There has also been some concern that prolonged use of stimulants to treat childhood ADHD can retard growth.

Psychiatrists most often use these medications to treat ADHD, narcolepsy, and refractory depression. Conservative measures are often sufficient to counteract the side effects of increased dopamine. When insomnia or nausea is a problem, changing the dose schedule can be helpful. Avoiding or reducing evening doses can alleviate insomnia; taking the medications after meals can lessen nausea and upset

TABLE 13.4. Medications that Enhance Dopamine Activity

Medication	Means of Increasing Dopamine (DA) Activity	Prominent Effects on Other Transmitters	Clinical Uses
Methylphenidate	Promotes DA release	⇑ NE	ADHD Narcolepsy Depression
Dextroamphetamine	Promotes DA release	⇑ NE	ADHD Narcolepsy Depression
Dextroamphetamine/ amphetamine	Promotes DA release	⇑ NE	ADHD Narcolepsy
Pemoline	Promotes DA release	None	ADHD Narcolepsy
Monoamine oxidase inhibitors	Blocks enzyme that inactivates DA	⇑ Serotonin ⇑ Norepinephrine	Depression Anxiety disorders Parkinson's disease ADHD
Sertraline	Blocks DA reuptake	⇑ Serotonin	Depression Anxiety disorders
Aripiprazole	Partial agonist of D2 receptors	⇓ Serotonin-2A ⇓ + ⇑ Serotonin-1A	Psychotic disorders Bipolar disorder
Pramipipole/ Ropinirole	Occupies DA receptor	None	Restless leg syndrome

stomach. When there is a concern about slowed growth, one can recommend that a child take periodic medication holidays from stimulants. We should add, however, that recent data indicates that delayed growth may be a symptom of ADHD and not necessarily a side effect of stimulants. In any event, monitoring growth on a growth chart is a useful exercise. When these measures fail to alleviate the problems, reducing the dose or switching to alternative medications may be helpful. For example, clonidine can be used both to augment stimulants in the treatment of ADHD and to counteract stimulant-induced insomnia and tics.

13.3.2 Side Effects of Dopamine-Blocking Medications

The predominant mechanism by which currently available antipsychotic medications interfere with dopamine activity is by blockade of dopamine receptors on neurons innervated by dopamine nerve terminals. Of the five types of dopamine receptors, all antipsychotics share in common the fact that they block the dopamine type 2 receptor, also known as the D2 receptor, to a varying degree. Some of the atypical antipsychotics also block other dopamine receptors (see Table 13.5). The role of blockade of D1, D3, D4, and other dopamine receptors in the therapeutic effects of antipsychotic drugs remains unclear. Aripiprazole is an exception to this in that it is a partial agonist at the D2 receptor.

TABLE 13.5. Medications that Reduce Dopamine (DA) Activity

Medication	Means of Reducing Dopamine Activity	Prominent Effects on Other Transmitters	Psychiatric Uses
Typical antipsychotics	Blocks D2 receptor	⇓ Acetylcholine ⇓ Histamine ⇓ NE alpha-1	Psychotic disorders Agitation Delirium Tourette's disorder
Clozapine	Blocks D2, D4 receptors	⇓ Serotonin ⇓ Histamine ⇓ NE alpha-1	Psychotic disorders Bipolar disorder
Risperidone	Blocks D2 receptor	⇓ Serotonin ⇓ NE alpha-1	Psychotic disorders Bipolar disorder
Olanzapine	Blocks D2, D4 receptors	⇓ Serotonin ⇓ Histamine ⇓ NE alpha-1	Psychotic disorders Bipolar disorder
Quetiapine	Blocks D2, D4 receptors	⇓ Serotonin ⇓ Histamine ⇓ NE alpha-1	Psychotic disorders Bipolar disorder
Ziprasidone	Blocks D2, D3, D4 receptors	⇓ Serotonin ⇓ Serotonin-2 ⇓ Norepinephrine	Psychotic disorders Bipolar disorder
Aripiprazole	Partial agonist of D2 receptors	⇓ Serotonin-2A ⇓ + ⇑ Serotonin-1A	Psychotic disorders Bipolar disorder

Antidepressants that increase serotonin activity can also indirectly decrease dopamine activity by inhibiting the activity of dopamine-secreting nerve cells. This effect on dopamine nerve cells is generally not of sufficient magnitude to treat psychosis, but it may explain why patients taking these antidepressants on rare occasions experience akathisia and other extrapyramidal side effects.

The Four Dopamine Pathways. There are four major dopamine circuits in the mammalian brain. They are known as the mesolimbic, mesocortical, tuberoinfundibular, and nigroneostriatal pathways. The mesolimbic pathway arises in the midbrain and projects to the so-called limbic structures. The mesocortical pathway arises in the midbrain and projects to frontal and temporal areas of the brain's cerebral cortex.

The tuberoinfundibular dopamine pathway is found in the hypothalamus and regulates the pituitary gland, controlling the release of the hormone prolactin. Prolactin has numerous effects but is perhaps best known for promoting milk production during breast-feeding. When dopamine release is increased from this pathway, it decreases prolactin production. Therefore, dopamine-blocking medications result in an increase in prolactin production. In women, the consequences of excessive prolactin secretion may include galactorrhea (abnormal milk production) and amenorrhea (the cessation of menstrual cycling). In men, elevated prolactin can lead to gynecomastia (breast enlargement). In both sexes, elevated prolactin can cause decreased libido and sexual dysfunction. These side effects should not be ignored, because they are a common reason for nonadherence with antipsychotic medication.

The fourth major dopamine pathway is the nigroneostriatal pathway. It arises in the substantia nigra and projects to the corpus striatum, also known as the basal ganglia. This pathway facilitates the production of smooth and coordinated muscle movement. In a moment, when you stretch your hand forward to turn this page, the motor area of your brain will send the signal through the pyramidal area of the brain stem down through the spinal cord and subsequently to the arm and hand to initiate this movement. Simultaneously, the nigroneostriatal pathway will take action and send signals through the brain stem and spinal cord to produce a coordinated movement as you stretch your hand forward to grasp the corner of the page and turn. In the brain stem, the signals from the nigroneostriatal pathway travel in an area just outside the pyramidal tract; therefore, this is called the extrapyramidal area.

Of course, nothing in the brain is quite that simple. Dopamine is not the sole neurotransmitter in the nigroneostriatal pathway. Acetylcholine also regulates this pathway and works in harmony with dopamine. Maintaining a balance between dopamine and acetylcholine is of paramount importance. When disease strikes this pathway, it disrupts the balance between dopamine and acetylcholine activity, producing readily noticeable changes in physical movement. Two such diseases are Parkinson's disease and Huntington's chorea. Several well-known celebrities have Parkinson's disease including Muhammad Ali, Janet Reno, and Michael J. Fox. When Parkinson's disease strikes, the level of dopamine activity falls off dramatically, leading to an imbalance in which dopamine activity falls abnormally low relative to acetylcholine activity. When this happens, the classic symptoms of Parkinson's disease emerge including a tremor, stiffness and rigidity, a stooped posture, a mask-like expressionless face, and a slow shuffling gait.

Huntington's disease is at the opposite end of the spectrum and affects the brain in several ways, but one of its principal effects is within the nigroneostriatal pathway. In contrast to Parkinson's disease, Huntington's disease triggers an excess of dopamine activity. The result is again an imbalance in dopamine and acetylcholine activity; however, in this case, dopamine activity is abnormally high relative to acetylcholine activity. This causes a variety of abnormal and involuntary movements known as dyskinesias. This can include involuntary thrusting of the tongue, facial grimacing, and rhythmic movements of the arms and trunk (choreoathetosis).

Now with Parkinson's and Huntington's diseases in mind, what effect might we anticipate a dopamine-blocking antipsychotic to have in the nigroneostriatal pathway? Of course, it lowers dopaminergic neurotransmission relative to acetylcholine activity and, therefore, has the potential to produce side effects that very much resemble Parkinson's disease. Patients taking classical antipsychotics can exhibit a shuffling gait, a mask-like face, a rigid body, and a resting tremor.

In addition to parkinsonism, another extrapyramidal side effect is the so-called acute dystonic reaction in which muscles (usually of the face or neck) go into an acute spasm. A dystonic reaction is painful and unpleasant, usually occurs early in treatment, and sometimes occurs after the very first dose of an antipsychotic. Another extrapyramidal symptom is akathisia, a restless inability to relax and sit still. Akathisia can range from a mild restlessness to extreme agitation. Rarely, patients have been known to attempt suicide during severe episodes of akathisia. It is easy to overlook akathisia, because it can easily be mistaken for a worsening of psychosis or anxiety.

One final side effect of dopamine-blocking medications relative to the nigroneostriatal pathway is tardive dyskinesia. These are involuntary movements similar to those experienced by patients with Huntington's disease. Tardive dyskinesia only arises when a patient has taken a typical antipsychotic drug for long periods of time. In fact, a patient is most likely to experience tardive dyskinesia after having taken a high potency antipsychotic at high doses for a long time. The message here is that if one is exposed to long-term dopamine receptor blockade, there is a risk of developing tardive dyskinesia. A rough estimate is that each year of taking an older style typical antipsychotic increases the risk of developing tardive dyskinesia by 10%. Therefore, after 5 years, there is about a 50% chance of developing tardive dyskinesia. One might reasonably ask how do medications that block dopamine receptors cause symptoms resembling Huntington's disease, a disease in which dopamine activity is too high? The current hypothesis is that with prolonged use of classical antipsychotics, dopamine receptors in the nigroneostriatal pathway become supersensitive. As a result, the little dopamine that still makes its way through the pathway triggers an exaggerated response and thus dyskinesias.

Let's examine a sample case study. A patient who has been taking haloperidol (Haldol) 10 mg a day for several years may well have developed tardive dyskinesia. What would happen if the dose were increased to 20 mg a day? When we see the patient a few days later, would the abnormal movements be worse, better, or about the same? In the short term, the involuntary movements would most likely either diminish or go away altogether, but this is only a temporary solution. In time, the sensitivity of the dopamine receptors in the nigroneostriatal tract would again be increased to adjust for the new dose of haloperidol. When that happens, the tardive dyskinesia would resurface.

Typical Versus Atypical Antipsychotics. We discussed at length in Chapter 5 just what makes a typical antipsychotic typical and what makes an atypical antipsychotic atypical. We'll spare you a rehash of that lengthy discussion; however, it is important to note that all typical antipsychotics are not created equal. Although they all work by blocking the dopamine D2 receptor, their potency at this receptor varies up to 100-fold. In addition, antipsychotic side effects are not due solely to dopamine receptor blockade. In many cases, the most troublesome side effects result from blocking other receptor types including histamine, acetylcholine, and the norepinephrine alpha-1 receptor system.

Typical antipsychotics can be divided into three groups: low potency, medium potency, and high potency. The relative strength of groups differs by about a factor of 10. In other words, a medium potency antipsychotic is about ten times stronger than a low potency antipsychotic on a milligram per milligram basis. A high potency antipsychotic is about ten times stronger than a medium potency antipsychotic. The most commonly used low potency antipsychotics are chlorpromazine (Thorazine) and thioridazine (Mellaril). The medium potency antipsychotics include loxapine (Loxitane) and perphenazine (Trilafon). Among the high potency antipsychotics, haloperidol (Haldol), fluphenazine (Prolixin), thiothixene (Navane), and trifluoperazine (Stelazine) are most commonly used. Side effects from dopamine blockade are most common and most severe among the high potency typical antipsychotics. Conversely, dopamine-blocking side effects occur less often with low potency antipsychotics. However, problems due to antihistamine, anticholinergic, and alpha-1 blockade are typically more problematic with the low potency antipsychotics.

Atypical antipsychotics are less apt to cause side effects associated with dopamine receptor blockade. Three theories may explain this. For one, blockade of the serotonin type-2 receptor attenuate the dopamine blockade in the nigroneostriatal pathway just enough to decrease the extrapyramidal side effects. Another theory is that the preference of some atypical antipsychotics to preferentially block D4 receptors instead of D2 receptors may reduce the degree of dopamine blockade in the nigroneostriatal and tuberoinfundibular pathways. Most likely, atypical antipsychotics are less apt to cause extrapyramidal side effects and tardive dyskinesia because they occupy no more than 65–75% of the D2 receptors at therapeutic doses, considerably lower than the percentage of D2 receptors blocked by the typical agents or, occupy the D2 receptors for a relatively brief duration (clozapine and seroqrel) or, are partial agonists at the D2 receptor (aripiprazole).

Nevertheless, some dopamine-blockade side effects can still be found with the atypicals. Prolactin elevation still occurs, particularly with risperidone. The risk of tardive dyskinesia is still there although it appears to be diminished by at least tenfold, and there are sporadic reports of dystonic reactions, akathisia, parkinsonism, and neuroleptic malignant syndrome.

Prolactin Elevation. In the remainder of this section, we will discuss the management of dopamine receptor blockade related side effects, namely, elevated prolactin, sexual dysfunction, amenorrhea, galactorrhea, and gynecomastia. One could theoretically prescribe a dopamine-stimulating medication to counteract the effects of elevated prolactin, but this essentially would be defeating the purpose of using an antidopaminergic agent for a psychotic illness. Thus, in psychotic illnesses, a dopamine-enhancing medication such as bromocriptine, L-DOPA, or a psychostimulant might reverse the elevated prolactin, but it would also tend to worsen the psychosis.

Given that limitation, the only ways to counteract elevated prolactin are to lower the dose of the antipsychotic or to switch to another antipsychotic that does not elevate prolactin. We prefer switching (especially if the problem has been encountered with an older style typical antipsychotic) to an atypical antipsychotic if side effects of elevated prolactin become problematic. Most atypical antipsychotics, with the exception of risperidone when used in high doses, do not elevate prolactin. There are few compelling reasons to use a typical antipsychotic compared to the newer atypical agents.

Acute Dystonic Reactions. When extrapyramidal side effects occur during treatment with an antipsychotic, there are countermeasures that can be taken without changing the medication or reducing the dose. Acute extrapyramidal effects occur when an antipsychotic reduces dopaminergic activity relative to acetylcholine activity. To compensate for this effect, a drug that reduces acetylcholine activity can be prescribed. By administering an anticholinergic medication, the normal balance of dopamine and acetylcholine activity in the nigroneostriatal pathway can be reestablished without compromising antipsychotic efficacy. The inherently greater anticholinergic effects of the lower potency typical antipsychotics such as chlorpromazine most likely explain why extrapyramidal symptoms are less likely to occur with these agents as compared to the higher potency drugs such as haloperidol.

The appropriate level of aggressiveness to treat the extrapyramidal side effects depends in large part on how problematic the symptoms are. When a patient experiences an acute dystonic reaction, immediate treatment is needed. In extreme cases with severe facial and neck spasms, which may include laryngospasm, the patient may not be able to safely swallow an oral medication; therefore, we recommend an intramuscular injection of an anticholinergic medication. Most commonly used are diphenhydramine (Benadryl), which can be given at 50 mg, or benztropine (Cogentin), which can be given at 1–2 mg. The patient's symptoms usually resolve within a few minutes after the injection; however, observation of the patient for a few hours is important because as the anticholinergic dose wears off the dystonic reaction may reemerge. When this happens, or if the dystonic reaction does not resolve within a few minutes of the first dose, then it is safe and appropriate to administer a second dose. Once the patient is stabilized, (s)he can return home but should be prescribed a daily oral dose of an anticholinergic. At this point, it would also make sense to consider switching to an atypical antipsychotic. When a patient has experienced a dystonic reaction, it may be difficult to convince him/her to continue ingesting the medication that triggered it. In addition, there is some evidence that acute extrapyramidal side effects may ultimately place patients at risk for tardive dyskinesia.

Parkinsonism. Less acute in presentation but nonetheless discomforting are the parkinsonian extrapyramidal side effects including tremor, rigidity, shuffling gait, stooped posture, and a mask-like facies. These can be controlled to some extent by routinely administering an anticholinergic along with the typical antipsychotic. Typical regimens are diphenhydramine 50 mg at bedtime or benztropine 1–2 mg once or twice daily. Trihexyphenidyl (Artane) and amantidine (Symmetrel) can also be used. Although anticholinergics can reduce or even remove parkinsonism, they do not reduce the risk of ultimately developing tardive dyskinesia.

Akathisia. Akathisia is yet another extrapyramidal side effect. The approach to treatment depends on its severity. For mild restlessness, dose reduction or dividing the daily dose to reduce the peak plasma levels of the medication may be successful. If mild akathisia remains a problem, it may be preferable to add a medication to treat this side effect or preferably switch to another antipsychotic or antidepressant that is less likely to cause akathisia.

When akathisia is severe, immediate and aggressive therapy is indicated. The first-line treatment for akathisia, like the parkinsonism described earlier, is the administration of an anticholinergic medication. However, anticholinergic medications are less effective when treating akathisia than other extrapyramidal side effects. When the akathisia does not resolve after two or three doses of diphenhydramine or benztropine, one might consider adding a medication that interferes with norepinephrine activity such as propranolol. In these cases 10 mg of propranolol given three times a day is often sufficient until the akathisia resolves. In extreme cases of akathisia, the patient may also need to be treated briefly with a benzodiazepine. We highly recommend that once your patient has experienced akathisia on an antipsychotic (or a serotonin-boosting antidepressant), serious consideration should be given to switching to another medication less likely to cause akathisia. The risk of recurrent episodes of akathisia will certainly undermine any benefit of treatment. Atypical antipsychotics are the choice to replace typical antipsychotics. When akathisia occurs while taking a serotonin-boosting antidepressant, switching to an antidepressant that acts primarily on norepinephrine or dopamine systems or to a different member of the same class are all potential strategies.

Tardive Dyskinesia (TD). As mentioned previously, TD is a potential side effect of long-term treatment with typical antipsychotics; it is believed to be very rare but possible after atypical antipsychotic treatment. Although we now know that TD is not irreversible in all patients, about half will recover after discontinuation of the antipsychotic and the passage of several months time, others will exhibit the symptoms of TD for the remainder of their lives. Reducing the dose of the antipsychotic not only fails to alleviate the problem, but it is often associated with a worsening of TD symptoms, at least temporarily.

A host of medications have been used to treat TD including medications that block norepinephrine activity (clonidine and propranolol), dopamine-activating medications (bromocriptine), benzodiazepines, acetylcholine-activating medications, calcium channel blockers, and monoamine oxidase inhibitors. In addition, vitamin E supplementation and atypical antipsychotics including clozapine have been used to treat TD.

Of all these treatments, the only consistent improvement is seen with the atypical antipsychotic clozapine (Clozaril). Treatment-resistant TD is in fact one generally accepted indication for using clozapine. However, because of the expense of this drug, the risk for granulocytopenia, and the requirement for biweekly blood draws, other measures should first be tried.

Among the benzodiazepines, long-acting clonazepam (Klonopin) is sometimes effective for TD. Unfortunately, after several months of treatment, tolerance to its beneficial effects often develops and the TD reemerges. When this occurs, clonazepam should be discontinued for a few weeks. It can then be restarted and may again lessen TD for a few more months.

Vitamin E supplementation has produced highly variable results. The most recent and largest study suggests that vitamin E is not beneficial for most patients with TD. It remains to be seen whether certain subgroups of patients with TD may yet be helped by vitamin E. Two things are clear: vitamin E is inexpensive, and it is generally considered a benign treatment. If the patient's family physician is consulted and is in agreement, vitamin E supplementation is usually worth a therapeutic trial.

The success of clozapine makes it reasonable to try it or one of the other atypical antipsychotics. Although we know that the atypical agents are far less likely to cause TD, other than clozapine, we do not currently know enough about how well they treat preexisting TD.

In summary, if a patient develops TD, we recommend switching to an atypical antipsychotic if this has not already been done. One can also try coadministering clonazepam and/or vitamin E. If these measures fail, a trial of clozapine is warranted, despite the risk of agranulocytosis.

13.4 SEROTONIN-RELATED SIDE EFFECTS

13.4.1 Side Effects of Serotonin-Boosting Medications

Probably the greatest advances in psychiatric medications of the last 15 years have involved the neurotransmitter serotonin. First was the arrival of serotonin-specific antidepressants with fewer side effects and greater safety than their predecessors. More recently, atypical antipsychotics have highlighted the importance of serotonin–dopamine interactions in the optimal treatment of schizophrenia and other psychotic disorders. While these are indeed significant advances, medications that alter serotonin activity are not without their own side effect burden.

Psychiatric medications enhance serotonin activity in one of four major ways. First, many drugs block reuptake of serotonin into the neuron that released it. This is the way that the so-called SSRIs work, but they are not alone in this regard. Some, but not all, of the older tricyclic antidepressants, with clomipramine the most potent and desipramine the least potent, block serotonin reuptake as well. In addition, venlafaxine (Effexor) and duloxetine (Cymbalta) are inhibitors of both serotonin and norepinephrine reuptake. Sibutramine (Meridia) inhibits the reuptake of serotonin, norepinephrine, and dopamine. Nefazodone (Serzone) and trazodone (Desyrel) are weak serotonin reuptake inhibitors. Serotonergic neurotransmission is also enhanced by blocking the enzyme that metabolizes serotonin. This, of course, is the mechanism by which the monoamine oxidase inhibitors enhance serotonergic, noradrenergic, and dopaminergic neurotransmission as well. Third, medications can also selectively enhance certain serotonin pathways by directly activating one or more serotonin receptors. Buspirone (Buspar) acts in this way by stimulating the serotonin-1A receptor. Finally, medications such as fenfluramine and dexfenfluramine (both removed from the U.S. market) stimulate the release of serotonin from presynaptic nerve terminals (see Table 13.6).

Compared to the older antidepressants, those that specifically enhance serotonin activity are safer and, in general, much easier to tolerate. However, like all drugs, they do have some nagging side effects. When a patient initiates therapy with a serotonin-enhancing medication such as a SSRI, (s)he may experience headaches, nausea or loose stools, increased anxiety, and sleep difficulties. Many patients, both male and female, can experience sexual dysfunction. The sexual side effects of these medications include a loss of sexual desire, difficulty achieving orgasm, and erectile dysfunction. Finally, too rapidly escalating the dose of a SSRI, particularly in combination with certain other drugs, can produce an illness known as serotonin syndrome. This is most likely to occur with a combination of a monoamine oxidase inhibitor and a SSRI or SNRI. Serotonin syndrome can leave a person very ill and in rare extreme cases can be life-threatening. Fortunately, the serotonin syndrome is a relatively rare occurrence. Let us review how to manage/minimize some of the side effects of serotonergic medications.

GI Side Effects. Nausea, indigestion, diarrhea, and abdominal cramping can all occur when the patient first begins taking a medication that boosts serotonin activity. Serotonin receptors are found not only in the brain but also in the gut. Fortunately, the body usually adapts quickly, and these side effects are only transient. Before starting one of these medications, it is important for the patient to be aware that this may occur. To minimize the severity, many clinicians start at a low dose and gradually increase it to the therapeutic range over 1–2 weeks or longer. Taking these medications after meals also tends to make the GI symptoms milder. Finally, it is important to be patient because although the symptoms may be distressful, they will generally resolve rather quickly. Other strategies that appear helpful for some include the use of ginger tea or the coadministration of mirtazapine for a brief period of time exploiting the serotonin-3 receptor antagonist properties of this medication,

TABLE 13.6. Medications that Enhance Serotonin Activity

Medication	Means of Increasing Serotonin Activity	Prominent Effects on Other Transmitters	Clinical Uses
Tricyclic antidepressants	Blocks serotonin reuptake	⇑ Norepinephrine ⇓ Acetylcholine ⇓ Histamine	Depression Anxiety disorders ADHD Pain Insomnia
Monoamine oxidase inhibitors	Blocks enzyme that destroys serotonin	⇑ Norepinephrine ⇑ Dopamine	Depression Anxiety disorders Parkinson's disease ADHD
Fluoxetine	Blocks serotonin reuptake		Depression Anxiety disorders Bulimia nervosa
Fluvoxamine	Blocks serotonin reuptake		Depression Anxiety disorders
Citalopram	Blocks serotonin reuptake		Depression Anxiety disorders
Escitalopram	Blocks serotonin reuptake		Depression Anxiety disorders
Paroxetine	Blocks serotonin reuptake	⇓ Acetylcholine ⇑ Norepinephrine	Depression Anxiety disorders
Sertraline	Blocks serotonin reuptake	⇑ Dopamine	Depression Anxiety disorders
Nefazodone	Blocks serotonin reuptake	Blocks serotonin-2 receptors	Depression Anxiety disorders
Trazodone	Blocks serotonin reuptake		Depression Insomnia
Venlafaxine	Blocks serotonin reuptake	⇑ Norepinephrine	Depression Anxiety disorders
Mirtazapine	Blocks NE alpha-2 receptor	⇑ Norepinephrine ⇓ Histamine	Depression Anxiety disorders
Duloxetine	Blocks serotonin reuptake	⇑ Norepinephrine	Depression Anxiety disorders?

which it shares with a number of antiemetic agents used to treat the nausea associated with chemotherapy.

For a handful of patients, the GI side effects will be intolerable. When this happens, it is best to switch medications. Sometimes even switching from one serotonin-boosting medication to another, for reasons that are obscure, can resolve the problem.

Sexual Side Effects. Unlike the temporary GI side effects of serotonin-boosting antidepressants, sexual side effects tend to be longlasting. Therefore, waiting it out is usually not helpful, and countermeasures in one form or another need to be taken. The underlying philosophy to reducing sexual side effects is to interfere (at least temporarily) with serotonin activity. Several approaches can be taken to counteracting the serotonin effects, but each requires some degree of planning sexual activity. There are a wide variety of strategies that are undertaken to reverse sexual dysfunction and this represents the unfortunate reality that none of them are especially effective in a large percentage of patients.

The first and least intrusive approach is to change the dosing schedule. Sexual side effects of these medications tend to be most problematic when the medication levels are at their peak. Therefore, if the medication is taken at bedtime (i.e., just *after* most sexual activity), then levels will be at their lowest during the evening hours when patients are most likely to engage in sex. This simple change can adequately alleviate the sexual side effects for some patients and is certainly worth a try. Of course, there is some risk that taking the medication at bedtime will accentuate other problematic side effects such as insomnia. When this measure fails, more extensive steps must be taken.

The choices include skipping doses of the medication, adding a second medication as a potential antidote to counteract the side effect, switching to another antidepressant that is less likely to produce sexual dysfunction, or, in the presence of an adequate response to the medication, trying to gradually reduce the dose in order to strike a balance between effectiveness and tolerability. At this point, the decision depends in large part on just how successful the antidepressant treatment has otherwise been. In other words, if the current antidepressant has provided an excellent treatment response, then one may decide to go to greater lengths to avoid having to switch antidepressants. On the other hand, if the antidepressant had shown little or no benefit, then the decision might more appropriately be to switch antidepressants before resorting to the addition of a second medication to counteract side effects.

When staying with the current antidepressant rather than switching, we prefer to try decreasing the dosage first and then if needed adding a second medication rather than skipping doses. We have found that taking frequent medication holidays may be counterproductive and often unsuccessful in any case. From a behaviorist perspective, we end up reinforcing poor medication adherence by rewarding skipped/missed doses with the ability to perform sexually. Medications that are believed to be helpful in counteracting this side effect are thought to do so by interfering with serotonin activity and one or more serotonin receptors or activating the noradrenergic/dopaminergic system. The ideal medication for this purpose would be one that blocked the serotonin receptor that mediated this side effect without affecting the serotonin receptor(s) that mediate clinical efficacy. Several medications including cyproheptadine, yohimbine, amantidine, methylphenidate, and buspirone have been tried to treat antidepressant-induced sexual dysfunction.

Some medications are taken on an as-needed basis in anticipation of sex. For example, cyproheptadine should be taken 1–2 hours before anticipated sexual activity at doses ranging from 2 to 16 mg. Yohimbine can be taken 2–4 hours before sexual activity at doses ranging from 5.4 to 16.2 mg. When these medications work successfully, the benefit can appear quickly. By contrast, buspirone must be taken every day. These antidotes are helpful for some patients but are not always reliable.

One additional medication that has recently been studied is sildenafil, which is more commonly known by its trade name Viagra. Sildenafil is taken at doses from 50 to 100 mg per dose about 1–2 hours before sex. Sildenafil is sometimes effective but its expense and potential complications in patients with heart disease limit its usefulness. It can be quite useful in males who experience erectile dysfunction, though it does not improve delayed ejaculation.

Another widely practiced strategy to treat sexual dysfunction is the addition of pro-noradrenergic or pro-dopaminergic medications such as dopamine agonists or psychostimulants. The addition of bupropion is also believed to be effective but its mechanism of action remains obscure.

In cases where the antidepressant response has not been resounding, we prefer switching antidepressants to avoid sexual side effects. The options include bupropion, nefazodone, and mirtazapine, which all effectively treat depression but produce minimal effects on sexual function. Sometimes, if a patient has responded well to one antidepressant but experiences a side effect such as sexual dysfunction, switching within the same class can be a useful approach.

13.4.2 Side Effects of Serotonin-Blocking Medications

When we talk about serotonin-blocking medications, a point of clarification must be made. In most cases, medications do not block overall serotonin activity but instead block the activity at one of the many serotonin receptor types. For example, the antidepressants trazodone, nefazodone, and mirtazapine increase total serotonin activity yet they block certain of the serotonin receptors. Mirtazapine increases both serotonin and norepinephrine activity by interfering with the alpha-2 receptor. By also blocking the serotonin-2 and serotonin-3 receptors, mirtazapine avoids the sexual dysfunction and GI side effects commonly experienced with other serotonin-boosting medications. We cannot truly call these serotonin-blocking medications, because they are serotonin-boosting medications that selectively block certain serotonin receptors.

As noted in the previous section, buspirone produces both serotonin-boosting and serotonin-blocking effects by stimulating the serotonin-1A receptor. These mixed effects produce an overall milder serotonin-boosting effect that limits it potential side effects but also results in a more limited range of clinical uses than is available to other serotonin-boosting medications. Clearly, we cannot really say that buspirone blocks serotonin activity in the same way that antipsychotics block dopamine activity.

Finally, many of the atypical antipsychotics act, at least in part, by blocking activity at the serotonin-2 receptor. This may lessen the potential for extrapyramidal side effects and contribute to reducing psychotic symptoms. Atypical antipsychotics do produce side effects, but there is no clear evidence that any of their common side effects are due to their action on serotonin systems.

The closest things to true antiserotonin medications used by psychiatrists are those used to treat serotonin-induced side effects. In particular, cyproheptadine has an overall serotonin-blocking effect. With repeated use, this medication can theoretically cause depression and anxiety, and there are case reports of recurrence of depressive symptoms following frequent administration of cyproheptadine.

13.5 GABA-RELATED SIDE EFFECTS

13.5.1 Side Effects of GABA-Boosting Medications

Gamma-aminobutyric acid (GABA) is an inhibitory neurotransmitter. By inhibitory, we mean that once released it causes neighboring nerve cells to be less active. For this reason, medications that increase GABA activity tend to have a calming effect. Therefore, they make excellent treatments for anxiety, insomnia, and agitation. Currently, the largest group of GABA-stimulating medications is the benzodiazepines. This group includes diazepam (Valium), alprazolam (Xanax), lorazepam (Ativan), and clonazepam (Klonopin) as well as others. Older medications including chloral hydrate, meprobamate (Miltown), and the barbiturates (e.g., phenobarbital, secobarbital, and pentobarbital) also stimulate the GABA system, but they have largely been abandoned in favor of the much safer benzodiazepines.

One newer agent, tiagabine (Gabitril) acts in a distinct manner by blocking GABA reuptake. Gabapentin (Neurontin) and pregabalin (Lyrica) are structurally similar to GABA and were once thought to be GABA-stimulating medications but are now known to act primarily on calcium channels. They are principally used by neurologists to manage epilepsy. Alcohol is also known to stimulate the GABA system.

GABA-enhancing medications have many uses. They are used to treat anxiety disorders including generalized anxiety disorder, panic disorder, social anxiety disorder, and PTSD. They are also used to treat agitation in patients with depression, bipolar disorder, psychotic disorders, and personality disorders. They have long been used to treat seizure disorders and to detoxify patients from alcohol. Finally, one GABA-enhancing medication, midazolam (Versed), is used to achieve conscious sedation during complicated medical procedures like colonoscopy and cardiac catheterization. Through conscious sedation, a patient is awake but drowsy and calm during the procedure. As a result, they are able to follow instructions and cooperate during the procedure but have no recollection of what transpired once the procedure is complete and the medication has worn off. Finally, GABA-stimulating medications are used as muscle relaxants to provide relief to patients with muscle spasms such as those associated with acute back pain.

GABA-boosting medications are in general well tolerated but not without side effects. They cause sedation and drowsiness, anterograde amnesia, and impaired motor coordination. Some of these effects provide an excellent example of how a side effect in one setting can be beneficial in another. For example, anterograde amnesia can be very frightening when you wake up the morning after taking a medication, and you can't remember what happened the day before. But it is precisely this property that makes it useful for conscious sedation during medical procedures. Likewise, drowsiness can be a big problem, but this also makes GABA-enhancing medications effective treatments for acute insomnia. Because tolerance usually develops to their sedating properties, benzodiazepines are poor choices for long-term treatment of insomnia. It all comes down to the therapeutic goal when prescribing the medication.

The most troublesome side effects of these medications are drowsiness and poor motor coordination. Impaired coordination can be quite dangerous for elderly patients who are prone to falls or those who take the medication before driving an automobile. We recommend following these steps to manage daytime drowsiness and poor coordination caused by GABA-enhancing medications. First, advise the patients before starting these medications that they should not imbibe alcohol. Alcohol and GABA-enhancing medications have potentially synergistic effects that when taken together can lead to extreme sedation, blackouts, and severely impaired motor coordination. Second, a review of the patient's list of medications is indicated to ensure that other sedating medicines are not being taken. Third, we recommend taking these medications at bedtime when possible, though as mentioned earlier, benzodiazepines can be used successfully for the treatment of anxiety disorders with a standing dose schedule (two to three times per day) because tolerance to the sedation does develop.

When all else fails, the patient may need to switch to another medication. Serotonin-boosting antidepressants are a reasonable alternative to benzodiazepines for patients with anxiety disorders. Likewise, there are several options for the bipolar patient who cannot tolerate GABAergic medications.

13.5.2 Side Effects of GABA-Blocking Medications

The only medication that blocks GABA activity is flumazenil (Mazicon). Flumazenil is used only in the emergency room or in an inpatient hospital setting to treat benzodiazepine overdose. It quickly and reliably reverses the toxic effects when a patient has accidentally or purposefully taken an overdose. Restricted to emergency situations, flumazenil is never used on a routine basis.

Flumazenil's one problematic side effect is that it can trigger benzodiazepine withdrawal including increased pulse, increased blood pressure, shakiness, anxiety, and seizures. Because it is only used in the hospital, supportive medical care is, by definition, available if this occurs.

13.6 ACETYLCHOLINE-RELATED SIDE EFFECTS

13.6.1 Side Effects of Acetylcholine-Boosting Medications

Medications that enhance acetylcholine activity are the mainstay of treatment for Alzheimer's disease and other dementias. They have found little other use in

TABLE 13.7. Medications that Enhance Acetylcholine Activity

Medication	Means of Increasing Acetylcholine (ACh) Activity	Clinical Uses
Donepezil	Blocks enzyme that destroys ACh	Dementia
Galantamine	Blocks enzyme that destroys ACh	Dementia
Rivastigmine	Blocks enzyme that destroys ACh	Dementia
Tacrine	Blocks enzyme that destroys ACh	Dementia

psychiatry. In addition to memory processing, acetylcholine is the primary neurotransmitter of the parasympathetic nervous system. As a result, the most common side effects from acetylcholine-boosting medications result from exaggerations in parasympathetic activity. Such side effects include slowed heart rate and a variety of gastrointestinal symptoms including drooling, nausea, indigestion, and diarrhea. A series of refinements has produced newer medications that are not only more effective but are also less prone to these troublesome side effects (see Table 13.7).

The key to managing the side effects of acetylcholine-enhancing medications is first and foremost using medications that are more easily tolerated. Second, these medications should be started at low doses and slowly increased over a period of several weeks.

13.6.2 Side Effects of Acetylcholine-Blocking Medication

The only typical use in psychiatry for acetylcholine-blocking (or anticholinergic) medications is to counteract extrapyramidal side effects. Diphenhydramine (Benadryl) and benztropine (Cogentin) are the two anticholinergics most commonly used for this purpose, though trihexyphenidyl (Artane) is available as well. Although psychiatrists have little use for acetylcholine-blocking medications, this does not imply that anticholinergic side effects are not a significant problem for patients taking psychiatric medications. A wide variety of psychiatric medications interfere with acetylcholine activity. Among antidepressants, the tricyclics are notorious for causing anticholinergic side effects. This is particularly prominent with amitriptyline and imipramine. The newer antidepressants are less prone to anticholinergic side effects, though paroxetine is mildly anticholinergic. Antipsychotics also block acetylcholine receptors, the worst offenders being the low potency antipsychotics, chlorpromazine (Thorazine) and thioridazine (Mellaril). This is less of a problem with the high potency antipsychotics such as haloperidol and fluphenazine, but the need to use anticholinergic side effect medications to offset extrapyramidal side effects can contribute to the burden (see Table 13.8).

Anticholinergic medications can produce a variety of side effects. They can cause dry mouth and dry skin. Dry mouth is not only a nuisance but can lead to rapid tooth decay as well. Anticholinergic medications can also cause blurred vision and

TABLE 13.8. Medications that Reduce Acetylcholine Activity

Medication	Means of Reducing Acetylcholine (ACh) Activity	Prominent Effects on Other Transmitters	Psychiatric Uses
Tricyclic antidepressants	Blocks ACh receptor	⇑ Serotonin ⇑ Norepinephrine ⇓ Acetylcholine ⇓ Histamine	Depression Anxiety disorders ADHD Pain Insomnia
Diphenhydramine	Blocks ACh receptor	⇓ Histamine	EPS Insomnia
Typical antipsychotics	Blocks ACh receptor	⇓ Histamine ⇓ Dopamine (D2) ⇓ Norepinephrine alpha-1	Psychotic disorders Agitation Delirium Tourette's disorder
Benztropine	Blocks ACh receptor		EPS

difficulty urinating. In extreme cases, particularly in men with enlarged prostate glands, this can trigger acute urinary retention that can be a medical emergency. Anticholinergic medications also produce gastrointestinal side effects, most notably constipation. Finally, these medications can impair memory and cause confusion and even delirium. The memory effects are most troublesome for older patients who may have less functional reserve brain capacity. In other words, a young person may be able to withstand the impact of an anticholinergic medication on brain function, whereas an older person may be more susceptible to problems.

Whenever possible, anticholinergic medications should be avoided or kept to a minimum. This is an important consideration because a wide variety of medications, psychiatric and otherwise, possess some acetylcholine-blocking properties. When a patient is using several medications, it is important to review the relative anticholinergic contribution of each medication. Taking one mildly anticholinergic medication may not be a problem, but taking three or four can have additive effects that do become problematic.

13.7 HISTAMINE-RELATED SIDE EFFECTS

13.7.1 Side Effects of Histamine-Blocking Medications

Diphenhydramine is the antihistamine that is most widely used by psychiatrists, and it is most often used more for its acetylcholine-blocking effects than its histamine blockade. This is not to say that histamine-blocking effects are not problematic. In fact, a wide variety of psychiatric medications block histamine receptors. The tricyclic antidepressants as a group are potent antihistamines. Doxepin (Sinequan) is among the most potent antihistamines ever made, considerably more potent than diphenhydramine, and available in a topical form that can be applied to allergic skin rashes. Among the newer antidepressants, trazodone (Desyrel), nefazodone (Serzone), and mirtazapine (Remeron) are all rather potent histamine blockers. Some antipsychotics also block histamine receptors. Among the typical antipsychotics, low potency medications have the strongest antihistamine effects. Conversely, the high potency antipsychotics such as haloperidol and fluphenazine have the least histamine-blocking effects. Among the atypical antipsychotics, olanzapine, clozapine, and quetiapine block histamine receptors (see Table 13.9).

TABLE 13.9. Medications that Reduce Histamine Activity

Medication	Means of Reducing Histamine Activity	Prominent Effects on Other Transmitters	Psychiatric Uses
Tricyclic antidepressants	Blocks histamine receptor	⇑ Serotonin ⇓Acetylcholine ⇑ Norepinephrine	Depression Anxiety disorders ADHD Pain Insomnia
Mirtazapine	Blocks histamine receptor	⇑Norepinephrine ⇑Serotonin	Depression
Nefazodone	Blocks histamine receptor	⇑Serotonin	Depression
Trazodone	Blocks histamine receptor	⇑Serotonin	Depression Insomnia
Diphenhydramine	Blocks histamine receptor	⇓Acetylcholine	EPS Insomnia
Typical antipsychotics	Blocks histamine receptor	⇓Acetylcholine ⇓Dopamine (D2) ⇓Norepinephrine alpha-1	Psychotic disorders Agitation Delirium Tourette's disorder
Clozapine	Blocks histamine receptor	⇓Serotonin ⇓Dopamine (D2, D4) ⇓Norepinephrine alpha-1	Psychotic disorders Bipolar disorder
Olanzapine	Blocks histamine receptor	⇓Serotonin ⇓Dopamine (D2, D4) ⇓Norepinephrine alpha-1	Psychotic disorders
Quetiapine	Blocks histamine receptor	⇓Serotonin ⇓Dopamine (D2, D4) ⇓Norepinephrine alpha-1	Psychotic disorders

The most significant problems with antihistamines are sedation and weight gain. Except for stimulants, there are no medications that counteract these effects. We do recommend the use of a stimulant to counteract antihistamine effects.

INDEX

Principles of Psychopharmacology for Mental Health Professionals
By Jeffrey E. Kelsey, D. Jeffrey Newport, and Charles B. Nemeroff